WHEN SLOW IS FAST ENOUGH

Educating the Delayed Preschool Child

JOAN F. GOODMAN
Graduate School of Education
University of Pennsylvania

Foreword by Robert Coles

THE GUILFORD PRESS
New York   London

© 1992 The Guilford Press
A Division of Guilford Publications, Inc.
72 Spring Street, New York, NY 10012

Printed in the United States of America

This book is printed on acid-free paper.

Last digit is print number: 9 8 7 6 5 4 3 2 1

Library of Congress Cataloging-in-Publication Data
Goodman, Joan F.
    When slow is fast enough: educating the delayed preschool
child / Joan F. Goodman.
        p.   cm.
    Includes bibliographical references and index.
    ISBN 0-89862-793-1 (hard).—ISBN 0-89862-491-6 (pbk.)
    1. Mentally handicapped children—Education (Preschool)—United
States.   2. Special education—United States.   3. Mentally
handicapped children—Rehabilitation—United States.   I. Title.
    [DNLM: 1. Child, Preschool—education—United States.
2. Education, Special—methods—United States.   3. Mental
Retardation—rehabilitation—United States.   LC 4031 G653]
LC4602.5.G66 1992
371.92—dc20
DNLM/DLC   92-1416
for Library of Congress   CIP

To the teachers I met across the country,
whose attention to the small details
of each child's care displayed
the largeness of their hearts.

Foreword

As I read Joan Goodman's persuasive and poignant book I remembered a family my wife, Jane, and I used to visit in Atlanta, at the height of the civil rights struggle in the South. The family was black and poor. One of its members, a young black woman of 15, had initiated school desegregation in a previously all white high school, and the result had been plenty of personal anguish for her, plenty of tearful ostracism prompting anxious apprehension and self-doubt. Still, she managed to get through the ordeal rather well, we thought—one of two blacks in a sea of a thousand white faces. Often, as we talked, she mentioned her younger brother, who had Down syndrome and was in a "special class" for such youngsters. She was not impressed by what was happening to this boy, and she several times compared his "troubles" to her own: "I've got lots to deal with, that's for sure—every day. The people who don't like me, they'd just as soon see me dead, if they could [bring that about]; but when I get real discouraged, I stop and think of my little brother, and all *he* has to put up with—it's no good. The school people, they're not paying attention to *him*; they're looking at Freddie as if he's another one of those 'retarded kids' (and you know *them!*), and you've got to get them 'in shape.' That's what they told my mom—that you mustn't expect too much from Freddie, and what we should do is get him in shape. When mom asked what that means, the teacher told her they were going to try to train him so that he listens and knows how to be 'obedient and cooperative,' that's what they say they want. Well, I guess everyone should be that—but it all sounds so familiar: you just keep in your place, and we're the ones who decide what that 'place' is! My mom said if you're not having a rough time because of the color of your skin, then you're having a rough time because the good Lord sent you here with the kind of mind He wanted you to have, and it's not the same as the kind the school folks have, and so they tell you to listen to what they say, and if you don't, then you'd better come see them, and when you do, you go there—well, they'll lecture you until you're ready to cry, or scream, or just say you surrender, and it's that [the last choice] they want, I'll tell you!"

So it can go for any number of children whose educational lives are judged not according to their own particular nature, but rather, in an all too categorical manner: you are *this* kind of person, and we have *this* kind of program in mind for you. It is the great virtue of this book that it takes on such a way of teaching (such a way of seeing the world) with great courage and a careful attention to what is really at stake: the destiny of individuals, of boys and girls who may, indeed, have difficulties with learning, with the usual educational challenges put to young people in our schools, but who are well worth our care, our concern, and our regard for exactly who they are, what they have to offer, and how they might best fulfill their various and unique destinies—as our fellow human beings, as our fellow citizens, and, as Freddie's mother would hasten to remind us, as "souls of God, put here to teach us something while we're trying to teach them something."

I can, even now, here those words being spoken, and they yet manage to say so very much; they also, I believe, make the same point Joan Goodman is trying so hard and so well to make in this sensitive, thoughtful, important book: that each of us is entitled to be considered as himself, as herself—yes, in need of various educational efforts, but not of a kind that ignores the particularity that is ours, ours alone. In a sense, then, the challenge so-called "retarded" children present to us is the age-old one, the still demanding and significant one—that we learn to stop and ask ourselves what we are doing, and why, on behalf of whom, and on the basis of which hopes and aspirations and purposes. This book, in its well-argued, lucid, gentle but firm way, helps address matters of importance not only to those who (as parents, as teachers, as friends and neighbors) work with "slow" children, but to all of us, who need to know not only our students and patients, whom we aim to assist, hand along in life, but ourselves—our assumptions and values. We stand or fall, after all, with respect to our overall usefulness in proportion to the kind of intellectual, moral, personal awareness we have managed to discover in those others whom we try to teach or lead, never mind in ourselves.

ROBERT COLES

Preface

Educators, like architects, develop large-scale plans and carry them out through detailed daily specification. Psychologists, like building inspectors, examine the constructions and judge their suitability for the well-being of children.

As a child psychologist, before undertaking this field study of programs for the preschool handicapped, I spent many years studying children suspected of developmental delays, probing their capacities, watching their reactions, and, finally, certifying their eligibility for early intervention services. Even as the director of an early intervention program, my eyes were so trained on the child—what she did when alone or with a parent, when given this or that toy, when touched or spoken to, when placed in one environment or another—that I barely registered the teachers' sequence of planned activities. Over time, I realized that while I fastened on the child's *responses,* the teacher was focused on the *stimuli*—what behaviors and knowledge she wanted to build into the child, the routines and schedules required to attain her goals.

Good education, of course, requires both perspectives. Educators are unlikely to succeed without a deep understanding of *whom* they are teaching as well as *what* they are teaching. But in the early "special" education programs familiar to me, the two perspectives did not seem well joined. Teachers, I found, were not sufficiently "psychologically minded." They were not tuned to the subtleties of the child's habitus. They did not sufficiently modify and vary their efforts to fit the children's worlds. Psychologists, for the most part, were but dimly aware of the demands on teachers to build into a group of heterogeneous and challenging children information and behaviors that would "ready" them by age 5 or 6 for the "regular" world.

As my interests increasingly shifted to "intervention," and

away from "diagnosis," I wanted to learn more about how these two perspectives played out in programs for young handicapped children across the country. To what extent and in what ways did teachers consider the psychological and developmental position of their children? What was the curriculum they wanted to and had to teach? What were their aspirations? What kind of children were "out there"? How did the children react to the programs? What pressures did families and the larger social context bring to bear? Was there a consistent set of overarching values that dominated programs? How much variability would I find in the structure, content, and ethos of programs?

This study is my answers to these questions, answers that I hope will be of interest to, and debated by, all those involved in the well-being of preschool children with special needs—teachers, parents, students, researchers, and policy makers. More broadly, because the fundamental question raised—How do we formulate and carry out socialization and educational policies with children?—transcends a particular population, I hope the book will be of interest to all those who reflect upon the care of young children, as that care increasingly is done outside the child's home.

The book has been a large undertaking lasting 3 years, and I had a lot of help along the way. Simply finding and scheduling the programs to visit was a major task enormously aided by Jill Greenberg, a doctoral student. Once on site, I found, without exception, that those associated with the programs, including administrators, teachers, and parents, gave willingly of their time and of their sober reflections. Early intervention attracts generous, hospitable people, and I met many of them. My greatest debt of gratitude goes to the teachers who permitted me to watch, videotape, and talk with them; who introduced me to parents, and shared with me their understanding of and written materials about the children in their rooms. I trust that they, and the equally helpful administrators, will understand that my admiration for them is in no way diminished by my concerns about our early intervention efforts.

Back at home, I am indebted to all the handicapped children and their families from whom I have learned so much about hurt, anger, denial, patience; about the joy of small attainments, the miniaturization of beauty; but, most of all, about the capacities of the human spirit to rebound after disappointment. The families have sustained my emotional and intellectual interest in this field for 27 years.

The many colleagues who have worked closely with me in the

educational, clinical, and academic settings where professionals meet handicapped youngsters have provided stimulation, "reality testing," and friendship. I thank those who have read drafts of the manuscript and shared their reactions: Maxine Field, Jean Fridy, Susan Hoban, Marvin Lazerson, Elizabeth Pollak, and Leslie Rescorla. My thanks to students past and present with whom I have discussed these matters time and time again—particularly Lori Bond, Jill Greenberg, Jeanne Liebman, Mark Pellico, Jerilynn Radcliffe, Linda Spungen, Susan Mayes, Marjorie Waxman—and to Tawn Stokes and Virginia Sutton for their valuable technical assistance.

Finally, every member of my family has been involved in, and supportive of, this project, and I have profited from their reactions. When I was not away in body, I was away in mind. For not just putting up with my preoccupation, but sharing in it, I thank my children—Lisa, Ellen, and Jonathan—and my son-in-law William Weinreb. Most especially, thanks to my husband, Frank, and son, Barak, but for whose critical comments on early drafts, this book would have been completed some time ago!

JOAN F. GOODMAN

Contents

CHAPTER ONE

Introduction

I listened as Adam recounted, like a videocassette playback, the blow by blow of his day. The hours existed for him as a series of unrelated acts, connected neither by analysis nor by critical perspective, uncolored by like or dislike, undistinguished by incident. As I nodded, inviting him to continue, I yearned to put words in his mouth, to break through the barrier of his plodding progress, to find in him some spark of sarcasm or wit . . . This was my problem, not his. When did I stop wanting, demanding, feeling that Adam had been cheated? When did I let go, quell my passion to power his life, direct his interests, think his thoughts? I was not proud of my complaints; they had long since ceased to do Adam much good . . . I confirmed his world, and that's all he wanted. The desire for more came only from me.

—DORRIS (1989, pp. 260–261)

CHOICES WE MAKE

Cleveland General Hospital, 1960: After years of waiting, the moment has come. John Molloy tightens his grip on Mary's hand as he watches the doctor cut the cord and free his newborn son. Overflowing with feelings of relief, tenderness, and awe, he barely notices the stillness that settles over the hospital room as the child is washed and readied for the newborn nursery. An hour later, rested and refreshed, Mary asks to have her son brought in. The nurse puts her off: the sleeping baby should not be disturbed; the pediatrician wants to examine him; the nursing staff is tied up with an emergency. Still later, now joined by John, Mary demands again to see their child. A flustered nurse returns with an obviously uncomfortable doctor who awkwardly announces that their child, quite certainly, has Down syndrome. The grim faces of the professionals leave no doubt that this is very bad news. When the word "mongoloid" slips out, Mary loses control. "How can this be?" she cries. "How can they know so soon? . . . The pregnancy went so well . . . I felt him active and kicking for months . . . The doctor assured me . . . Our family has never had defective children . . . I want to see the baby."

John is silent, sullen, paralyzed by the sudden emotional stab: After years of trying and waiting, this is his bitter fruit. The doctor commiserates—his own younger brother is retarded—but firmly resists Mary's entreaties to see the child: "Better not to see him, better not to get attached," he says. "Your baby will be placed in an institution that is capable of caring for him. After a while, you can visit him there. Children like your son can never be independent, never learn to read or write, have no hope of becoming normal or even close to it. If you keep him home, you and John will have to care for him the rest of his life, or at least the rest of yours—and after that, what then? You will have sacrificed everything, and for what? No, it is best not to become attached now."[1]

Cleveland General Hospital, 1990: *Rose and Jack Melina are the parents of a new baby girl. Brought to them soon after birth, the baby rocks gently in Rose's arms. The doctor and nurse drop by for a talk. Sitting at the bedside, the doctor strokes the child's head, inserts a finger into her clenched fist, and asks Rose how she is feeling. Jack says proudly he can tell already this is a "good baby." So far not even a whimper. Rose, with a trace of concern, wonders why she cannot keep the infant's head upright without a great deal of support. "She seems so floppy," Rose remarks.*

Taking advantage of the opening, the doctor agrees that the baby is more floppy than most. Has Rose noticed a few other abnormalities—the differences in the shape of the baby's eyes, tongue, hands? These are signs, the doctor says, that their child probably has Down syndrome. He will not be able to say for certain until chromosome tests are completed, but he hopes the Melinas will not despair. Observing their puzzled look, he goes on to explain: "The condition used to be called mongolism and was associated with severe mental retardation. But that word fell into disuse as scientists began to understand these children better. There has been a revolution in the care of children with Down syndrome. They are no longer placed in institutions and, thanks to early intervention services, can look forward to a promising future in the community.[2] A great variety of publicly financed services are available to you and your child. Therapists—physical, occupational, developmental, and speech—can come to your home im-

mediately. They will teach her how to move and play. They will also teach you how to increase her body tone, keep her active and communicative. She will be eligible for a center-based program, even as an infant, and will continue in school until she is 21. At least once a year professionals will ask for your input into a treatment plan. If at any time you are dissatisfied with your child's education or progress, there are procedures in place for resolving disagreements. You will have access to support groups where you can share experiences and swap advice with others living through the same experience; to respite care which brings experienced workers into your home so that you can get a break for hours or days; to counseling services if you want professional advice. This is not a tragedy. There is every reason to be optimistic. It would be a mistake to put any ceiling on your hopes and expectations and, at the very least, it is reasonable to expect that your daughter will be self-sufficient." The nurse then offers the Melinas names and agencies to contact for immediate help and parents who are on call to pay a hospital visit to the family.

The differences between these two messages bespeak the great progress made in the treatment of retarded children over the last 30 years. The Molloys go home with anger, shame, despair, and no child. The Melinas go home with hope and two baskets—one stuffed with books, pamphlets, programs, and toys; the other, gaily decorated by the hospital staff, containing their baby. Once shunned and put away, retarded children are now in plain view, trained for jobs in ordinary life. We see retarded children exulting in their triumphs at the Special Olympics. We see a Down syndrome child living a full and happy life on a network television show. It is a reform the country can take pride in, especially in a time when the well-being of children generally has declined. The pledge not to give up on the handicapped speaks well for this nation.

Yet in reality, how different are these doctors' messages, separated by three decades of experience and research into retardation? The message to both the Molloys and Melinas is that their child is a social misfit who must be shipped off or fixed up. The Molloy child, judged incurable, is to be removed from society for the benefit of his family; the Melina child, judged remediable, is to be immersed in treatment so that she can be integrated (or, in contemporary lingo, "mainstreamed") into society.

One could imagine a third scenario. The doctor might have said to the family: "Your child has Down syndrome. That means it is highly probable that he will be mentally retarded, though the precise degree varies substantially from child to child. I know this is a crushing disappointment, and I do not want to minimize your loss in any way. However, I hope you will believe me when I tell you that over time your grief will recede as you come to know your child and discover that he is so much more than his retardation. Slowly all of us are learning the lesson that a retarded child has just as much to offer his family, community, and country as anyone else, and just as good a chance for happiness. I can assure you that society at large is also much more accepting of mental retardation than it was 30 years ago, when we were infants. Today, retarded people, like other minorities, are less burdened by stigma and repudiation. Society is struggling to meet them halfway, demanding what they can accomplish and accommodating to what they cannot. You see daily how curbs are cut, ramps built, and bathrooms enlarged to meet the needs of those in wheelchairs; how TV broadcasts use sign interpreters for the deaf; and how elevators use braille to mark floors. Though less visible, society is also creating new opportunities for the retarded. Businesses that formerly would never have hired any problematic worker now provide assistance ('supported employment') to retarded employees with job-related problems. And right from the start, early intervention programs will respect who your child is, his natural developmental pace, without neglecting his potential."

It is unlikely that parents of retarded children* will hear this speech from early interventionists who prefer the optimistic nonlabeling approach of the Melinas' doctor. In both word and deed, at least during the preschool years, we stress acceleration of growth over acceptance of delay. A retarded child like the Molloy or Melina baby is perceived and treated by the adult (professional) world as impaired. It is somehow insufficient to protect and accept him, to watch over his development, giving guidance and support

---

*The word "retarded" may not have the same meaning to all readers. Indeed, professionals continue to debate the definition of the term; often they avoid using it, particularly with young children; and frequently they substitute more neutral words (e.g., "slow" and "delayed"). In this book I accept the conventional definition (American Psychiatric Association, 1987; Grossman, 1983). A child is mentally retarded if his intelligence and adaptive function are two or more standard deviations below the mean (usually a score below 70, with 100 being average). The category is further divided into mild (approximately 55 to 70), moderate (approximately 40 to 55), severe (approximately 25 to 40), and profound (below approximately 25). The diagnosis is made without regard to cause (medical or social) or prognosis.

as he probes his universe, albeit a diminished one. We feel obliged to act, to prod and coerce, to take charge of his behavior, to repair the damage. It does not feel right to relax our demands on retarded children and set up simplified environments. The message today is to make them do it our way, not to indulge their way. Waiting out the child's slow-paced growth, following and reacting to his minimal overtures, it is now believed, wastes valuable time—time we should use to stimulate his achievement. The possibility that our forceful intrusion might have negative consequences, that supportive rather than directive intervention might produce a better outcome, appears cold-hearted, perhaps even negligent. Where nature lags, nurture must do double time.

The question of how much we try to fix up and how much we allow to let be is part of a greater, ancient dispute about rearing children. And, because it engages questions of serious social and personal values, it is as intractable as it is fundamental. So long as families, schools, and other socializing agencies disagree on what is "good" and "right" behavior in children, the balance they strike will vary. In our society many parents believe it wrong to inhibit the free and natural ways of children. They make every effort to minimize conformity and obedience to an adult culture. They intentionally create a special culture for young children that gives great latitude for self-expression and postpones entry into adult life. Their homes are permissive, sometimes anarchic; their schools progressive, without clear schedules and curricula. At the other end of the spectrum are families who value, above all, control and discipline. They want children who do as adults tell them to do; who will learn quickly to inhibit infantile behavior in favor of more restrained, more civilized ways. Their homes are orderly and rule-bound, their schools are traditional, more teacher-directed and instructional.[3]

The balance between the expressive and repressive mode, between freedom and restraint, is conditioned by societal demands as well as parental values. In a complex and regulated society like ours, which requires a fair degree of conformity, the dispute is narrower than it would be in a wide-open culture with vast choices in life style. We want all citizens to be literate, vote, pay taxes, and live by laws and customs that powerfully restrain instinctual behavior (particularly aggressive and sexual). Every child, therefore, must learn specific skills and rules, must inhibit or sublimate a number of drives. On the other hand, we all agree that the younger the child, the greater the permissible freedom. Little children wear diapers, suck their thumbs, eat with their fingers, cry, bang, throw, dump, and make messes. As they get older, they give up these childish ways. The disagreement we have is over just what minimal behaviors a child must acquire, to what extent, by when; and what allowances can be made for distinct groups of children such as the mentally retarded.

The debate, moreover, involves questions of fact as well as of value, of means as well as ends, of practice as well as principle. While the value issues are unresolvable, we can ask of psychology and education, what are the costs and benefits of our interventions? What difference does it make if we instruct a child to use a potty, eat with utensils, find a hidden object at 1, 2, or 3 years of age? If we want a child to sit in a chair for 10 minutes at age 6, when do we start our sit-still demands? Is there a best age to teach manners, bike riding, reading, baseball, piano playing—that is, a time when the child learns with greatest ease, and parental time and effort are minimized? This is the question of critical periods, about which we know rather little but which, in principle, we could answer through carefully constructed research.[4]

If we reach agreement on a set of goals—for example, eventual reading competence (sixth-grade level) or honesty—then by varying amount, kind, and onset of instruction, we can empirically investigate how to accomplish our goals most effectively. Alongside the question of how best to achieve the desired benefits, we must also ask whether our interventions will produce damage. If we give too much instruction too early and thereby restrict a child's spontaneity, are there unforeseen costs to the child? For example, does early training create disciplined habits in children or suppress curiosity and imagination?[5]

The dilemma—part moral, part practical—in balancing our wishes to support children in their natural spontaneous impulses, yet impose upon them the necessary cultural restraints, is heightened in a deviant population. For normal children there is the comfort of knowing that the self-righting mechanisms of growth will correct, within a wide margin, the excesses of parents. The child's natural endowment and the influence of other social forces further buffer the impact of any particular philosophy of parenting. Given decent opportunities, the child with strict parents may well in the end look a lot like the child of lenient parents; both, predictably, will make adequate adjustments. We cannot be so optimistic about the development of an abnormal population. A mentally retarded child will probably not self-right. For this reason there is more pressure to intervene, and with such pressure comes a complex calculus of costs and benefits, rights and responsibilities. Few would advocate accommodating to the blindness of a child whose sight can be restored easily by surgery, or accommodating to a child's retardation that could be corrected by changes in diet. But when interventions are prolonged and their outcome uncertain, when there is no quick fix, we have to consider more carefully the competing alternatives. It is very human, but not necessarily wise, to redouble our efforts in the face of disappointing performance. In the case of disabled youngsters this reflexive response means doing more and more at younger and younger ages.

Our reformist enthusiasm toward the retarded finds a parallel in the history of deaf education. Until recently deaf education was controlled by "oralists," who insisted that vocal speech was the right goal for deaf children and that sign language, their natural form of communication, must be suppressed. Oralists, like early interventionists, wanted "to fashion them [the deaf] into the likeness of common men" through integration with the hearing (Howe, cited in Lane, 1989, p. 312). Alexander Graham Bell, a leading oralist, believed, mistakenly as it turned out, that after a few years of special education the deaf could be mainstreamed with the hearing. Samuel Gridley Howe, another prominent oralist, wanted to advance the deaf by limiting their contact with one another (a precursor of today's philosophy that the retarded, placed in mainstreamed classes, will model themselves after the nonretarded). In pursuit of this overly ambitious and largely futile goal, teachers assumed a dominating and authoritarian role, relegating children to a repressed, passive, and acquiescent one. In hindsight, as Leo Jacobs (1989) argues, this policy was disastrous: When deaf children are born to hearing parents (substitute retarded children born to nonretarded parents), there is a profound shock and an equally profound desire "approaching an unreasoning obsession, that their deaf child should also act normally—that is, behave like a hearing child" (p. 24). Educators of the deaf had the same obsession. Rather than aiming for the development of "happy, well-adjusted and productive deaf citizens, the hearing persons who have been in the saddle of authority have placed the greatest emphasis upon molding deaf children into acceptable facsimiles of hearing people, i.e., themselves" (p. 46). Out of this desire to normalize, and in disregard of children's problems and needs, was created a system of education that "has been a blight upon the educational practices for the deaf for the more than 170 years that we have had formal educational programs in the United States" (p. 30). Jacobs continues in offended outrage:

The most reprehensible thing about foisting a pure oral philosophy of communication upon a deaf child is its repressive character. It is extremely distressing to observe a hefty adult clamp-
ing a little deaf child's jaws so that the child cannot look in any
direction other than directly at the perspiring grown-up in order
for the adult either to demonstrate to the child how a word
should be spoken or to compel the little being to read the adult's
lips and get what he or she was trying to tell the child. This
practice has given some deaf youngsters such a psychological tic
that they find it impossible to look directly into anyone's eyes.
(p. 40)

Because the objective was too hard for most deaf students,
instruction was reduced to highly repetitive drills in narrow
phonetic skills. Teachers, by subdividing each task into tiny components, deceived themselves that progress was occurring. In fact,
between the ages of 10 to 16, the average gain in reading was less
than 1 year (Jacobs, 1989, quoting a 1959 study by Wrightstone,
Aronow, & Muskowitz). Today it is generally conceded that this
prolonged attempt in oral fluency was a failure and a disservice to
the deaf community.[6]

Much the same, I believe, is happening in early intervention.
We, too, desire "to fashion them [the retarded] into the likeness of
common men." We do our utmost to ready the preschool handicapped for participation in regular kindergarten. Our goal is their
inclusion, to the extent possible, in "regular education programs"
(Public Law 94-142, p. 13). To prepare 3- to 5-year-old children,
naturally progressing at half their chronological age, to fit in with
normal 5-year-olds, teachers must squelch their toddler-like immaturities, drill them in a narrow range of acceptable behaviors
and required skills. The pressure to accelerate development—
coming from yearning parents, the law, the nature of schools, the
history of special education, and powerful social mores—forces
teachers of the delayed, like teachers of the deaf, to regulate and
control, rather than support the child's own timetable. Inevitably
these teachers, too, become authoritarian, the children docile. And
when children fail to learn, these teachers, too, resort to repetition
of tasks and infinitesimal gains as evidence of success.

The nature of our intervention is, of course, a balancing act,
not an either–or choice. For the deaf, who have a useful, easily
learned alternative to oral language, it is very hard to justify
extensive amounts of time spent learning oral speech. What the
retarded may gain or lose in our drive for acceleration is more
subtle and varies from one subgroup to another.[7]

The purpose of this book is to consider if and when more becomes less—if and when our well-meaning efforts to mend tear into the integrity of a developing child; our attempts at hot-housing leave the child less adaptive; and whether everyone might be better off with a change in goals and modes of intervention. The question of whether we can accelerate development is one of the enduring controversies in psychology and education that may never, and probably should never, be resolved. America is a country that does not take kindly to limits. We will always try to reverse destiny. But that spirit benefits the handicapped if, and only if, expectations are not unrealistically grandiose and the efforts to change children not unduly harsh.

These issues have become especially timely as early intervention programs rapidly gear up to serve all handicapped children from ages 0 to 5. The enterprise raises broad and fundamental questions of social value: To what extent does compassion mean modifying the child to fit his surroundings or the surroundings to fit the child? Should we become more tolerant of diversity or encourage conformity by leaning hard against a child's nature? In the societal tension between the concepts of pluralism and assimilation, where do the retarded fit? What exactly do we mean by "improved outcome"? There are more specific child-rearing and educational questions: Is it better to have a child emerging from 21 years of schooling able to read a preprimer or to generate leisure-time activities? Is it better to turn out an individual who can obediently follow orders or to sacrifice some obedience for initiative? What trade-offs do we want to make between conformity and self-expression? There are, in addition, questions of a more practical or empirical character: What expectations for a developmentally delayed population can we reasonably meet? If we adopt a more responsive rather than a proactive mode, what will be the outcome? Do the various subcategories within the retarded population respond differently to our interventions? Are the children more responsive to acceleration in some developmental areas but not others? Assuming agreement on the "product" we are trying to achieve, how do we best (most humanely and efficiently) achieve it? What interventions are best introduced, and when? Does an early introduction of cognitive skills or early requirements for social conformity accelerate, retard, or have no effect on eventual outcome? If a goal is adult employability and self-care, what early experiences head the child in that direction? What are appropriate academic expectations?

One might reasonably ask: Why explore issues that cannot be

answered without prior agreement on values and without more empirical data? My justification is fourfold: First, we have plunged into a very large undertaking without sufficient discussion of our goals and methods. Our recent national decision to offer education and related services to children with developmental disabilities starting at birth is an extraordinary commitment. It will be an expensive undertaking. States already educating handicapped preschoolers (mostly 3- to 5-year-olds) have found that the cost is more than double (2.1) that of educating regular children in prekindergarten through Grade 12 (Moore, Strang, Schwartz, & Braddock, 1988).[8] Projected expenses for early intervention (birth to 5) are two to four times the cost of Head Start. To stay ahead of the critics and avoid a backlash requires vigorous self-scrutiny. Second, legislative decisions have already prematurely and inadvertently propelled the enterprise in a single direction; we must deliberate now if we want to put other models in place. Third, there are important discrepancies between what the service providers and the research literature have to say about the nature and development of the handicapped. This disagreement should be addressed. Fourth, although early intervention is a circumscribed undertaking with its own regulations, personnel, and objectives, the issues raised go well beyond it. The fundamental assumptions about the nature and needs of children, about how much and in what way adults should interfere, are of concern to educators and parents of all children, whatever their aptitude. As families increasingly surrender their children to educational institutions at ever younger ages and for longer hours, we must ask, what exactly does it mean to "care" for children?

In my judgment, despite the generous motives of society and committed able personnel in the field, our early intervention efforts, broadly speaking, have taken a wrong turn. In our eagerness to transform the retarded, we have adopted an extreme position on the freedom–restraint continuum. We cultivate these children as we would bonsai plants, leaving nothing to nature lest weeds emerge. But for all our fastidious attention, we are not getting bonsai results. The gain we seek, normal function or a close approximation thereto, is not offset by the pain we inflict in subjecting small retarded children to a restrictive regime "for their own good." There is no doubt that these children (and their families) need help; they have heavy burdens to carry. But it is help that will enable them to develop a comfortable sense of themselves; a sense of their own competence, individuality, dignity, and rightful place in the community. I hope to persuade the reader that a redirection is in order. We must widen our goals, reduce our demands, diversify our methods, and enlarge the degree of individualization. This expanded approach closely mimics the way in which parents acculturate "normal" young children—a blending of reactive and proactive strategies, the balance depending upon the child and the specific objective.

To narrow the discourse a bit, I have chosen to focus on 3- to 5-year-old children with moderate retardation (functioning very roughly between a third and a half of their chronological age) who are participating in early intervention programs. Even within this category, the children I have studied are a heterogeneous group. In addition to delay, many of them have other disabilities—autism, cerebral palsy, hyperactivity, distractibility. And, because early intervention classes always have mixtures of children, I have not completely excluded from observations children below age 3, nor the more and less severely retarded. I targeted a particular group only to make the issues concrete.

CHAPTER PREVIEWS

There are many possible approaches to a review of this sort. I chose to do a field study, sacrificing the orderliness and objectivity that one achieves through systematic measurement of separated variables for the chance to observe the pattern of events and reflections that emerge when different sorts of players—children, teachers, parents, administrators, and the paying citizenry—make common cause. The rationale for this approach is discussed in Chapter Two.

Chapter Three examines the values, practices and assumptions of early intervention in terms of three theoretical models that have become traditional in the literature of preschool education: the behavioral or cultural transmission model, the developmental or progressive model, and the romantic or libertarian model. Each of these embodies a set of goals, a methodology for accomplishing them, and a theory about the nature of children. In terms of the prior discussion, the behavioral model is associated with adult direction and a controlled, predetermined treatment approach; the developmental model, with a greater degree of child direction and a supportive, indeterminate treatment method; the romantic model, with full child self-determination and a permissive, open-ended mode of treatment. These models informed my observations of classroom activities and discussions with families and staff.

I considered the extent to which each program was committed to one or another theoretical model, and how the choice of models fluctuated depending upon the particular curriculum task and set of children. The reader, impatient of theory, who wants to interpret an early intervention program through her own prism, may wish to read Chapter Four before Chapter Three.

Chapter Four describes a morning in a fictional early intervention program, Midwood, attended by the kind of children I targeted for observation—moderately retarded 3- to 5-year-olds. It is meant to be a composite, a representative distillation that captures the main motifs of most programs. Midwood is not representative of every school, but it contains major elements found in most. (Only 1 program out of 20 did not resemble it to a significant extent.) Readers who have a different overall impression of the typical early intervention program may, nonetheless, find the description and analysis that follows applicable to parts of programs.

Using Midwood as a foundation, but supplementing it with field notes, I expand in Chapter Five on the early intervention culture: what is being taught, and how children are responding. The main point here is that the distance between the position of teachers and their charges is vast, the material too difficult and too remote for them to absorb. Despite my great admiration for the professionals in these programs—for their genuine devotion to the welfare of handicapped children, their impressive skills and resourcefulness, their warmth, kindness and modesty—I believe that they are stuck with a set of instructional objectives and teaching methods inappropriate to the children's developmental level. Acquisition of skills is the dominant ideology, control by teachers the dominant methodology. Unable or disinclined to modify these objectives, they are forced to use a number of restrictive techniques, discussed in Chapter Six. While on the surface it may appear that programs run smoothly and that teachers are gentle in their handling of retarded children, a closer look reveals a structure that is highly authoritarian for all its seeming benevolence.

The pressures for acceleration and teacher control, for bending the child to the procrustean demands of the culture, rather than the reverse, originate in sources often remote from the classroom. As discussed in Chapter Seven, the federal legislation mandating special education explicitly states that the funds are justified by the promise of acceleration. The law requires teachers to write an Individual Educational Program (IEP) for every child that sets out a year in advance (sometimes early intervention programs use a 6-month interval) exactly what objectives will be attained. These objectives must be monitored and their accomplishments verified objectively. Only an extraordinarily ingenious teacher can be child-directed and flexible, yet conform to the IEP law. The placement of small children in elementary school buildings and the ambition to mainstream them add further pressure. Chapter Eight reviews the nearer forces that also push for acceleration within a narrow behavioral realm. These include the high expectations of parents, the intimate relationships between teachers and parents, the traditions of special education practice, and the view of teachers that retarded children are different from the nonretarded.

Chapter Nine summarizes the psychological literature on the nature of mentally retarded children and the relationship of this literature to developmental principles. It explores the discrepancies between the research findings and the assumptions underlying most real-world special education practice. It argues that the evidence, though far from conclusive, is at least consistent with a less didactic, more individualized and flexible approach that would better fit the complexity and variety of children attending early intervention programs.

That approach, which I call a "parental" model, is outlined in Chapter Ten. It would promote, to the extent possible, a reciprocal rather than a directive relationship between teachers and children. As with parents, teachers must tailor both the amount and kind of their intervention to the characteristics of each child and the nature of each educational objective. For some children whose problem is largely one of developmental rate (often those with Down syndrome), we need to back off and create an environment supportive of their natural rhythms. For them, expectations must be delayed, not accelerated. For other children, such as those with autism, we need to offer heavy adult intervention, or they will remain stuck "in a world of their own." For some attainments (e.g., toileting) adult direction is required for all children, whereas for other attainments (e.g., curiosity) no amount of direction will be of benefit. How to accomplish all this is illustrated through a newly launched Midwood II.

For most of the moderately retarded, catching up to normal kindergarten children during the preschool years is not a realistic goal. Instead of drilling them in preacademics, we should use our time to encourage other avenues of growth, responding to and expanding upon their interests and overtures. Parents do not expect a 2-year-old to behave and learn as a 4-year-old. Neither should educators expect a child *functioning* as a 2-year-old to act like a 4-year-old. Yet parents of both 2- and 4-year-olds impose certain behavioral requirements on their children—for example, toileting, eating, and sleeping routines. Educators, too, must choose the areas where authority should be brought to bear and those in which freedom should be allowed to flourish, recognizing that, like families, educators will (and should) continue to debate how much we accommodate the handicapped and how much the handicapped must accommodate us.

CHAPTER TWO

Methods

The essence of perception is that it is selective; there is no
value-free mode of seeing . . . All description is in some
degree evaluative inasmuch as only a fool would choose to
describe the trivial. All evaluation is interpretive to the
degree that one seeks to make some sense of what a situation
or an experience means.

—Eisner (1985, pp. 222, 230)

EVALUATIVE, OBJECTIVE, AND QUALITATIVE

The double purpose of this field study was to describe and
evaluate what is happening in early intervention programs; it is
thus both objective and judgmental. Although I have tried to keep
some separation between the two purposes—for example, when
describing Midwood, I refrain from analysis, leaving the reader
free to formulate his or her own—they are in fact symbiotic. There
can be no observations without prior and subsequent judgments,
no judgments without observations. All observations originate
from a point of view about what is, and is not, important to
investigate. Without a value orientation we would be stymied by
the infinite number of possible observables. Once the data are
collected, we again rely on a point of view for interpretation. Our
assumptions, therefore, bracket our observations.

Take, for instance, the question of a child's academic progress.
Investigators of different ideological persuasions have a number of
options. One investigator believes learning is equivalent to knowledge attained and is displayed by questions answered correctly.
She develops an observational schedule and codes the child's responses to the teacher's demands. When the child does poorly she
may, depending on her beliefs, determine that the demands were

excessive, or insufficient, or unrewarding, or insensitive to competing child interests, etc. Another investigator, with a different perspective, believes learning is equivalent to increased curiosity and is demonstrated by questions asked or diversity of ideas generated in a discussion. She will have a different set of observational categories and a different set of judgments. A third investigator objects to framing the question in terms of child outcome without first asking if the curriculum is appropriate.This requires expanding the observations from questions asked and answers given to a more molar look at the activities of child and teacher. The broadened investigation might conclude with a set of interpretations that address a child's and teacher's motivations, culture, and family attitudes.

Implicit in any study of learning are numerous assumptions about outcome and methods: What do we mean by academic progress (e.g., better reading skills, better analytic skills, greater scholastic interest, better citizenship)? How is it best displayed (e.g., use of leisure time, participation in intellectual activities, projects completed, teacher judgments, standardized tests)? What conclusions should we draw from the data (e.g., need more field trips, parent involvement, child choice, discovery, study guides, recitations)? The bias of the researcher is both inevitable and indispensable. Without it there would be no insight. Because all research is (and should be) infiltrated with values, it is more useful to expose and justify one's perspective than to try to eliminate it in some vain attempt at pure objectivity.

The role of an educational researcher, as Elliot Eisner (1985) has aptly illustrated, is analogous to that of an art critic. As an expert (connoisseur), the critic is finely tuned to subtleties others may miss. Her cultivated eye is trained by an aesthetic, a set of standards about what is good, and a way of organizing the subject matter. The critic, by enabling others to see more profoundly, acts as a "midwife to perception" (p. 217). To have credibility, Eisner stresses, the critic must be objective (empirical), the qualities she notes observable to others. There is no incompatibility between holding a point of view, an aesthetic, and objectivity; indeed, they are complementary.

In carrying out a study, the choice between qualitative or quantitative methods, or a combination of the two, depends upon the piece of reality under investigation and the trade-offs one is willing to make. Returning to the previous example, quantitative methods would be very appropriate for investigating a child's question-answering or question-asking behavior, qualitative ones better suited for the match between a teaching environment and child status considerations. Even though every investigative tool reflects a point of view, quantitative methods that rely on standardized instruments have certain advantages: they are more "observer proof" than less determinate methods of observation, more replicable, and comparisons are more precise. But one does not always want to bind the investigator to rigid predetermined schedules of interviewing and observation. As Eisner has put it:

> We tend to take it for granted, or we seem to believe that with the use of an observation schedule the problem of seeing what goes on in classrooms is cared for. This is simply naive. What is significant in a social setting might have little to do with the incidence of a particular activity or statement but a lot to do with a single act or statement or with the organizational structure of the classroom or with the character of an assigned task or with the way in which a reward is given. Observation schedules are tools that can guide one's attention, but their mechanical use can blind one to what is significant. (1985, p. 220)

In any complex multidetermined situation—such as a classroom—aggregating the individual parts does not necessarily produce a verisimilitude of the whole. Identical incidents may have very different meaning depending upon context, and "context" includes what is valued as well as what is occurring. For instance, lack of compliance with a teacher's suggestion may be important or not depending on whether suggestions are genuine take-it-or-leave-it ideas, disguised orders, teacher expectations, or classroom conventions. Without some grasp of the classroom culture, an investigator would not know how to weight noncompliance.

For this field study, qualitative methods (or what Lightfoot, 1983, has called "portraiture techniques") were more appropriate to the broad focus—what is going on, how is it working, what causal forces are operating, what are the implications? Qualitative methods leave more elbowroom to incorporate the unexpected, shift perspectives, respond to relevant data and new ideas as they emerge. They are more sensitive to unpredicted patterns and relationships—for example, between staffing patterns and teaching methods, or between school setting and curriculum—that a more restricted investigation ignores. That's the upside. On the downside, they enlarge the possibility of distorting what's out there to fit preconceptions. How can the reader be assured that the investigator is using her viewpoint as a lens to facilitate perception, rather than as a radar to attract only confirmatory material?

There is no totally satisfactory response to this concern. Precautions can be taken against arbitrariness by using at least a loose structure for observation, videotaping and sharing observations, and providing redundancy through multiple sources. In the last analysis, however, the investigator, like the critic, must persuade the reader with sufficiency of documentation. The findings have to click with the experiences of others exposed to the same subject matter.

PERSUASIONS AND PROCEDURES

A Point of View

As previously mentioned, I chose to observe early intervention programs through traditional models—behavioral, developmental, and romantic (although there is little loyalty to, or evidence of, the third)—because, at least according to Lawrence Kohlberg and colleagues (1987), these models bring together a psychology, epistemology, set of moral constructs, and educational objectives. (We will consider in the next chapter whether the models truly are this inclusive or whether they permit mix-and-match possibilities.) The breadth of the models was appealing and forced me to consider not only what transpired between teachers and children but also how teachers conceptualized the nature of retarded children (psychology and epistemology), what they wanted to accomplish, and why (educational objectives and moral constructs).

From my prior experience with early intervention I expected to find, and did, that the behavioral model was dominant. I had no vested interest in that outcome, however, and the observational lens should not have clouded my observations. I was not out to "prove" that early intervention has gone behavioral. Instead of inventing a prototypical program for the reader, I could have presented a variety of programs. In fact, I had planned to do just that. As it turned out, I found a fair degree of heterogeneity in teachers' stated allegiances and in their manner with children, but considerable homogeneity in the daily experiences of children, due to standard goals and curricula.

I might have chosen to emphasize the dissimilarities. In addition to variations in schedules, services offered, teacher personalities, groupings of children, and equipment, there were real differences in the amount of freedom children were given, inclusion of parents, adherence to the IEP, stated philosophy, etc. I was,

tally retarded" children, the initial response is usually, "we don't use that word." If one then suggests "developmental disabilities," the variety of children produced is so vast that it is hard to discuss them as a group. But if one says "children with Down syndrome and others at about their level," there is a higher probability of agreement on the population. Second, children with Down syndrome were included because they are a clearly identifiable, fairly large group, and the subject of a substantial literature. Third, and most importantly, the moderately retarded, who cannot be assimilated easily into the normal category, force us to confront the issues in this book. There is a developmental chasm between a 4-year-old at a 4-year level and a 4-year-old at a 2-year level. Even the most enthusiastic integrationist agrees that the latter will require heavy doses of extra help to keep up with a curriculum for normal 4-year-olds. So the hard question cannot be avoided: whether to lower the objectives or work harder to accomplish them. In contrast, however, to many of the severely and profoundly retarded, a large percentage of moderately retarded children do make slow developmental progress without intensive training.

I spent a minimum of 3 days in each program, studying it from multiple angles to achieve as full a picture as possible. One cannot understand a program merely by looking at classroom activities. In contemporary lingo, programs exist in an ecology of everwidening influences. I tried to thread my way by speaking with teachers, administrators, and parents, reviewing state and local policies, and then supplementing the data I accumulated by a review of federal law and the relevant research literature on development and education.

For the few hours the children were at school, I sat in the classroom with them. In each school I usually observed three sessions with one teacher and, for those schools on split schedules, I also observed a second classroom less intensively. My procedure was to concentrate on one moderately retarded child for a halfday, while tracking the activities of the entire group. I tried to capture the flow of events as experienced by that child and, most especially, the encounters between child and adults. At the same time I wanted to understand the day through the teacher's position, so I shifted back and forth between teacher and target child. With only six children in a class and many total group activities, it was not too difficult an observational task. I kept running notes of the class activities with time notations when they shifted periods (e.g., from circle, to art, to gross motor), again trying to capture in detail the teacher–child encounters. I also did some videotaping at each center, largely to keep the reality present when I sat down to make interpretations.

At the noon break, or after school was dismissed, I interviewed teachers (32), administrators (24), and parents (41, usually mothers whom I generally saw at their homes in the late afternoon). The basic purpose of these interviews was to understand how the central players perceived the programs—their purpose (moral constructs), content (educational objectives), methods (epistemology), and perception of the children (psychology). Interviews lasted about an hour—somewhat less with teachers, more with administrators and parents. Names of parents were generally given to me by the teachers, and I contacted them to make the interview arrangements. Because they were preselected I cannot be certain that their enthusiasm about early intervention is characteristic of parents at large.

I asked a set of routine questions to make sure the same issues were covered at each interview. Although at the start I had hoped to code and categorize at least a few of the responses, I found that it was generally impossible to understand what an answer meant except by extended follow-up questioning, and often a point relevant to one question was given as a response to another. The topic of early intervention is full of slogans and cliches. There are "good" words like "developmental," "individualized," and "mainstreaming" and "bad" words like "labeling," "retarded," and "segregated." It took probing and rephrasing to uncover just what these words and others (e.g., "functional skills," "behavioral," "sensorimotor stimulation") meant to the speaker.

I started each interview with parents by asking them to tell me their child's history—how did they find out he had a disability, when did intervention services begin, what sort of services had they received? No matter how often parents had given their story, I found they were usually glad to tell it again to a sympathetic listener. Their sad, brave, and often lonely tales could never be coded but were critical to hear. They helped me understand that far beyond their instructional role, the programs were places where, after great affliction, parents found friendship and understanding. After hearing an account of the child's history, I asked parents what they thought the program was trying to accomplish—its overall objectives, teaching methods, specific instruction for their child—and their reaction to it. I asked them what changes they would like to see and their views on mainstreaming.

Finally, I asked them what personal benefits they had, and had not, received and what they had learned about their child and how to manage him.

With teachers I started by asking about their professional backgrounds. Then came questions related to their philosophies and curricula: the educational models they espoused; whether they thought these children learned differently from normal children, and if so, in what way; how central was the IEP to their programs and how did they develop the IEP; what was their planning like (for the day, week, month, year); and what were their objectives for a typical child and family—what was the youngster like on entrance and what changes would you aim for? The next set of questions concerned methods: To what extent were the methods directive versus permissive (i.e., to what degree did the child or teacher set the agenda); how did they control children, and for what behavior; how did they conceptualize and carry out individualization; and how should they (and *did* they) incorporate parents? Finally, I asked them for their personal responses: What were their sources of satisfaction and dissatisfaction; what would they like to see changed; what personal growth had they experienced or desired, and what were their views on mainstreaming?

I asked administrators all the same questions, plus another set about the structure of the program—funding and transportation, nature and use of the setting, population served, frequency and duration of attendance, services provided, grouping and scheduling, provisions for parents, use of volunteers, characteristics of the staff (qualifications, salaries, turnover), and adult–child ratios. I also asked them a set of questions about evaluation: How were the children evaluated initially for admission, for their IEPs, and how were teachers, administrators and programs evaluated? In my discussion of the results I have collapsed teacher and administrator responses to the questions on philosophy and curriculum, methods, and personal attitudes because, somewhat surprisingly, I did not see systematic differences. Quotes from interviews are exact except for modest corrections of incomplete and ungrammatical sentences.

In every program I collected as much written documentation as possible: regulations, newsletters, lesson plans, data sheets, and always IEPs for a number of the children. Altogether I gathered 180 IEPs. To understand goal progression, I obtained two or more sequential IEPs for 24 children (at least two from each program) .

REPORTING THE DATA

The following chapters are an analysis, not a summary, of early intervention. I rejected an initial plan to present, separately and in sequence, classroom observations; parent, teacher, and administrator interviews; IEPs; etc., in favor of a layered interpretation supported with documentation. I have provided, first, a background review of the major early childhood models, including discussion of their relevance to the retarded. Next is a preliminary description of a prototypical program (Midwood), followed by a broader and deeper look at programs noting, in particular, those tensions created by the contrasting positions of teachers and children and how such tensions are handled. Then, I move beyond the programs themselves to their operational constraints and, pulling back still further, to a review of the psychological premises supporting them. Last, drawing upon the analysis, I offer a suggestion for program modifications. Much of the material collected (e.g., extensive data on the regulations and expenditures of different states, child and staff evaluation, teacher backgrounds, the different experiences of children in mainstreamed and nonmainstreamed settings, the nature and administration of therapies, etc.) is irrelevant to the line of argument and so has been omitted. Reporting this additional material would distract and burden the reader without changing the perspective. Aside from the events and characters of Midwood, all references to incidents and statements by participants are factual.

A word on terminology. Throughout the following chapters I have not flinched at using the term "mental retardation" for children functioning in that range *regardless* of whether they carry other diagnoses such as autism, cerebral palsy, behavioral disorder, attentional deficit disorder, etc. That means children with behavioral and/or emotional disorders who *function* in the retarded range may be called retarded as well as autistic, hyperactive, or whatever. In doing this I am following the definitions developed by the major professional organizations concerned (American Association of Mental Deficiency, American Psychiatric Association, International Classification of Diseases). I also write of "retarded children" rather than the sometimes preferred "children with retardation," although I conform to the latter formulation when it is not dreadfully awkward. The former expression fits much of our other speech patterns—slow children, smart children, sick children. Of course this does not mean that I think a retarded child is defined by his retardation. If there is a single message in this book, it is that they are children first and foremost, and it is their childishness that we must support. Finally, I have stayed with "retarded"–"nonretarded" (or normal) and away from the buzz words of today—"atypical" and "typical." While I appreciate that use of obfuscating terminology is designed to protect children against self-fulfilling prophecies, it is also a barrier to clear communication and research. More importantly, if greater social acceptance of mentally retarded children is a goal, then this acceptance must begin with a desensitization to the term. Obviously I do not want to offend by using the "MR word," but neither do I want to indulge in a deception, promoted by waffling terminology.*

Another controversial issue of terminology has to do with the choice between "handicapped" and "disabled." Many in the field of special education advocate the exclusive use of the latter on the grounds that the former "describes a condition or barrier imposed by society, the environment, or by one's own self. Handicap can be used when citing laws and situations but should not be used to describe a disability" (*Guidelines* . . . , 1990, p. 4). This preference is reflected in the recent Congressional action changing the title of Public Law 94-142 from the Education of the Handicapped Act to Individuals with Disabilities Education Act (Public Law 101-476, Education of the Handicapped Act, Amendments of 1990). Although both terms are used in this book, I generally prefer "handicapped"; it seems to me a gentler term, implying disadvantage rather than ultimate incapacity. I do not share the opinion that "handicap" should be reserved for "a condition or barrier imposed by society," an arbitrarily restrictive definition that finds no support in general usage.

A word about prototypes. The morning at Midwood is meant to be "prototypical" of early intervention programs, not average.[4] There is no such program as Midwood but, to a greater or lesser

---

*Throughout the book I refer to "teachers" rather than "teachers and aides." Even though there are important differences between the roles, the general comments made about teachers include aides as well. I have also favored the feminine pronoun over either the masculine or the combined feminine and masculine. The world of early intervention is predominantly female. In the schools I visited, all but one teacher and one aide were females, and, although I spoke with several fathers, most of the caretakers were also female.

degree, Midwood is in almost every program. Each incident described in Midwood I and Midwood II is typical of a large number of related incidents, but none actually occurred in the manner portrayed. The combination of incidents is meant to be a distillation of the early intervention culture—its usual patterns of social interaction and types of activities. Why representative and not average? Because, assuming one could actually enumerate all the variables and determine the average of each, the composite still might not be a good reflection of the institution. For example, the average classroom, unlike Midwood, may not have both an autistic and cerebral palsied child, or an inexperienced and older, experienced teacher; but these combinations and the dynamics they produce illuminate central features of early intervention. Prototypes are ideals that embody the essence of a category, but do not have all its attributes. They permit one to select pieces which, when joined, exemplify what early intervention is all about and most clearly separate it from other cultures such as home, hospital, day-care, or nursery school. It is in this sense that Midwood is a prototype; it represents the essence of the category *early intervention,* even though the particular combination of people and events may not be average. But before describing the prototype, let us examine the three models used in this study to observe, interpret and evaluate programs.

CHAPTER THREE

Educational Models and the Nature of Children

The history of educational theory is marked by opposition between the idea that education is development from within and that it is formation from without; that it is based upon natural endowments and that education is a process of overcoming natural inclination and substituting in its place habits acquired under external pressure.

—DEWEY (1938, p. 17)

THREE ORIENTATIONS

The historic battle between child-centered libertarian and teacher-centered authoritarian schooling is at bedrock a dispute about human nature and human development. Lawrence Kohlberg and colleagues (Kohlberg & Mayer, 1972; Kohlberg et al., 1987) have given us a useful conceptual framework for understanding the controversy. Kohlberg identifies three contending schools of thought. The first, or "romantic," school—which traces its lineage to the French 18th-century philosopher Jean Jacques Rousseau—holds that human nature is good and should be allowed to unfold without adult interference: they educate best who govern least. At the other extreme, the "cultural transmission" or "behavioral" school—which is associated with the British 17th-century philosopher John Locke—maintains that human nature is plastic, its development subject to social shaping: they educate best who govern most. Finally, a more recent and intermediate tradition—identified with 20th-century thinkers Jean Piaget and John Dewey—is what Kohlberg calls the "progressive" or "de-

27

velopmental" school; its representatives believe that while innate structures control the pace and stage of a child's development, her psychological growth depends upon interaction with the outside social and physical world: they educate best who govern jointly.

The three orientations are, according to Kohlberg, fundamentally incompatible. From each view of human nature sprouts a cluster of related and necessary beliefs. The romantic school is committed to a maturational psychology in which children's mental growth, like their physical growth, is controlled by an internal clock that ticks steadily and reliably if not interrupted; a theory of knowledge that is existential or phenomenological (truth means self-awareness); a morality that equates the good with the natural (whatever it is the child wants is what she should want); and, as an educational objective, the pursuit of mental health, self-confidence, curiosity, self-discipline, self-actualization—what Kohlberg calls an arbitrary "bag of virtues."

The cultural transmission school is committed to the psychological principles of behaviorism, according to which children's actions are shaped not by the gradual unfurling of some internal scroll, but by external experiences; a theory of knowledge as exclusively a product of experience and sensation; a relativistic morality which defines virtue as conformity to existing social values (good is found in consensus); and, as an educational objective, the satisfaction of standards set by the community and measured by tests and grades.

The progressive school cuts a path between the other two: a child's behavior is determined by the interplay between an internal script and encounters with the outside world; knowledge is dialectic, neither objective nor internal, but the product of a child's actions upon a given problem; morality lies in development and in the virtues of inquiry, reflection, freedom, and democracy; and the aim of education is to assist the child in an intellectual and moral journey through the stages, with ever greater differentiation, integration, and responsible autonomy.

Each of these schools likewise has a different notion of how children are motivated. For the romantic school, the child's motivation is internal and can only be dampened by outside meddling. For the cultural transmission school, children are motivated by parents' and teachers' strategic deployment of experience and reinforcements. For the progressive school, children are motivated internally to understand and create meaning, but that rich soil must be fertilized through external experience.

Kohlberg makes his distinctions thoughtfully: three models,

three choices, and one—the progressive school—that is psychologically and morally correct. But, as we shall see, he exaggerates their incompatibility. The visions held by the original philosophers on children's nature and proper nurture overlap to a significant extent; they differ in emphasis and degree, and the attempt to present them as sharply contradictory models is oversimplified.

The Distinctions

"Everything is good as it comes from the hands of the Creator; everything degenerates in the hands of man" (Rousseau, 1964). Thus opens Rousseau's *Emile*. The faults of children that we wrongly impute to nature are, instead, the result of bad training; nature itself makes no mistakes (although, admittedly, it is not evenhanded in its distribution of mental capacities and dispositions). Children, like plants, are "the natural products of a soil" whose growth requires support, not reshaping; society should provide "nutriments" for the child's "inclinations." Adults should "leave the child the use of his natural liberty" and exclude from their vocabulary the words *obey* and *command* (Rousseau, 1762/ 1969). If we try to thwart nature in educating children, we will either turn them into tyrants by indulging imaginary needs or enslave them by exercising excessive power. Children will become strong, independent, even courageous, if we leave them to experience the delights, as well as the bruises, of liberty. Young children learn best from raw encounters with the world, not from adult pampering or prohibitions.

Not so, argues Locke (1693/1927). The young child is by nature a "brute," lacking in both reason and understanding; free will is not the expression of natural, uncultivated drives but the mature, knowledgeable, and restrained exercise of liberty. The mind of the young child must be "made obedient to Discipline, and pliant to Reason, when at first it [is] most tender, most easy to be bow'd." Until maturity, therefore, children are "to be under the absolute Power and Restraint of those in whose Hands they are." They "should look upon their Parents as their Lords, their absolute Governors, and as such stand in awe of them," for fear and awe are the means by which we gain control over their unruly minds. Only those who have become accustomed as children to "submit their Desires, and go without their Longings, even *from their very Cradles*" will be able to exercise their freedom responsibly as adults.

Indulge a child, fail to curb him, and you will create an undisciplined irresponsible adult. "He that is not us'd to submit his Will to the Reason of others *when* he is *young*, will scarce hearken to submit to his own Reason when he is of an Age to make Use of it."

Rousseau's philosophy of freedom (according to Kohlberg et al., 1987) finds its modern-day expression in A. S. Neil's school, Summerhill. Neil (1960), too, believes children are good and should be left to grow freely, surrounded by the natural world. Class attendance at Summerhill is entirely voluntary; healthy children, Neil assumes, will want to learn and, in any case, cannot be forced to do so. Freedom, however, is not license. Adults must have a limited authority to safeguard the freedom of others and to protect children from experiences they are too young to handle (e.g., coping with traffic, tools, a hot stove). This minimal use of authority, claims Neil, produces independent happy people; it avoids the errors both of the overdisciplined home where children have no rights and of the spoiled home where they have nothing but rights. The ideal home is one in which children and adults have equal rights. And the same applies to school.

A contemporary version of Locke (according to Kohlberg et al., 1987) is found in B. F. Skinner's utopian community, Walden II. Although Skinner the behaviorist, speaking through his character Frazier (1948/1976), denies the existence of free will—insisting that all actions, indeed all motives, desires, and wishes are the consequence of "behavioral engineering"—he contends that the *feeling* of freedom (essentially, the awareness of choice) is the result of, not the precondition for, learning. At the outset of life the child, restrained by adult control, therefore feels unfree. Gradually, by systematically exposing the child to various degrees and kinds of temptations and adversities, the adult teaches the child habits of resistance and self-control. As the child accepts the rules of the society—and all moral training is completed by age 6—adults relax these external controls, confident that the child is now destined to grow up socially responsible. The child then feels free.

The progressive tradition blurs the distinction between natural endowment and environment by adopting a constructivist position. Human nature, according to the progressive school, is rooted in biological structures and passes through predestined stages, but the content and expression of these structures and stages is formed by interaction with the environment. "The world is not sat in by the child, it is made by him" (Kessen, 1965, p. 58). According to this tradition, children, at every moment, are acting on their external world, reshaping and defining it, while it simultaneously changes them. Adults do not imprint the meaning of objects and ideas on a child, as Locke believed, for unless the child already has a will and reason capable of acting upon and responding to the outside world, she will find it meaningless. Nor would a child's free expression of will and reason, without external stimuli, lead to intelligence, as Rousseau maintained. Even a potential genius will be less than human if raised in a dark closet. Children must have constant, vital interplay with their physical and social environments to achieve their potential. Understanding emerges from the child's repeated, although initially inept, forays into a world of evanescent properties, from which he gradually constructs a meaningful reality.

As we consider how to educate children whose will and reason are impaired, it is important not to skip lightly over the principle of knowledge-through-action, fundamental to Piaget's theory (see, e.g., Piaget, 1952, 1970).[1] According to Piaget, a child knows an object only when it is assimilated through movement; mere looking does not make it yours. To "know" something is to understand how it feels when you touch, clasp, or swipe it, how it gratifies or displeases you, the functions it performs. A bottle is to suck, a cord is to pull, a rattle is to shake. The earliest mental representations of objects are not figurative copies of what is "really" there, but mental diagrams derived from our sensorimotor encounters with the "reality." It is only through manipulation that objects become real, substantial and permanent. Piaget (1954) gives this example (one of many): At 8 months of age Jacqueline, his daughter, takes her father's watch while he holds onto the chain.

> She examines the watch with great interest, feels it, turns it over . . . I pull the chain; she feels a resistance and holds it back with force, but ends by letting it go. As she is lying down she does not try to look but holds out her arm, catches the watch again and brings it before her eyes . . . If I pull the object progressively (a little farther each time she has caught it) she searches farther and farther, handling and pulling everything that she encounters . . . But this permanence is solely the function of prehension. If, before her eyes, I hide the watch behind my hand, behind the quilt, etc., she does not react and forgets everything immediately; in the absence of tactile factors visual images seem to melt into each other without substance. (p. 21)

Dewey, though less a student of development, is like-minded. Learning occurs only when "interest" and "experience" are activated.

The child's own instincts and powers furnish the material and give the starting point for all education. Save as the efforts of the educator connect with some activity which the child is carrying on of his own initiative independent of the educator, education becomes reduced to a pressure from without. It may, indeed, give certain external results, but cannot truly be called educative. Without insight into the psychological structure and activities of the individual, the educative process will, therefore, be haphazard and arbitrary. If it chances to coincide with the child's activities it will get a leverage; if it does not, it will result in friction, or disintegration, or arrest of the child's nature. (1897/1959, p. 20)

Unless a teacher begins and ends with a child's interests, her instruction is "dead and barren" (Dewey, 1902/1959, p. 106). Just as food is inert and useless until digested by the child's body, so too is instruction dead until animated by the child's interest and action.[2]

The Overlap

At first blush the models, with their apparently distinct understanding of human nature and learning, do indeed seem irreconcilable. But that is true only if we accept the mutually exclusive assumptions about the nature of children. *If* a child is born good, his life ready to unroll like a long scroll, then it follows that adult intervention threatens to upset the blueprint. *If* he is born indeterminate, ready to learn but not predisposed in any direction good or bad, then to withhold authority is irresponsible. There is no obligation, however, to accept the extreme either–or assumptions; it is not illogical—in the sense that a form cannot be both a circle and a square—to combine the assumptions. Suppose that the mind is more complex; that it is *both* partially inscribed and partially empty, partially virtuous and partially neutral? Then it becomes possible, even necessary, to blend the traditions without violating a child's basic nature, and to think of the schools as ideal types from which to draw. A closer look at Locke and Rousseau suggests that they, as well as Piaget, adopt this composite perspective. Locke did not envision the child without a predisposing nature, nor Rousseau a society without educational responsibility.

The originators of both the romantic and cultural transmission schools accept the psychological premise that children possess an innate inquisitiveness that propels development. Rousseau claimed that just as the body seeks activity, so, in due time, will the mind seek knowledge. Even Locke (1693/1927) believed in the importance of children's curiosity, which "is but an Appetite after Knowledge; and therefore ought to be encouraged in them, not only as a good Sign, but as the great Instrument Nature has provided to remove that Ignorance they were born with." As adults we should appeal to their interests. "A Child will learn three times as much when he is *in Tune,* as he will with double the Time and Pains when he goes awkwardly or is dragg'ed unwillingly to it." And nearly three centuries later, Skinner (1948/1976) advised adults to "appeal to the curiosity which is characteristic of the unrestrained child . . . appeal to that drive to control the environment which makes a baby continue to crumple a piece of noisy paper."

Both philosophers accept the limitations on body and mind imposed by nature. Rousseau dismissed nature's mistakes out of hand. "I would not undertake the care of a feeble, sickly child, should he live to four score years . . . If I vainly lavish my care upon him, what can I do but double the loss to society by robbing it of two men, instead of one? Let another tend this weakling for me" (Rousseau, 1762/1969). Even Locke, the protobehaviorist, saw that "God has stamp'd certain Characters upon Men's Minds, which like their Shapes, may perhaps be a little mended, but can hardly be totally alter'd and transform'ed into the contrary . . . For in many Cases, all that we can do, or should aim at, is, to make the best of what Nature has given" (1693/1927). Therefore, *"lunatics and ideots . . . [who] cannot possibly have the use of right reason to guide themselves, have for their guide, the reason that guideth other men which are tutors over them"* (1690/1980). Because they never achieve the rationality necessary for free will, their lot is permanent subservience to adults.

Both philosophers see a virtue to childishness which should not (and effectively cannot) be repressed. Rousseau railed against precocious instruction in language and reading, indeed anything the adult, but not the child, considers worthy: "Nature provides for the child's growth in her own fashion, and this should never be thwarted. Do not make him sit still when he wants to run about, nor run when he wants to be quiet" (Rousseau, 1762/1969). He urged adults: "Do not save time, but lose it." Even Locke preferred play for the immature child to forced instruction. "For all their innocent Folly, Playing, and *childish Actions, are to be left perfectly free and unrestrain'd* as far as they can consist [*sic*] with the Respect for those that are present; and that with the greatest Allowance" (1693/1927). Children should not be made to do things "but when they have a Mind and *Disposition to* it." And "none of the Things they are to learn, should ever be made a Burthen to them, or impos'd on them as a Task"; under pressure they will turn away forever.

Both recognized the difference between parroting and learning. Young children, being docile and eager mimics, can easily be taught without really understanding. Rousseau (1964) noted that "the delicate texture of their brains reflects like a mirror every object which is presented to them," but he objected to "the mass of ill-digested and disconnected information with which we load the frail brains of children . . . [that do] more harm than good to the understanding." Locke (1693/1927) echoed these sentiments: "And here give me leave to take Notice of one Thing I think a Fault in the ordinary Method of Education; and that is, the charging of Children's Memories, upon all Occasions, with *Rules* and Precepts, which they often do not understand, and constantly as soon forget as given."

On the other hand, both men realized that the weak and helpless child cannot be left entirely to nature. Even Rousseau (1762/1969) warned parents to be wary of their children who, finding the possession of power very pleasing, will take a mile if given an inch. "The child's first tears are prayers, beware lest they become commands; he begins by asking for aid, he ends by demanding service . . . the more he cries the less you should heed him. He must learn in good time not to give commands to men, for he is not their master." Parents must understand that their advantage in strength and knowledge enables them to control children with a light hand. Far better that they leave the child alone to learn through the "heavy yoke of necessity" than that they interfere with suggestions and prohibitions. A good parent maneuvers a child's opportunities so that he enjoys "well-regulated liberty," liberty regulated, that is, in accordance with parental wishes. The child "ought only to do what he wants, but he ought to want to do nothing but what you want him to do. He should never take a step you have not foreseen, nor utter a word you could not foretell." The natural consequences that follow from a child's unruliness are the best discipline against it: "He breaks the windows of his room. Let the wind blow in day and night; do not mind his catching cold. It is better that he should catch cold than that he should do such silly things" (Rousseau, 1964).

Neither philosopher was a radical ideologue. Rousseau, though anti-authoritarian, anti-establishment, and pro-peasant education, did not extol primitive man, while Locke, albeit appreciative of good breeding, was no repressive martinet. They shared the belief that education should prepare children (alas, boys only) to take their place in society and perform its functions; should inculcate virtue, not mere book learning; and should establish a limited personal freedom, what Rousseau called "well-regulated liberty" and Locke (1693/1927) the "Rules and Restraints of Reason." The major difference was that Rousseau believed in the school of hard knocks; the best lessons, he thought, are taught by experience, by the consequences of natural, self-generated activities (in a preplanned environment). In contrast, Locke believed in the discipline of adults; through deprivation and praise children acquire "esteem," "shame," and "disgrace," the glue that binds them in awe and reverence to their parents. "If you can once get into Children a Love of Credit, and an Apprehension of Shame and Disgrace, you have put into 'em the true Principle, which will constantly work and incline them to the right" (1693/1927). Both forswore use of the rod.

Thus, returning to early childhood, we see that the original patriarchs permit us to imagine how perspectives can be reconciled and combined without self-contradiction. Take, for example, a preschool program that aims to train children in socially acceptable behavior, to help them understand reality through their own constructions, and to allow them simple fun. Why not? The combined objectives do not violate any original-nature assumptions as long as one assumes a nature that is at once imitative, responsive to adult molding, *and* curious, eager to engage the environment.

One way to combine the schools would be to select according to a child's age: for example, romantic for the infant, developmental for the toddler, cultural transmission for the older child. Any doubts about the viability of combining models along these lines should be put to rest by the brilliant success of the Japanese educational system. The American public is now well aware that Japan is producing the world's best-educated students (at least according to conventional criteria) who yet remain socially compliant, group-oriented, responsive to authority, and trained in formal traditions. Yet these hardworking, successful, conforming students, well indoctrinated in the values of their culture, spend their early childhoods in a sanctuary of indulgence, the envy of any hedonist.[3]

Another way to combine the schools would be to match according to educational content. Piaget's theory, as applied to the preschool context by Constance Kamii and Rheta DeVries (Kamii

& DeVries, 1977; DeVries & Kohlberg, 1987), identifies three different types of knowledge—physical, logico-mathematical, and social-conventional—each requiring its own form of instruction. Teaching a child to go to the potty is not accomplished through the same methods as teaching her about spatial relations or the meaning of numbers. Social-conventional knowledge is arbitrary; it can be taught by rote as a series of skills or rules, regardless of whether the child understands them. Physical knowledge (properties of objects and how they affect each other) can only be acquired by acting on objects and finding out how they respond. Logico-mathematical knowledge (abstract systems of symbolic operations not inherent in objects), however, is not directly teachable; it must be constructed through "reflective abstraction" from the child's experiences with objects.

The objectives we seek in educating children determine the models of instruction we use, and these, in turn, will determine (at least in part) what kind of child emerges. As Kohlberg points out, when you buy into cultural transmission values, you are more or less locked into behavioral instruction and call forth the imitative conditionable child. Thus, if the toddler is to be toilet-trained, eat with a fork, or recite numbers by a predetermined time, the adult must take charge, direct the instruction, control the responses and rely on the child's adult-responsiveness to get results. Without this careful choreography of example and reinforcement, the child is unlikely to learn these behaviors on schedule. On the other hand, if one wants a child to invent, to make discoveries, the adult must recede and hope the child's native initiative will surface. So it may come down to this: To the extent a teacher limits and specifies objectives in advance, she is forced into a didactic role that relies on behavioral teaching; to the extent she leaves objectives indeterminate, up to the child, she is free to adopt the progressive or romantic approach.

Like other distinctions made in this chapter, these, too, fade a bit on inspection. If the teacher is a follower of Piaget rather than Neil (Summerhill), she may choose to give nature a boost: encourage development by asking questions, praise a child's discovery, or set up a more challenging environment. These techniques are behavioral in the sense of shaping responses, but still they do not demand a *specific* response or involve direct instruction. We could call this "soft behaviorism" and oppose it to classical behaviorism, where a designated outcome is assigned and elicited by an instructor.

With this concession, it seems fair to say that, while one can select multiple objectives, those objectives, once chosen, limit the methods used and the aspect of the child's nature enlisted. The more specific the goal, the more control must be exerted over the response. And this added control shifts the motivation from intrinsic—I want to do it because I am curious—to extrinsic—I want to do it to please you.

One's decision to choose a mix of objectives and models assumes, once again, that children can adapt to a range of teaching styles—teacher-directed, child-directed, or combined. But what if some children have no initiative or curiosity? For them, presumably, the progressive or romantic traditions are ruled out. A child without interest in his environment requires teacher mediation to learn. Yet another way to combine models, then, is to distinguish a particular child's receptivity to one or another form of instruction. Particularly among troubled youngsters with developmental difficulties, one group (e.g., the autistic, or the severely retarded) may benefit more from a particular regime (e.g., behavioral) than another. This brings us to an important question—Is human nature somehow altered in the mentally retarded?—and to an important juncture where the three orientations we have been discussing meet up with conceptions of the retarded child.

EDUCATIONAL MODELS AND THE NATURE OF THE RETARDED

Special Education Models

Although the extremes represented by Summerhill and Walden II are rarely encountered today, preschools do vary considerably in educational objectives and methods of instruction, reflecting basic disagreements on the nature and needs of the child. There are progressive programs working on the assumption that, because meaning cannot be delivered to children but must be constructed by them, the best adults can do is to provide for, and protect developmentally, appropriate play opportunities. Through play, through the exercise of individual choice and imagination, children gratify their natural curiosity, master the objects and their world, grow in confidence and competence. The teacher responds to inquiries but avoids direct instruction, since any attempt to accelerate development beyond a child's stage is doomed to failure (e.g., instruction in numbers before a child reaches the stage of concrete operations, age 5 to 7, and grasps the principle of reversibility).

This is the strongly held position of the National Academy of Early Childhood Programs (Bredekamp, 1987), which advises programs seeking its endorsement to stress child-initiated, child-directed, and teacher-supported play and to minimize staff-initiated group instruction periods during which children are expected to be quiet and listen. The Academy maintains that self-selected interactions with the world benefit a child far more than meeting social criteria of excellence.

> Finished products or "correct" solutions that conform to adult standards are not very accurate criteria for judging whether learning has occurred. Much of young children's learning takes place when they direct their own play activities. During play, children feel successful when they engage in a task they have defined for themselves . . . Such learning should not be inhibited by adult-established concepts of completion, achievement, and failure. (p. 3)

Special education professionals working with handicapped children tend to enlist in the competing (cultural transmission) camp. Since its inception, special education has been dominated by a diagnostic–prescriptive model under which specific deficits in children's abilities and skills are identified and measured, behavioral objectives then established and remediation attempted. Teachers cannot leave cures to a child's natural evolution but must adopt a strongly prescriptive and directive role (Anastasiow, 1978; Bailey & Wolery, 1984; Carta et al., 1991; Hanson & Lynch, 1989; Heshusius, 1982; Mahoney, O'Sullivan, & Fors, 1989; Mowder & Widerstrom, 1986; Neisworth & Bagnato, 1987).

Preschool special education, though still in its infancy, has followed in this tradition, but with a twist: Professionals in the field often advocate a separation between *objectives*, which they say should be developmental, and *methods*, which should be behavioral (Bagnato, Neisworth, & Munson, 1989; Bailey & Wolery, 1984; Berkeley & Ludlow, 1989; Fewell & Kelly, 1983; Garwood, 1983; Linder, 1983; Mirenda & Donnellan, 1987; Neisworth & Bagnato, 1987; Peters, Neisworth, & Yawkey, 1985)—the very separation previously criticized. The disagreement, however, turns out to be largely semantic, a confusion in the use of the term "developmental." To special education professionals "develop-

mental" means merely that objectives are selected from a sequenced inventory of developmental milestones; for example, a
child is not asked to speak unless he has some verbal understanding, or to run unless he can walk. The "developmental" objectives,
however, are in fact behavioral—that is, are specific, clearly defined, observable, and measurable; they are set up in advance to be
accomplished over a period of time with a teacher directing instruction and monitoring progress. Using the word "developmental" for this yoking of milestones to behavioral interventions may be more in line with the child's nature (maturational status) than not using milestones, but it still falls in the
cultural transmission camp: ends are highly specified rather than
open-ended, methods are teacher-directed and the psychology relies on children's pliancy (conditionability), not on their curiosity.
It is at odds with the "progressive–developmental" (Piaget–Dewey)
meaning of the word in which objectives must be kept indeterminate because learning is child-initiated, with only a supportive or suggestive role for the teacher.

The dominance of the cultural transmission model for retarded preschoolers, but not for the nonretarded, maps nicely onto
a "medical" model of education: children, unable to keep up, are
seen as pathological, in need of "treatment." If a child has a gallop-
ing infection, the physician does not wait for the child to resolve
the illness through his own interest and efforts, but isolates and
aggressively treats the infection. The progressive–developmental
school can be accepted only if the handicapped child is perceived
as normal-but-slow, with the personal resources to make meaning
of the world at his own delayed pace. He is not sick, he requires
only patience and support. And, finally, the hands-off romantic
school is unacceptable unless one regards the retarded child as
either a gift of God, specially endowed, or as hopeless, unremedi-
able. There are few advocates of this school left in these reformist
times.[4]

Retarded Children: Defective or Delayed?

One's position on the nature of the retarded child is obviously
critical to the choice of a school. When planning an intervention
with a retarded child, do we think of his mind merely as a younger
version of a normal child's, or as unlike other children's of any
age? The question, oversimplified, boils down to a choice between
mental delay and mental defect: do the wheels turn slowly or are

they jammed? Within the retarded population is there a mix of types, some defective and some delayed, and, if so, are there operative principles for deciding who belongs to which group? Although the defect view has always had the upper hand (Cicchetti & Beeghly, 1990; Hodapp, Burack, & Zigler, 1990), in recent years, largely through the influence of Edward Zigler and his colleagues at Yale University, a combined "two-group" approach has become increasingly popular (for good discussions see Hodapp et al., 1990; Zigler & Balla, 1982; Zigler & Hodapp, 1986). Through their influence, and spurred by advances in the field of developmental psychology, developmental concepts have infiltrated some intervention programs (e.g., Hohmann, Banet, & Weikart, 1979; Meisels, 1979).

According to the two-group theory, 75% of children whom we classify as mildly retarded (with IQs roughly between 50 and 70) nevertheless fall within the normal distribution of intelligence; they go through the same sequences in the same way as other children, only they proceed at a slower rate and reach a lower ceiling. They are "essentially normal individuals, in the sense that they fall within the normal variation dictated by the gene pool" (Zigler, 1969, p. 537), hence "delayed." They come from low socioeconomic backgrounds and show no evidence of organic impairment. The second group, usually (but not always) with IQs below 50, are physically damaged, hence "defective." They come from all income levels and are likely to have a different structure of intelligence (Zigler, Balla, & Hodapp, 1984). It is "illogical," say these investigators, "to extend developmental principles to individuals with organic defects, whatever their IQs may be" (Zigler & Hodapp, 1986, p. 29) since there is no reason to believe the same cognitive processes are operative. Low functioning children, most of whom are "defective," seem less able than the mildly retarded to generate concepts on their own; they tend to fixate on an external or internal stimulus so that behavioral techniques are called for (Zigler & Hodapp, 1986). Recently, these authors have modified their position by reducing the psychological distance between the two groups. Even "defectives," they now suggest, go through the same Piagetian stages as do other children (similar sequences), but within a stage they show more variability from one domain of accomplishment to another (dissimilar structures). Children with Down syndrome, for example, have more difficulty with language than with social skills (Hodapp et al., 1990; Hodapp & Zigler, 1990).

Others who believe that there are two groups of retarded

children divide them according to functional level rather than causation: Those with IQs below 50 (largely the same as Zigler's organic group) show defect characteristics, those above 50 are delayed but otherwise normal. Like Zigler, they believe the lower the level and older the child, the more appropriate a cultural transmission approach (what they call functional or skill-based) (Bailey & Wolery, 1984; Linder, 1983; Zigler & Hodapp, 1986).

Lining up against the two-group view on one side is a long tradition of researchers who believe *all* retarded children suffer from a defect more profound than mere delay (Anastasiow, 1978; Bailey & Wolery, 1984; Brinker & Lewis, 1982; Fewell & Kelly, 1983; Hanson & Lynch, 1989; Linder, 1983; Naglieri, 1989; Whitman, 1990). The assumption of defect calls for cultural transmission instruction. According to Bailey and Wolery (1984), it is not clear that a Piagetian approach fits the retarded who

> may not be as likely to explore as nonhandicapped children. Second, handicapped preschoolers may not learn through simple manipulation; reinforcement and other artificial feedback may be necessary to teach desired details. Third, handicapped youngsters may not independently engage in exploratory behaviors to best facilitate long-term growth . . . In general, handicapped youngsters really do need a more structured program. (p. 107)

Most of the qualities that presumably mark the retarded are subsumed under what could be called general mental inertness—they are passive, purposeless, low in initiative, ideation, and planning, forgetful, inattentive, repetitive, inflexible, narrowly concentrated. But it has also been noted, paradoxically, that they are distractible, impulsive, and overactive. The very child who insists on the same plate, same hat, same story each day, and who cannot be budged from repetitively running a car up and down a ramp, will also stop listening to a story the moment another child walks past his line of vision, stop drawing if he drops his crayon, and dart away from the group when he spies snacks on a shelf.[5]

In 1935 Kurt Lewin, who along with Heinz Werner was one of the first great theorists on the psychology of retardation, explained this peculiar combination of characteristics. According to Lewin, the psyche can be thought of as having regions with firmer or weaker boundaries between them. Retarded differ from normal children in having fewer regions (little psychological differentiation) and firmer boundaries between the regions (rigidity). Consequently, a normal child with open fences between numerous regions can move between psychological lots aware of, but not interrupted by, the surrounding field. With his mental flexibility and dexterity, he also can create new fields by selecting and joining similar components from different regions (a flexibility basic to concept development). The retarded, by contrast, have solid walls, not open fences, between their psychological regions; when they are in one lot, they do not "see" the other lots and are at the "mercies of the momentary situation" (Lewin, p. 216). This makes them rigid and single-minded. Introduce a small change, however, and the child's organization will be disrupted. He is thrown into another psychological region and totally forgets what he was doing; hence the distractibility.

Put another way, the retarded are excessively concrete, they lack the "abstract attitude" (Scheerer, Rothman, & Goldstein, 1945). With little mobility of thought, they cannot reorganize their current "field" to incorporate a new stimulus, nor can they select the common components from a confused field. A retarded child, for example, is momentarily absorbed in the repetitive pounding of Play-Doh with a plastic hammer (rigid). Someone grabs the hammer away and the child quits, wanders about the room, and finds nothing to do (distractible). He does not have the imagination (a form of abstraction) to consider changing either his means or ends by substituting another tool on his table for the hammer, or by doing something else with the Play-Doh other than pound. He is locked into the specifics of his immediate field and cannot regroup, even though in past experiences with Play-Doh he has used different implements and had other purposes. Then, when he leaves the table, his new field is large and confused, a big open psychological space that he cannot structure.

To make the same point once more, there is inadequate separation between the slow child and his activity, as well as a merging of differentiated regions within his environment. He is "at the mercies of the momentary situation" because he cannot reflect upon what he is doing. The flip side of being immersed in the field—also characteristic of nondelayed children but, says Lewin, to a lesser degree—is an inability to impose a framework, see options, exercise choice, monitor one's actions. Other researchers have called this a failure of the "executive function" and use the finding to explain the persistent failure of retarded children to learn and recall material effectively. It produces a cognitive (sometimes physical) passivity and randomness, a child without purpose beyond his present engagement who flits or commits to narrow stereotypical acts.[6]

Opposed to the two-group theory from the other side, is a newer developmental tradition that emphasizes the basic similarities between the retarded and nonretarded (Cicchetti & Beeghly, 1990; Kopp, 1990; Motti, Cicchetti, & Sroufe, 1983). Organically impaired or whole, IQ above or below 50, all are basically the same. The retarded are just what the name implies, slow to develop, but not deviant. They go through the same stages in the same sequence as normal children, albeit at a different rate. They have initiative and ideas, they can learn and be shaped at the level of other children who have *the same mental age*. This is important. When the developmentalists use the term "normal" to describe the retarded, they mean that the mind (and behavior) of a retarded 4-year-old, functioning at a 2-year level (IQ about 50), is similar to that of an average 2-year-old (functioning at the 2-year level, IQ about 100). The only special intervention the retarded child requires is an adjustment for mental age.[7]

Although it matters a lot whether one thinks of a child as defective or delayed, once again we have two positions that are not entirely incompatible. Within a retarded population, all of whom are "organic" or have IQs below 50, there may be some children most accurately described as delayed, others as defective. And, just to complicate matters more, a child most accurately described as delayed is apt to show a few defective characteristics, if only because she learns more slowly even than the younger nonretarded child of her own mental age. Because the 4-year-old with her 50 IQ will learn in 1 year only half the fare of a nonretarded 2-year-old, she is sluggish in her moment-to-moment processing. Still, her basic being-in-the-world—actions and reactions—may be very "2-ish" (for more about the nature of the retarded, see Chapter Nine). Putting aside etiology and IQ cuts, it is obvious to anyone who has visited an early intervention program that some children blend into the normal–younger population and others do not. If the child with Down syndrome is the paradigm of the primarily delayed (as writers like Cicchetti and Kopp have documented), the child with autism is the exemplar of the primarily defective, though both are organic and likely to be moderately retarded.

The defining characteristics of autism, as identified by Leo Kanner in 1943, are a set of deviant traits: inability to relate and extreme aloneness (often marked by avoidance of any eye contact with people); obsessive desire for the maintenance of sameness (insistence on routines or furniture arrangements); ritualistic habits (such as spinning); absence or peculiarity of language (e.g., echoing what others say, failure to use first-person pronouns); and often a spread of abilities (e.g., excellent rote memory with weak communication skills). Although more recent research has concluded that most autistic children are retarded, the spikes (splinter skills) are not uncommon and contribute to the distinctiveness of these children.[8]

No one has described the autistic child as merely delayed or advocated leaving her (like the child with Down syndrome) to follow a natural developmental course (Volkmar, Burack, & Cohen, 1990). Unfortunately, autism is a resistant disorder; it yields, if at all, only to the most rigorous intervention, as illustrated by the work of O. Ivar Lovaas (1987). In a massive behavioral intervention study—perhaps the most successful ever reported—Lovaas recruited 19 autistic youngsters under 4 years of age to be treated by therapists in their homes 40 hours a week. Parents were trained to be co-therapists so that the children were under treatment "most of their waking hours for many years" (p. 3). A control group of 19 children received 10 hours or less of one-to-one treatment. Results were impressive: "Forty-seven percent of the experimental group achieved normal intellectual and educational functioning in contrast to only 2% of the control group subjects" (p. 7). This is a good example of a defect group that responded to the cultural transmission school.[9]

If the population labelled "retarded" is not adequately described either as defective or delayed, if within the category we find both types and combinations, then in thinking about early intervention we must consider not just blending schools, depending upon the objectives sought (e.g., physical, logico-mathematical or social-conventional knowledge), but choosing different schools for different children (e.g., those with autism, Down syndrome, severely or mildly delayed).

SUMMING UP

We began with the three models Kohlberg has called romantic, cultural transmission and progressive. Each starts with its own psychological vision of the child—virtuous by nature, requiring only freedom; unformed and pliable, requiring social instruction; biologically prestructured, but requiring appropriate environmental interactions for development. From each psy-

chological vision follows a set of objectives and methods of instruction.

On close inspection, however, the simple trichotomy yields to
a more complex picture of the nature of children. Rousseau, Locke,
and Piaget all recognized that on the one hand, children are pliable, imitative, and responsive to reinforcement. Even Piaget
noted this quality: "But let there be no misunderstandings. Memory, passive obedience, imitation of the adult, and the receptive
factors in general are all as natural to the child as spontaneous
activity" (1970, pp. 137–138). They will sit, recite, and obey adults;
they will go to the toilet and eat with a spoon when trained. On the
other hand, children also have drives to explore, discover, and
make their own meaning out of the chaotic stimuli that surround
them. They will walk, stumble, get up and walk again, endlessly
repeating the cycle until they have mastered the skill. (Even if
endlessly reinforced for sitting, would they not get up defiantly
and walk again?) They become acquainted with the world by
handling and moving objects about; a drawer presents an irresistible invitation to search and remove, no matter what the consequences.

The models, therefore, must be combined if they are to do
justice to the child's complex nature. Educators may select models
on the basis of a child's age, instructional content area, or child
characteristics. Yet there are limits to the mixing-and-matching of
models. Selection of a particular objective locks one into a method
of instruction and an appeal to one or another aspect of the child's
psychology. If the goal is acquisition of a particular skill, adult-
direction and behavioral methods would seem unavoidable; if,
instead, the goal is self-expression or discovery, child-centered
open-ended instruction seems called for. Progressive school adherents (e.g., Kamii & DeVries, 1977) suggest choosing a model
according to the kind of knowledge one wants to have children
acquire: precise objectives and behavioral methods for social-
conventional knowledge, but not for the physical and logico-
mathematical realms.

The choice of models becomes more complicated when the
task is to educate the handicapped. In the contemporary literature
there are two schools of thought about the retarded, plus one that
partakes of both. The common belief, subscribed to by most authorities in the field, is that the retarded are "defective." They have
qualities of mind not characteristic of normal children, such as
passivity, rigidity, concreteness; but also distractibility, impetuos-
ity, and overactivity. More recent investigators have argued that

retarded children are primarily "delayed," very much like younger normal children in their habits of mind. Still others say both visions are correct. Those with very low IQ are defective, whereas those with higher IQ and unimpaired biology are normal but delayed.

But the cut by IQ or "organicity" does not quite work, for within the moderately retarded population—the group that concerns us in this book—there are children both with Down syndrome, the standard example of delay, and children with autism, the classic example of defect. Models, therefore, may have to be matched to individual (or classes of) children, as well as to specific objectives (e.g., children with Down syndrome could be exposed to different "schools" depending on the goal, but children with autism might receive only behavioral interventions).

To view the retarded as defective assigns them to the cultural transmission model. Adherents of this position want teacher-directed programs with specific objectives taught and monitored through behavioral techniques. To view the retarded as merely delayed assigns them to the progressive model. It calls for a child-directed intervention that supports children's interests and choices but awaits their timetable. Early interventionists suggest uniting models by combining "developmental" objectives (sequenced achievements drawn from inventories) with behavioral instruction, but the term "developmental" in this context is untrue to the Piaget–Kohlberg meaning. We can mix approaches by matching a model to an objective (behavioral with toilet training, developmental with play development) or to a learning domain (social-conventional versus logico-mathematical), but the selection of an objective pretty much determines the methodology of intervention. A third conceptualization of the retarded as uniquely blessed or cursed by nature, but in either case unmodifiable, subjects them to the romantic view but has no contemporary currency. It would be consistent either with no early intervention or an open environment where teachers protect the impulses of the retarded child from interference.

The models of education and various views of the retarded also map onto the three original vignettes in Chapter One. The first, providing institutionalization, assumes a defective as well as preformed child. It is an essentially romantic model—leave the child alone by separating him from society (or, equally consistent, leave him at home without special treatment). The second, calling for aggressive treatment, assumes a defective but pliable child. It is essentially a cultural transmission model—the more and the sooner we intervene the better. The third, providing a modified environment, assumes a normal-but-slow child. It is essentially the progressive model—the child will develop slowly through supportive interactions, but his own timetable controls the pace and shapes the form.

In the following chapters we will investigate *how* early intervention programs align themselves with these alternatives, and *why* they have adopted one set of goals and methods over another. Practice, after all, rests on moral values as well as on psychological theory: What, given a set of psychological assumptions regarding the child's nature, do we want to produce and how do we produce it? This takes us back to the general freedom–restraint issue raised in the first chapter, but again complicated by our special population.[10]

Most of us, it is safe to say, value freedom for young *normal* children; we believe they profit both intellectually and psychologically (through feelings of confidence and effectiveness) from mucking about in the world without a lot of restrictive adult authority. But for the retarded, some argue, freedom is a luxury we cannot afford; their painfully slow development and/or (depending on one's orientation) cognitive defects demand strong adult direction. Freedom as the exercise of choice requires, in this view, a self-consciousness not available to the retarded child, while freedom as the expression of primitive impulses is vulgar, crude, and uncivilized, not in the child's best interest.

Others disagree. They maintain that although IQ level may control the amount of protection a child needs, it should not determine the amount of freedom allowed him. Retardation should not put limits on liberty. How much freedom we grant, to whom, under what conditions, is a fundamental issue for early intervention that we must confront. This much is clear: "The problem is rarely one of total freedom versus total control but rather what the balance is, and to what end, and in light of what alternative" (Cremin, 1976, p. 44).

In every program one finds a complex mix of assumptions about educational objectives, pedagogy, moral values, and pragmatics. They, in turn, are linked to notions about the capacities of children, how they learn, where they should be headed, and what is feasible. The next chapter, depicting a prototypical program, gives the reader a chance to make her own tentative analysis and judgment about the values, assumptions, and practice that reign at Midwood.

CHAPTER FOUR

Midwood School

To see a world in a Grain of Sand,
And a Heaven in a Wild Flower,
Hold Infinity in the palm of your hand,
And Eternity in an hour.
A Robin Redbreast in a Cage
Puts all Heaven in a Rage.
— WILLIAM BLAKE, "Auguries of Innocence"
    (1803/1950, p. 18)

THE SETTING

It is 8:30 on a gray Monday morning in November, the air is damp and chilly. A number of school buses and family cars line up along a crescent driveway, and 32 children trundle out headed for four special education preschool classes. The eight children we will follow, assigned to teacher Teresa's class, arrive in three different buses and two family cars.* Defying the harbinger of dark cold wintry days ahead, the teachers and aides cheerily greet the children: Look at Molly's new red shoes, aren't they pretty?" "Austin, you're looking so handsome today; how about a good morning smile for Teresa?" "Doreen said 'hi.' Good talking, Doreen."

The preschoolers, ranging in age from 3 to 5, will spend 2½ hours 5 days a week at Midwood, a midwestern, middle-class, suburban public elementary school. Another group of 32 children

*To help the reader identify the participants at Midwood, names of the children and teachers begin with the same first letter as their status marker—for example, "t" for teacher and Teresa. Names of children and teachers have been changed in all the vignettes and interviews that follow.

48

arrive at 12:30 for the afternoon programs. The four classes, brought to Midwood a year ago from overcrowded schools elsewhere, are the only ones in the building for preschoolers and the only ones for special-needs children of any age. The other 400 children at Midwood are distributed fairly evenly in grades kindergarten through sixth. Teresa and her three special education colleagues are both professionally and socially faculty outliers. Teachers of the "regular" children, Teresa believes, feel estranged from the special ed group and resent what they perceive as perks— small enrollments, aides, fancy and plentiful equipment— particularly when contrasted to their own stripped-to-essentials budgets. Further, Teresa senses, many of the "regulars" truly think that educating young handicapped children is a poor use of scarce resources.

But the matter is not up for debate. Early intervention for handicapped preschoolers has been a state entitlement for the past 5 years. When the two sets of teachers meet, infrequently, they avoid talking about the controversy that divides them; conversation is kept to a pleasant but innocuous level, tensions are left unaddressed. However, weeks can go by with no contact. The special ed classes are on a different schedule; they use the playground when no one else is on it, they don't go to the cafeteria. Administrative arrangements increase the separation; the four special teachers report to a district director of early childhood special education. The building principal has loose oversight, but more good will than expertise. He occasionally drops in to "jolly" the children, but does not (and would not want to) evaluate teachers, make suggestions, or interfere with the classroom in any way.

After debriefing the bus driver regarding the children's behaviors (no notable incidents, but Heather, uncharacteristically, slept for most of the ride), the adults collect their charges and the first challenge of the day is on—traversing the corridors to class. Midwood, built in the 1950s, is designed in an "L" shape with two rows of classrooms off long hallways. The special ed rooms are clustered together at the end of the hall. They share a large bathroom with open toilets (so that children can be assisted) and tables for changing diapers and clothes. *L*arry (age 5, *l*anguage delay, from a marginal, possibly abusive, family), *M*olly (age 4, diagnosis unknown, *m*oderate delay) and *D*avid (age 5, *D*own syndrome, moderately retarded) walk hand-in-hand with *A*lice (teacher *a*ide). Accompanying them through the door, but then racing noisily down the corridor, is *H*eather (age 5, *h*yperactive–distractible, moderately retarded) with *A*nita (second teacher *a*ide) in hot pursuit. Teresa puts Carl (age 3, cerebral palsy, severely retarded) into the red wagon she has brought from her room, assigns Stephen (age 4, speech delay, mild motor immaturity) to help her pull it and asks Doreen (age 3, Down syndrome) to hold her hand. Austin (age 5, autistic), with his left hand continuously grazing the left wall, walks more or less abreast of Teresa. When the hall breaks into a small foyer (entrance to a third-grade classroom), he follows the perimeter, tracing the three foyer walls with the tips of his fingers. Intermittently Austin delays the groups' slow progress to make guttural noises accompanied by intense hand flapping. Either spontaneously or at Teresa's admonition—"It's time to walk now, Austin; good walking"—he moves forward again.

The small procession continues its spasmodic pace down the corridor. That is, until midway, when Doreen stages a "sit-down." A walker for only the past few months, Doreen is fiercely independent. Like any toddler, she is less interested in the group's destination than in her more immediate surroundings; right now, it is the backpack slipping from her back down her arm. With delight she watches it fall—finally the flap is accessible to her roving hands—and immediately flops down to join it on the floor. Teresa, now faced with increasing confusion—Austin walking on, oblivious to this disruption, and Doreen planted solidly in the middle of the hallway contentedly pulling at a diaper in her bag— does a quick risk–benefit calculation. Torn between Austin and Doreen, she decides that the odds favor Austin getting to class on his own over Doreen's willingness to follow if she tries to keep everyone moving. Uneasily, Teresa lets Austin go, but she cannot allow the red wagon (that Stephen is pulling with Carl inside) to proceed without her supervision. If the wagon tips, Carl, with his poor self-protective reflexes and metal leg braces, might well be injured. So Teresa tells Stephen: "We need to stop, Stephen. We need to help Doreen now." On past days following a Doreen sit-down, Teresa has successfully remobilized her by remarks like: "It's time to walk now. Teddy Bear is waiting to see you; he has missed you this weekend."

Today, having successfully extracted the diaper from the bag, Doreen is unresponsive to her teacher's cajoling. Looking most content, she responds to these entreaties with a negative shake of her head and exclaims, "Me sit."

Teresa is in a quandary. She appreciates Doreen's joy in practicing her newly developed walking competence and believes it is her task as a teacher to provide as much support as possible. The physical therapist has explained to her that walking is a threshold skill. Once mastered it will permit Doreen to make more rapid progress in other motor areas such as climbing, throwing, catching, and chasing, but right now lots of practice is needed to strengthen her flaccid muscles. To pick her up or to threaten her—"Either you walk or I'll carry you"—would contradict the objective of encouraging motor growth. It would deflate her enthusiasm and "motor initiative." It is also very alien to Teresa's way of addressing handicapped children. Like most special ed teachers, Teresa is highly averse to confrontations and often goes through elaborate circumlocutions to avoid them. Rather than directly criticizing children by telling them what they are doing is wrong (e.g., "You must not play with the diaper now. You must not sit on the floor."), she has been trained always to put messages positively. So she tries again: "Can I help you put away your diaper, Doreen? It's time to walk now." No response. "Floors are for walking on, Doreen. We can play in our room."

Doreen looks up untouched. "Me play." Teresa has run out of time.

Stephen, on remarkably good behavior thus far, is tipping the red wagon up–down, up–down, with Carl inside near panic. Alone with three children, none of whom is cooperating, and with a potential accident looming, Teresa reaches down to pick up Doreen—"Doreen wants help today; Teresa will help you get to class"—and puts her into the wagon with Carl. Doreen immediately wails in protest. Carl joins in the crying and flails at Doreen. Teresa, grabbing Stephen by one hand and pulling the wagon with the other, rushes down the remaining corridor with three very unhappy children. And so Teresa enters the classroom to see, with relief, that Austin has made it along with the other four. She puts Carl onto the floor (he is able to move by rolling) and tells the children they may play.

Not an easy way to start a gray Monday morning.

Teresa, at 38, is teaching preschool handicapped children for her eighth consecutive year. As someone who drifted into the field—"I was not one of those do-goody people always volunteering at church and school"—she is surprised by the longevity of her teaching career. Teresa is the second of six children from a working-class Catholic home. Growing up she had responsibilities for the care of younger siblings and did some baby-sitting for a family with a handicapped child. But, as a mediocre student in a strict parochial school, she dreamed of becoming a dancer, not a teacher. Her attraction to small children dated from a college course in developmental psychology that required intense observation of an infant, and from the birth of her first niece. "I don't know why, I suddenly loved playing with babies and toddlers and discovered I was good with them, knew instinctively what they wanted and how to quiet them." Her inquiries revealed that the only way to make a living working with a preschool population was through special education. Happily, the state university she attended offered certification in preschool education, special education, and preschool–special education. By graduation she had completed both special and preschool–special and moved into the classroom where she had done her practice teaching. With the exception of 1 year—when she was switched to a primary special education class—she has been with preschoolers in the same district ever since. She is delighted with the large, well-equipped rooms at Midwood, although having toilets 50 feet down the hallway and access to a playground even further, present her with daily struggles.

Teresa's room is large, bright, orderly, and filled with objects designed for preschoolers. It follows an organizational pattern familiar to those working in early childhood: areas separated by hinged wood cupboards and shelving to create the appearance of small enclosures within a large room. In one corner of the room lined up against the wall is a miniature stove, refrigerator, sink, cabinet, doll-sized crib, stroller, rocker, clothespole, bureau, small circular table covered with a cloth, brooms, dustpans, and a mirror standing on the floor at child height. On and around the pole are dress-up clothes; on the stove are pots and pans; in the cabinet are plastic dishes, cups, utensils, and realistic foods (hamburgers, fruits of all sorts, vegetables, bread, cake, drinks, baby bottles, etc.); in the bureau are more hats, shoes, aprons, blouses, pants, skirts, and dresses; on the table are phones, an adding machine, and baskets. The rocking chair is tipped by the weight of a large teddy bear. In and around the crib are scattered an array of hard and soft black and white dolls and blankets.

An adjacent larger area is equipped for gross-motor activities with a set of kindergarten wood blocks neatly stacked on shelves. The illustration of each block form is attached to the shelf lip so children can readily find (and return) what they want. The symbol system is followed for all play material in the room. In addition to the large blocks, there are smaller colored blocks, cardboard blocks, train tracks, trucks and cars. Another enclosure is set aside for fine-motor activities. Six shelves are stacked with plastic see-through boxes containing different size Lego blocks, parquetry blocks, blocks for stacking, form and number sorting blocks, beads for lacing and sequencing, snap-lock beads, cubes for nesting,

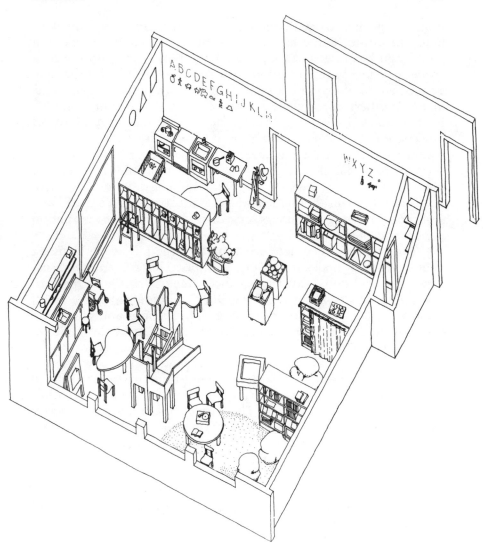

Midwood I.   Drawing by Felix Drury.

multiple pegboards with their inserts, farm animals, and doll-house furniture. Lying loose are a large set of vinyl dinosaurs, a half-dozen bean bags, a couple of "busy boxes," pop-up boxes, a "roller coaster" wire formation with small colorful beads that can be pushed up, down and around, a miniature house, garage, and farm. Another set of shelves, covered with a curtain, contains board games, lotto and bingo games (for matching pictures of objects, colors, forms, numbers, sizes, animals, sequences, form completion, etc.), a couple dozen puzzles ranging from single insert forms—triangle, square, circle—to multiple interlocking pieces (no missing pieces), a large flannel board on an easel with boxes of felt forms, animals, and story illustrations, cans of Play-Doh, scissors, Magic Markers, crayons, glue, glitter, construction paper, and paint.

Then there is a "quiet corner" with large pillows, a beanbag chair, a rack of books (on colors, numbers, letters, animals, seasons, and traditional favorites such as *Babar; The Cat in the Hat; Goodnight, Moon; Harry the Dirty Dog; The Little House*), a small table with a tape recorder, phonograph, records and children's instruments (bells, tambourine, rhythm sticks, triangles), and an adult rocker. This part of the room is carpeted. Deeper inside the room is a plastic table on legs for water, sand or rice (now empty), a small climbing structure with attached slide, two kidney-shaped tables surrounded with small chairs. Behind each chair is a child's printed name and a symbol. (The same symbol and name adorn the cubbies where children store their clothes and bags.) Free-standing is a two-sided easel permitting a painter on each side, Carl's walker, and a wheelchair for one of the afternoon children. An adult sink, with a stool for children, over which are strung shelves for canned juice, dry cereal, and crackers, and a large storage closet (with trikes, push toys, more books, records, manipulatives, games, and art supplies) line the remaining perimeter of the floor. Everything looks newly minted, available, inviting. It is a catalog of preschool fun come to life.

The walls are just as carefully organized. One large section is a combination of blackboard, magnetic board, Velcro strip, and corkboard. Posted on the white magnetic board is a calendar for the month, depiction of weather conditions (a sun, clouds, rain, snow, hot perspiring child, cold shivering child), individual photographs of the children under which are printed their first names, and illustrations of "our songs" (a bus for "The Wheels on the Bus," a monkey for "Ten Little Monkeys," a farm for "Old MacDonald Had a Farm," a boat for "Row, Row, Row Your Boat," and a child with a lifted leg for "Hokey Pokey"). Above the board is strung a colorful paper train, each car having a child's name and birthdate. Another section of wall space is devoted to colors, shapes, and letters: Large circles exemplify the primary colors; triangles, squares, and more circles, the basic shapes; and pictured objects, the letters of the alphabet that begin their names. The decorative highlight of the room is a Thanksgiving scene, made by the teachers, of a pilgrim family sitting around a food-laden table, with trees dripping leaves in the background. Two sets of art projects brighten the walls: Fall paper leaves (cut out by teachers) have been pasted onto individual pieces of colored construction paper, and pumpkins made with paper plates (also by the teachers) have been given facial features, their misalignment—mouth above nose, eyes both on the same side of the face—revealing them as work of the children. The wall opposite the entrance is a bank of windows with opened blinds through which, on a good day, natural light floods the room. Today, however, the overhead fluorescents are needed.

ARRIVAL ACTIVITIES

While the trip down the corridor seemed endless to Teresa, it is only 8:35 when she unloads the wagon and organizes the class for "toileting and washing." She instructs Austin, David, Stephen, and Larry to sit by the door so Alice can take them to the bathroom. Three go voluntarily, but Austin, at the window fingering the blinds, doesn't pay the slightest attention. Alice, having anticipated the difficulty, immediately takes his hand and, pulling him away from the window, says, "Austin, you heard Teresa. You have to stop playing and go pee-pee now." With his eyes focused on the floor where a beam of light has struck, Austin passively takes Alice's hand and follows her lead. On a return trip she will take Molly, Doreen, and Carl, all still in diapers, for a change.

Alice, a 49-year-old woman with grown children and a high-school diploma, has been Teresa's aide for 2 years. Although she has taken a few college courses, Alice has neither the aspiration nor the funds to become a teacher. She, like all the aides, is paid an hourly wage ($7.50) and has no prospects for advancement. From habit and conviction, her style is more abrupt than Teresa's; she doesn't believe that the "positive speech only" credo is an effective means of managing children, particularly those who need "discipline" like Heather and Molly. However, she likes Teresa and usually follows her style without objection.

Meanwhile, Anita has taken Heather to the toilet. Heather is Anita's special charge and the reason Teresa was granted a second aide. At 5, Heather is a sturdy, stocky, altogether normal-looking child who must be watched continuously. In an effort to contain her, Teresa put covers on the door handles so she cannot bolt out of the room, attached a tray to her chair to keep her seated, put curtains over some of the toy shelves to make them less inviting, and purchased screens and a kiddie corral to enclose her in an area. Teresa's husband even constructed a large plywood playpen which, when partially filled with Styrofoam packing material or colored balls, briefly attracts Heather. But because she flings the balls all over the room, it has been put away. Small group work that includes Heather is almost impossible. Give her Magic Markers and a large sheet of paper, and before long she will be drawing on the table edges or legs. Give her interlocking Lego-style material, and after a couple combinations she may well begin hurling the pieces around the room. Give her a card with pictures to identify or point to, and she is likely to grab, bend, or mouth them. Heather has a favorite book (*Goodnight, Moon*), much of which she can recite by heart; but while seemingly absorbed in reciting and turning pages, she suddenly may rip them and then cry because she can no longer "read" the pages. Teresa has tried to understand what brings on Heather's impulsive moves: Do they result from teacher demands, frustration over failure, boredom with repetition, altercations with other children? After hours of observation she has concluded they just happen, without external provocation, intention, or regret; there is no rhyme or reason to Heather. When possible, Anita anticipates the next destructive or impulsive move and physically restrains or guides Heather. When she fails and Heather disrupts the group, hits a child, or destroys material, Anita directs her to the "timeout" chair located in a corner of the room. Although Heather goes to it willingly enough, Anita must monitor her in the corner, for the nearby books and toys are potential weapons.

Anita has been working with Teresa only since the fall. She attends a local community college at night and is thinking of a career with handicapped preschoolers. Because she is only 23 and new to the field, she waits for instruction from Teresa throughout the day. Teresa is pleased that after 2½ months Anita has learned the routine, knows how to handle children, particularly Heather, and shows a willingness to help out with end-of-the-day chores (e.g., cutting out stencils for the next art session, putting up completed projects on the wall, sponging the tables, resupplying diapers and foods from a utility room in another wing of the school, photocopying parent notes, placing supply orders, searching for missing puzzle pieces until they are retrieved). Just recently, Teresa noted with delight, she had the idea of making kites with the children. Her youthful good cheer is welcome in the room, but, in Teresa's experience the livelier a teacher begins, the quicker she is likely to fade out; the class will be lucky if she lasts the year. Given a choice, Teresa would always select an Alice over an Anita, but there is never any choice—aides are in very scarce supply.

While the aides are busy with toileting and washing, Teresa assists the children with jackets. This is an important moment for working on "self-help" objectives. Each child has a different level of competence in disrobing, and Teresa carefully distributes just the necessary amount of help. Austin, Stephen, Larry, and David are fully independent. Molly and Doreen can handle a zipper when it is visible, so Teresa unzips their jackets just halfway; they then take over. Only the first group of children attach jacket to hook, but all the children are expected to find at least their own cubbies. In the putting-away process, Teresa removes journals from each bag and reads the parents' messages. Heather's mother reports a restless night with frequent waking and a poor breakfast after a Sunday outing with her father, whom she had not seen for about a month. Teresa passes this notebook on to Anita with the comment: "This explains why she slept on the bus. She'll probably be tough today."

Doreen's mother writes that her child was dry all night and she is ready to start toilet training if the school will advise on the best approach. Carl's mother wants Teresa to talk with the physical therapist about how much Carl should be using his walker. There is some question about whether frequent use is good for his legs. Molly went to the zoo over the weekend, her mother writes, and when the monkeys grabbed the rails with their tails, just inches from the visitors, she said, "Monkey no bite me," a big sentence for Molly. Teresa makes a mental note to allude to monkeys during circle time and to call Doreen's mom about toilet training. No comments today from the other four parents. The notebooks are placed on Teresa's desk. Before the children go home she will write a notation in each.

It is 8:45 as Teresa surveys the room to see how free play is progressing. Austin, after returning from the bathroom, begins his daily to-and-fro routine between the beanbag chair in the quiet corner and the middle wall window. He wets his finger, and makes a vertical line on the glass pane (between the slats of the blinds). Then, with hands raised to shoulder height, he runs on his toes to the beanbag chair, where he licks the identical digit of the opposite hand, and presses it against the vinyl chair cover. Then back to the window and the same routine all over again: lick the finger, make a saliva mark on the pane, run to the beanbag, lick again, another finger impression, accompanied by excited screeches after each lick.

"Austin," Teresa directs from her desk, "It's time to find something else to do." No response; she tries again:

"Austin, why don't you play with the airplane?" Still no response, so she picks up an abandoned helicopter from the floor and brings it over to him. "Look, Austin, I can help you make it fly and land on the beanbag chair. This is fun."

After demonstrating, she places it in his hand. Austin raises the helicopter above his head and begins turning both it and himself rapidly around in circles, mumbling: "Fly the friendly skies of United, skies of United, friendly skies of United."

Teresa finds Austin to be her most difficult child. She has read his thick folder, filled with the terms "autistic," "autistic-like," and "pervasive developmental disorder," countless times trying to get an understanding of what makes him tick. None of the reports gives her insight into this child, whose heavy-lidded big brown eyes rarely make contact with hers. Occasionally, in a rare spare moment, Teresa will put on one of Austin's favorite audiotapes and rock with him in her lap. Then he may offer a responsive touch or glance, but it lasts only a second. For the most part Austin stays in his own world as he wanders about the room, grazing the shelves with his hands, staring out the window, reciting TV commercials, while Teresa interrupts these behaviors as much as she can. Perhaps Austin understands more of what is going on around him than others suppose. Teresa believes this, and so despite his resistance, she makes sure he is included in all activities. There is also the hope that he will pick up social skills just from being around the other children.

This is Austin's third year in early intervention and his second year with Teresa. As an infant he had been quiet, easy to care for, content to sit and watch the world go by. Since all his motor milestones were normal, his parents (father is a surveyor for an oil company, mother is a part-time paralegal) dismissed the remoteness and indifference as "temperament," rather a relief after their boisterous, demanding first child, now 7. Even at 2, the pediatrician they had consulted with mounting worry had cautioned them not to compare children; Austin would undoubtedly be all right. By the time Austin was 2½, however, the combination of limited language (repeating phrases addressed to him or heard on TV), fixations (only eating from one plate and insisting on a particular arrangement of his alphabet blocks), unvarying daily repetition of a few videotapes hour after hour, and resistance to all but the barest social contact convinced them something was very wrong with their son.

The diagnosis of autism from a children's hospital came as no surprise. With both her children in school, Austin's mother helps Teresa whenever she is needed (e.g., field trips, school parties, parent meetings) and is active in a local group of families with autistic children. She believes Austin has made significant progress at Midwood, especially with Teresa. He has weaned himself from diapers; acquired decent eating habits; follows some directions; will sit with the other children; and, although his speech is still not communicative, will pull an adult's hand to an object he seeks but cannot reach. Sometimes, when he wants an object very badly, he even utters a request. He is still ravenous for TV, particularly the ads, and still constantly insists on the repetition of a few videotapes.

The two children with Down syndrome are engrossed, as usual, in the doll corner. Doreen, face to face with a head-to-foot mirror, is putting on a fireman's hat, tilting her head, letting the hat fall, picking it up, and replacing it again. Never taking her eyes off her reflection, she moves a bit from side to side, forward and backward, twisting her head and angling her body this way and that as the hat slides around. When next it drops off, David, just waiting for this opportunity, seizes it. There is a brief tug of war not observed by the teachers. No matter, Doreen finds an even better hat—felt with a big, wavy feather—and continues preening and shifting it about her head. David is dressed in an oversized man's jacket, unintentionally put on backwards so that it resembles a straightjacket, with a tie wrapped several times around his neck and a baby in his arms. Putting on the fireman's hat, he announces: "I go work. You stay." Doreen is staying, all right, but not as pretend wife or mother. She continues moving the hat around her head, intermittently stopping to smile at the image. Anita, momentarily freed from supervising Heather, suggests to David that if he is going to work he should leave the baby behind and take his lunch.

"What kind of sandwich do you want to eat at work today, David?"

"No sandwich," David replies, "I take baby."

Anita, trying to be helpful: "You can drop the baby off at a day-care center and still take a peanut butter sandwich."

David answers, "OK, 'bye," and walks smartly away (with baby, but still no lunch) to the edge of the doll corner, then quickly returns.

Teresa, noting that Doreen is still preening in front of the mirror, asks Anita: "Can you help Doreen find something more productive to do?"

Anita lifts a baby from the crib and comments: "Doreen, you look like a beautiful Mommy in that blue hat. Let's take care of your baby here."

Doreen turns, and with a final nostalgic look over her shoulder into the mirror, joins Anita, who immediately gives her a bottle and suggests that she feed the baby. Instead Doreen takes her hat off and puts it over the unclothed baby.

"Oh, that's too big for baby," Anita observes, "It's *big*. We need something *small* because babies are *small*. Let's cover her with a blanket instead." She promptly hands Doreen a blanket removed from the crib. Anita then leaves, summoned by loud noises that can have emanated only from Heather. Doreen takes the blanket, partially covers the baby, then lies down next to the baby and tries to stretch the blanket over herself. This is tough. She cannot see her arm movements and is in an awkward position to spread a blanket over her body. Not one to give up easily, Doreen flings the blanket; it lands over one arm. No good. Another try and it is over her face. Definitely no good. She sits up and wraps the blanket over her legs, then lies down and tries to snuggle under it, but most of her body remains blanketless. Clearly this is not what she had in mind. So she sits up again, picks up the blanket, flattens it on the floor, and lies down on top of it with a triumphant smile. Not bad but, after a moment of reflection, not quite right, either. The smile disappears; she sits up once more to try another maneuver. David has returned. He immediately finds himself a blanket, sits down next to Doreen and, bringing two ends of the blanket up to either shoulder, manages to lie down with the blanket largely covering him. Doreen takes note and partially imitates this successful strategy; then she returns to the mirror.

Doreen is a first child of young parents (father is a high-school teacher, mother a musician who gives piano lessons).

"I knew the moment I saw her that she had Down syndrome," her mother related, "but it took over 24 hours before I could get a doctor to confirm it. I was furious at the doctors, furious at the nurses, furious at my husband, and too upset to pay much attention to Doreen. Then came the depression. I didn't want to go out of the house. I didn't want anyone to come in. I wanted to hide my child so no one would see her. I didn't want sympathy from family, from other parents, and definitely not from professionals who arrived offering advice on 'infant stimulation' a day after we got home from the hospital. But as time passed, I began to see I was not in this alone. In his silent way my husband was suffering terribly from the double whammy of a defective child and a wife gone bonkers. We began to talk and to love one another again. My spirits lifted. We decided that if we were going to raise a child with Down syndrome she would be the smartest, cutest, highest functioning one ever born. We would stop feeling sorry for ourselves and throw all our energies into helping her. It was then that I welcomed the therapists, spent every waking moment waving mobiles in front of her face, strapped rattles to her hands and feet, played music while she napped, and, most of all, talked, talked, talked to her. For the first year or so we thought we might pull off a miracle. You know, in the beginning these children keep up pretty well, but after a while, as I began taking her to the playground and noticing other children her age, my dreams of a super-Down's child began to fade. I'm not sure what to expect now. I know she isn't especially advanced, but she is learning. Since starting preschool last summer she has begun to walk and talk a little. With all the attention from Teresa, from her therapists (speech therapy, physical therapy, and occupational therapy), and from us, we still have high hopes. It's not as bad as it used to be for children like Doreen."

At school Doreen is a charmer. Stubborn, yes, but so delighted with her new motor emancipation, with the skills and appearance of her body, so confident that her accomplishments naturally will overjoy all adults, so even-tempered and amiable, that she is irresistible, even if she does regularly try to get her way. Teresa finds Doreen quite like other children she has had with Down syndrome: sociable, active, playful, engaging, and stubborn. David, the other child in her class with Down's syndrome, is quieter, more serious, more accomplished, and, at 5, 2 years older. He has a talent for preacademics: knows his colors, has made substantial progress on letters and numbers, even recites some letter sounds. He also has a long attention span and conforms to group routines. With his thick glasses, squat frame, and slow, lumbering gait he appears prematurely weighted down with worldly cares. Teresa is very proud of David's accomplishments and hopes that he, along with Stephen and Larry, will go into a regular kindergarten next fall.

But on this day, like most others, Heather commands attention. The loud disturbance that pulls Anita away from Doreen is Heather, dumping a can of Playskool wood blocks into the empty sandbox. The staff has developed a routine for this sort of incident.

Step 1: Anita asks, "Do you need help with the blocks, Heather? Anita can help you." No response. "We could build a tower, Heather, a nice high tower, and then you could knock it down. We could go 1-2-3-boom!" And she laughs.

Heather replies, "Play sand now. Me want sand."

Anita patiently explains, "We can't play with the sand today, Heather. We had the sand out Friday, and you dumped it all over the floor. Remember how hard it was to clean up? We swept and swept. So we had to put it away for today. When you can keep the sand in the sandbox and play nicely, then we will have the sand out more often, and I know soon you will stop throwing sand because you want to follow the rules. Isn't that right?"

"I be good, 'Nita. Sand now, please," Heather answers, running to the shelf where the sand toys are stored. Anita is sorely tempted to give in; a specific request like this is different from Heather's normal habit of plunging into whatever catches her eye, and may be a sign that she will be more respectful of the material. But no, they have to be consistent, and the policy is 2 days of no sand whenever Heather is thoroughly out of control, as she was last Friday; besides, there is still the matter of the blocks. "Heather, we will have sand another day. It's time to put away the blocks now."

Step 2 of the routine: Whether or not Heather resumes play, she still has to restore the environment to its original condition. Anita escorts Heather back to the abandoned blocks, now strewn in and around the sandbox, but not before Heather grabs a sand pail and shovel with her free hand. "Anita will help you put the blocks in the container," Anita says. "Then it will be almost time for circle. Here, I'll hold the box. You put in the blocks."

Heather, acting as if she has not heard a word, begins putting blocks into her sand pail, picking them up, and dropping them back in again. Anita, barely showing a trace of exasperation, repeats several times: "I will help you, Heather. Blocks must go in the box now." This time she takes Heather's hand in hers, closes it around a block, moves it over to the container, opens it to release the block, places it over another scattered block, and so on until the job is completed, all the while saying: "Good helping, Heather. You're doing a nice job. You're putting all the blocks away. I'm proud of you. Now let's find something else to do."

In a flash, the just-filled cylindric cannister is on its side, blocks dispersed. Was it Heather's clumsiness, had she done it on purpose, was she angry? Anita doesn't know. But this event triggers Step 3: "Oh, Heather, the blocks needed to stay in the box. Now we have to pick them up again, and then I think you need some quiet time to think about what you have done." After repeating once more the hand-over-hand return of the blocks, Anita gets the time counter, sets it for 1 minute, and sits Heather in a corner chair, her back to the room activities.

Heather immediately climbs onto the window ledge. "I sit here," she says. Anita puts her back in the chair, tightens the tray around her, and sits on the floor by her side.

At birth Heather (second child, father a building contractor and mother a part-time dental assistant) was the most animated baby in the newborn nursery, or so her parents thought. As an infant and toddler she was active, but not overly so, alert, curious, unusually sociable and joyous, a favorite in an extended family with mostly males. Then, at 18 months of age, she came down with a very high fever and extreme listlessness. For 2 days her mother administered cold baths and baby aspirin, assuming it was the flu. But the fever didn't abate; the listlessness got worse, and she stopped moving altogether. When her mother finally called the pediatrician, the doctor immediately suspected meningitis and sent them to the hospital. By the time they got there, Heather was comatose. After the long illness, she never regained full function.

For two years the family watched and waited, trying to be optimistic, celebrating every new word in her vocabulary and each motor accomplishment. In time she regained what she had lost, but at age 4 her mental and motor development were clearly compromised and the hyperactivity only increased. Mother, who had quit her job when Heather became ill, could not manage her She tried everything, playing endlessly with her on the floor, trying to find an activity that would sustain her interest, sending Heather to her room when she misbehaved, reinforcing her with food when she was good, proofing their home against her outbursts, routinizing all aspects of life, always informing Heather about what was going to happen next, and rocking and singing to her every night. But nothing she did seemed to help, and with the passing years Heather became more destructive. So Heather's mother hired a sitter and went back to work full time. Now, dejected, separated from her husband, overweight, looking more like 45 than 35, she does not communicate frequently with Teresa and shows up with her estranged husband only for the annual IEP conferences. Although Teresa has sympathy for all Heather's mother has endured, it is not in her nature fully to accept the never-ending mourning—tinged as it is with guilt. She keeps up the daily journal, asks questions about Heather's behavior at home (usually receiving cursory answers), and hopes that before the school year is over, she and Heather's mother will have a better working relationship.

CIRCLE TIME

Free play is over at 9:00 a.m. Ten minutes before, Teresa announces: "Soon it will be time to clean up." Five minutes before, she dims the lights and says, "It is time to clean up now. It is time to get ready for circle."

Before joining circle, she took a quick panoramic look around the room at the children's activities. Larry and Stephen spent their time in the building corner constructing a large roadway. (They are the highest functioning children in the class and, therefore, minor figures in this study. Both have immature language. Larry is from a marginal family who may have abused him early in life. He is supposed to be aggressive, but Teresa has not seen any behavioral problems. Stephen, who comes from a large working-class family, has fine-motor delays, in addition to articulation difficulties.) Carl (also a secondary figure because of his severe retardation), always attracted by group action, rolled over to join the road-builders. Though his diplegia prevents him from participating, he watched the boys and chortled frequently, particularly when the bridges and ramps collapsed. Molly, also seeking proximity, pulled the red wagon over to fill with assorted blocks from the shelf. Her collection was regularly raided by Stephen and Larry, who found it a convenient supply for their building. Molly did not mind—their invasions just left space in the wagon for more blocks, which she sometimes, heedlessly, picked up from the middle of the boys' roadway. With a "Molly, no. Leave it alone. That's our block," sometimes accompanied by a shove, one of the boys would snatch it back, and then all three children continued their separate and joint pursuits.

Austin presented more of a problem. After tiring of the helicopter play, he had begun roaming again. He liked to run his hands over the toy shelves, and this meant walking right through the roadway, displacing many blocks and ruining the layout. Alice, responding to the boys' complaints, took Austin to the doll corner to join David and Doreen. He picked up a plastic imitation Coke bottle, and began rotating it while chanting, "It's the real thing, it's the real thing."

Alice, in a small chair at the circular table, asked him: "Bring me corn, Austin, *yellow* corn. I'm hungry. Oh, Austin, I'm so hungry. How about bringing me some grapes, the *green* grapes?" After repeated requests, Austin finally brought her a pot. "No, Austin, the pot is for cooking. I need some food to eat." Austin, still invested in rotating the coke bottle, made no further moves to comply.

Clean-up proceeds uneventfully, with a few reminders to Molly and Doreen to be "all done." The children, except Austin and Carl, find their own chairs (name and personal symbol attached to the back) lined up in a semicircle facing Teresa's chair, which is backed to the wall boards. Alice carries Carl to his special orthopedic chair and then positions herself in a chair behind Austin. Anita latches a restraining tray across the armrests of Heather's chair and sits down behind her. Teresa brings Austin by the hand, removing the coke bottle in transit.

Teresa begins the welcome, rhythmically chanting and clapping her hands: "Larry, Larry, who came to school today, who came to school today?"

Larry, an ace at this routine, responds, also in a chant: "Larry came to school today," which prompts Teresa and the aides to sing, "Hello, Larry. Hello, Larry. Hello, Larry. We're so glad that you are here." Larry then finds and removes his name, located underneath his photograph on a strip of Velcro, and places it on another higher Velcro strip next to the calendar.

Teresa asks Larry, "Who else is here today?"

"Stephen."

Teresa corrects, "Stephen is here today," and Larry repeats the phrase. Teresa claps her hands and chants: "Stephen, Stephen, who came to school today, who came to school today?" Stephen, also skilled at this repartee, responds, "I came to school today," which signals another chorus of "Hello, Stephen. Hello, Stephen. Hello, Stephen. We're so happy you are here," at which point he finds his name and posts it, picks another child, and the cycle repeats.

Carl rolls up to find his name, tactfully placed low enough for him to reach it. Neither he, nor Molly, nor Doreen get out the sentence, "I am here today," even with extensive coaching.

Austin, when asked by Teresa, "Are you here today?", repeats the question. But when told to say "I am here today," he repeats it and then proceeds to read off, not only his own name, but all the other printed words posted on the oak tag—"sun," "cloud," "hot," "cold," etc.

Meanwhile Heather, very unhappy at being constrained, has been bouncing up and down while attached to her chair. Teresa wants to avoid putting Heather in "timeout" again, so she asks Anita to hold her on her lap. Doreen, seated next to Molly, is entranced with her neighbor's long, soft hair. She intermittently strokes it and wraps it around her fingers. Molly is indifferent, for she and David are alternating touches of each other's arms, legs, and clothes.

For a while, Teresa misses the byplay, but as soon as she notices it, in a gap between the "hellos," she reminds the children, "It is time to listen now. Doreen, and David, and Molly, where do we keep our hands? Hands need to sit on our laps, remember?" (Alice reaches around to place the children's hands on their laps.) Teresa continues: "That's better. I like the way you're sitting now. And you, too, Heather, that's nice quiet sitting in Anita's lap."

Teresa proceeds with the calendar and weather. "Who knows what month this is?"

Larry: "Winter."

"That's good thinking, Larry, but winter is the season. What is the month?"

Stephen: "Thanksgiving."

"Almost right, Stephen. This is November. Can you say November?"

"November."

Teresa: "And what day is today?"

Austin: "Day is days of the week, 7 days of the week, Saturday, Sunday, Monday . . ."

"Thank-you, Austin. That's right, today is Monday. Now what date is today?" No response. "Let's look up here" (she points to the calendar of the month attached to the magnetic board with hooks for numbers, now complete through 11). "It's time to *count* together, 1, 2, 3, 4." She stops at 11. "So what is next?"

David chimes in, "12."

"Good counting, David. That's right, today is November 12th. Can you find the right number and put it up, David?" He picks it from a row of numbers at the bottom of the magnetic board that currently start with 12 and go through 31, and places it on the calendar hook.

"Good, David. Now who would like to count *fast* to 12?"

Stephen volunteers and seems to get it approximately right, though his blurred speech makes it difficult to tell. "Good work,

Stephen. Now who would like to do the numbers *slowly* up to 12?"

Larry volunteers and is correct. Austin accompanies him but keeps going "13, 14, 15, 16."

"Thank-you, Larry," says Teresa. Pointing to the colored calendar, she asks, "Now, Austin, can you tell me what *color* November 12th is?"

"November 12th is green today."

"Very good, and is November 11th green?"

"November 11th is green today."

"No, Austin, November 11th is . . . ?"

David: "Red 11."

"Very good, David, I like the way you are using your words today." After some more questions about colors and numbers, Teresa shifts to the weather.

"Heather, look out the window and tell us what kind of day it is." Heather sprints over to the window and tries to open it. "No, Heather, just look out and tell us if it is sunny or cloudy."

"Cloudy."

"Very good looking, Heather. Now come back and find the cloudy face to put up by the calendar."

Heather bounds back, and using her two hands, pulls the cloudy *and* sunny faces from the magnetic board, turning both over to Teresa, who attaches the cloudy face on the board.

"Who can tell us if it is *cold* or *hot* out?" Aside from Austin— "cold or hot out"—no one comments. "Larry, you said it was winter. Actually, it is fall, but can you remember whether winter is hot or cold?"

"Cold."

"Very good remembering, Larry. Now come find the cold shivering child." Larry approaches the board looking back and forth between the two figures—one shivering, one sweating—and at Teresa for a hint. Tentatively he picks one, watching Teresa nod and smile as he does so.

While Teresa is busy with the calendar, Anita and Alice keep putting out brush fires. Molly, who has stopped playing with David's belt and with the pom-poms on her skirt, twists restlessly in her chair, making 180-degree turns. When she sees Heather get up to observe the weather, she, too, leaves the circle, crawls under a table, and sits down cross-legged. Her feet, now both visible and accessible, present an attractive diversion. Quickly she slides one foot out of a loosely clasped sneaker and begins to pull off her sock.

Teresa, taking note, says to Anita, "Molly wants you to help her sit."

Anita dashes over, gently reminding Molly, "It is circle time now, I will help you sit," and back they go. But Molly escapes again when Teresa asks Larry to find "the cold, shivering child."

After restoring Molly a second time and complimenting her for "good sitting," Teresa begins the songs. She has Carl roll up to the magnetic board and point to the illustration of his favorite. He picks "The Wheels on the Bus," the picture easiest to reach from his prone position. Teresa and the aides begin asking the children for verse suggestions.[1] This is a popular item, and several of the children participate at least partially. Doreen likes making the honk-honk-honk gesture and sound, which she begins as soon as they start singing and continues while the song proceeds to new verses. Teresa then has the children stand and puts on a tape of "Hokey Pokey," Heather's choice.[2] Again, Doreen is always about two gestures behind the verses, shaking her leg when it is time to wave her arms, jumping forward when she should be turning. Austin continues to turn in circles, through verse and chorus alike, until stopped by Alice. Heather, in a paroxysm of giggles, keeps stomping her feet. It is not precision dancing, but some of the children, particularly Larry and Stephen, are on target some of the time. None, however, can sing and move simultaneously, and most look to Teresa's example for their clues rather than following the vocalist on the tape. Four more songs follow and then a story.

For the last part of circle, Teresa produces a large, felt grab bag. She announces: "I've got a fun surprise for us. Inside this bag are lots of things that have to do with a Thanksgiving meal. I want you to put your hand in and find something in the bag. Then I want you to guess what it is before you take it out." She starts with David but has to fend off Heather who has slipped out from under her restraining tray and plunges both hands into the bag.

"Here. Me find stuff."

Teresa: "You'll have a turn in a little while, Heather. I know it is hard to wait, but it is David's turn now. David, can you find something?" He pulls out an apple. "David, you forgot. First you are supposed to feel the object and guess, then pull it out, OK?"

David: "It's an apple."

"Very good, David, and what *color* is the apple?"

"Red apple."

"Good, David. Is the apple *round* or *square*?"

Austin: "Apple juice is good for you."

David: "Apple gives us A."

Austin: "A, B, C, CBS, Channel 10."

Teresa gives her attention to David: "Yes, apple gives us A.

That's good remembering," and she points to the letter "A" strung above the board. She then repeats her question about shape, and David responds, "Red square."

Teresa, turning to Stephen, asks, "Is the apple *round* or *square*?"

"Round."

"That's right, Stephen. Now you find something else that is round in the bag." Stephen pulls out an orange and labels it. Teresa asks Stephen to identify the color, which he does. "What else is orange, Stephen? Can you find something in the room that is orange?" She stares at a leftover Halloween pumpkin.

Austin jumps up: "Orange juice is good for you."

Teresa again ignores Austin and asks Larry to find a rectangle in the bag. He pulls out a brown plastic table top but calls it a square. Teresa makes the correction. When she gets to the lower functioning children—Molly, Doreen, and Heather—she modifies the task by asking them to pull out an object and label it. Heather plunges into the bag, pulls out a potato, and hurls it. Molly finds the ice cream (plastic) and starts to lick it. Teresa reminds them, "It's time now to *name* the food." Among them they get "apple," "juice," "ice cream," "table," "spoon," and "cup," but miss "knife," "fork," "banana," "pie," "napkin," "turkey," "cranberries," and "potatoes." The spoon, cup, and apple are turned over to Carl to handle.

Teresa continues displaying two apples for the entire group: "Are these the *same* or *different*?" Different children give different answers. Larry gets it right. "Good, Larry. Now"—holding up an apple and a banana—"are these two the *same* or *different*?" Again Larry is correct. "Good, Larry. Now, David, which is *bigger*, the apple or the table?" David, uncertain, gets it right.

Heather corrects him. "Big apple, big, very big apple," and Austin adds, "Apple juice is good for you."

Teresa, hands opening wide as she talks: "Yes, an apple is *big* and good for you, but a table is much, much *bigger*."

This line of questioning (big, little, same, different, color naming) continues for a couple of minutes until Teresa, noticing the children squirming (it is now 9:20), announces: "We are going to make Thanksgiving pictures for all of you to take home." She sends the higher children (Larry, Stephen, and David) to one table with Alice, the lower children (Doreen, Molly, Heather, and Austin) to another with Anita. Carl is placed in his orthopedic chair (which has a tray attachment) and given some soft Play-Doh to finger.

The plan is that the first group will paste a precut table onto their individual sheets of paper; on top of the table they will paste two small paper plates, and on top of them, some food items. Place settings are to be mounted next to the plates. Most of the objects to be pasted have been precut, but the children will color the food, and a few will cut some of the easier forms from construction paper. The second group will be given white sheets of construction paper with tables already attached. Their task is simply to paste the food on top of the table. Teresa and Anita prepared the cutouts Friday after school, but the idea for the project was part of their monthly unit planning—in November the emphasis is on barnyard animals, Thanksgiving, and fall. The project is meant to serve several functions: it should be fun, it gives the children something of their own to share with parents, and it meets the matching and sorting IEP goals of several pupils.

ART TIME

In the transition between circle and art, Molly walks unnoticed to the cubby area. Along with the underside of tables, this is her favorite retreat. Normally she sits down in the cubby and plays with whatever is around—a jacket, mitten, or toy brought from home. But today she wanders over to Austin's bright blue backpack and pokes her hand into an opening. Out comes a shirt. After brief inspection, Molly carries this over to Doreen's cubby. There she pulls out a sock and, continuing on her treasure hunt, goes to Larry's. Finding his pack rather empty, she stuffs the shirt and sock inside. In doing so, she strikes gold—a candy bar. Molly, in order to shield herself from view, folds into a small ball, her back to the group, and quickly begins to devour her discovery, when Larry, uncannily sensing his candy in danger, pounces on her. Molly, much smaller but fiercely determined, lies on her back, raises her feet and kicks at Larry. He furiously lunges for the candy, but Molly protects it with her body. Anita comes quickly over to quell the disturbance. She removes the candy from Molly, despite howls of protest, and says, "I know you didn't mean to take Larry's candy, Molly. It was just a mistake. We need to learn better things to do with our hands. Larry, I know you are angry at Molly, but she didn't realize it belonged to you. She is sorry, aren't you, Molly?" Promising Larry he can eat the candy later, Anita walks both children back to their respective tables, unaware of the redistributed garments.

Four-year-old Molly is a "garden variety" mentally retarded child. Intellectually, and even perhaps physically, she could pass for a 1½- to 2-year-old. As is so often the case with such children, she seemed perfectly normal the first 1½ years of her life. At her first birthday party her parents, a beautician and beauty parlor owner, noted that she was just beginning to crawl, whereas her older sister was taking tentative steps at the same age. Then at 18 months, her parents realized she was very quiet and didn't do much beyond playing with her busy box. They asked Molly's maternal grandmother whether she thought something was wrong with Molly. The grandmother made light of the inquiry, reminding them of a cousin whose early development also had been slow. There was no reason to expect a problem, she pointed out, no history in the family of slowness, no problems with pregnancy or delivery, no health problems in the child. Molly was a cute, smiling, loving child developing on her own timetable. The family just had to be patient.

But at 2½ Molly began attending day-care 3 days a week, and the staff there, noting her total absence of speech, urged the parents to have her evaluated. Molly's diagnosis was "developmental delay," with a recommendation for early intervention. Molly's grandmother still does not see a problem. "When you were little," she tells her daughter, "we didn't have all the fancy evaluations and special schools, but kids grew up OK, and so will she." Molly's parents are very optimistic that she will catch up. They see impressive progress: she has started to talk and play with her sister and seems to have a wonderful memory (when Teresa told them of the candy incident, they did not accept her interpretation that Molly had stumbled across the prize, but thought pleasurably that she must have known Larry occasionally brought candy to school and recalled where he kept it).

Like Doreen, Molly is an active, playful, good-tempered child. But her elfin body, impish darting movements, and solo actions make her more invisible; teachers keep "losing" Molly even though she constantly gets into things, reorganizes objects and furniture, collects, deposits, and hoards materials. She rarely participates in group activities, her gaze remaining fixed on what is near at hand (her own clothing, neighboring children, an item she has secreted in her fist). She is impulsive and may, without warning, just up and leave an activity. Before the teacher responds, she has dumped a tub of toys. Molly, therefore, requires an unusual degree of supervision, but her behavior is easier to handle than Heather's.

The impulsiveness is not as extreme or violent. The staff believes that if they can get her to "use her words," she will be less rambunctious and more easily kept in group sessions.

As usual, Larry and Stephen understand the art project and, following Alice's prefabricated example, get busy on their own. Alice keeps them on track with continuous instructions: "OK, boys, I want you to find the cut-out table . . . Good, you found it. What shape did Teresa tell you the table was? Now put paste on one side . . . That's right, very good. Now paste the table onto your paper." She pauses to help Stephen, who has difficulty aligning the horizontal dimensions of the table and construction paper. "Now you need to find the plates. Each of you is to take two plates and paste them at each end of your table. David, look at what you are doing. How many plates do you have?"

David has three and counts: "1, 2, 3, 4."

"No, David, you have three, but you should have two. Now we are going to cut out the apples. What color paper will we use? " Before getting a response, she hands each child a piece of red construction paper with two apples drawn. Noticing that Stephen is having trouble cutting, she puts her hand over his, and they cut around the apple together.

From another table,Teresa suggests that Alice give Stephen a better pair of scissors. David requires additional instruction. He starts to paste the food directly onto the table (rather than onto the plate) and continues even after being corrected.

Alice demonstrates the correct placements directly on his paper: "Look, David, the paste goes on the apple. Then we turn the apple over and put it on the plate like this, not on the table. At home I know you wouldn't eat your food off the table. First you would put it on the plate like . . ." and she instructs him to continue. He starts out all right but requires additional direction when he begins randomly to paste foods and utensils in a pile.

Life is more chaotic at the other table. Austin wants to paste his objects in a line along the bottom of the paper without any relationship to his premounted table. Heather is grabbing up all the crayons and taking them over to the block shelves. Doreen is wriggling the paste brush around in one of the small paste jars (she should be coloring), while Molly is gouging the paste with a crayon saved from Heather's horde.

Teresa, who has joined Anita, realizes too much material is exposed. She removes the paste, despite Doreen's protests, redistributes the crayons, and remarks, "Heather, we need to share. There are plenty for everyone."

Teresa has the children concentrate on coloring. Austin does fine, but Heather colors outside the lines and has to be reminded by Teresa that, "We are coloring our food, *just* the food, so we can have a beautiful Thanksgiving meal." Doreen and Molly make chicken scratches. Teresa praises them all and brings back the paste. "These are going to be so gorgeous. Won't mommy and daddy be proud. Heather, what is it you are pasting now?"

Heather replies, "I paste now."

"But *what* are you pasting? Is it an apple?"

"Yes."

"Good talking, Heather. I'm proud of you."

Austin and Heather make progress with their pasting, though not always landing the food on the table, but Molly and Doreen just do not get it. Doreen's interest is in the brush. She rubs it on top of the food items but doesn't understand that the function of paste is adhesion. When told to turn the pasty food over so it will stick to the paper, she just bangs her hands on the objects. Noticing the paste on her hand, she begins to lick it. Molly also likes the feel of paste and, now that the crayons have been put away, plunges her fingers into the jar, smells them, and rubs them against each other, enjoying the sticky feelings. Removing the paste again, Teresa takes Doreen's "food," turns it over properly, picks up Doreen's hand and, pressing it down over the items, comments, "Now you are pressing the food onto the table. That's good pressing. The food will stick on the table now and won't fall off when you take it home."

SNACK TIME

It is 9:35, 5 minutes before snack. In a flurry of orchestrated activity, Alice cleans the first art table; instructs Austin, Larry, Stephen, and David to wash their hands; and attends to Carl's diaper change. Anita sets up the snack table with cups, cans of juice (apple and cranberry), and animal crackers, inviting Heather to help (which she does); then supervises Heather's hand washing. Teresa quickly finishes up Molly's and Doreen's art work and starts to sponge off the second table. Doreen fetches a small sponge from the doll corner: "Me do it, clean," she says. Teresa permits a couple of strokes and then brings both girls to the sink so she can complete the cleanup rapidly and not keep children waiting at the table.

Doreen and Molly are dawdling. Perched on a common stool,

they alternate putting their hands under the spigot, opening and closing their fists. They briefly fall into a hand-over-hand routine, taking turns until Doreen puts both hands under the flowing water and Molly starts to push her away. Teresa notices and comes over to expedite the hand washing.

When everyone is quietly seated around the table, Teresa announces she has two kinds of juices, apple and cranberry. She pours a bit of each into separate cups and asks the children to identify the colors. Cranberry is easy. Larry and Stephen yell out "red." Apple juice is tougher. Teresa withdraws the question and asks the children: "Where does apple juice come from?"

Austin responds, "Apple juice is good for you." Teresa ignores the comment and provides the answer.

She then asks each child which juice he or she wants. If one cannot, or does not, respond, she pushes a can forward and asks: "Do you want apple juice?" If they still do not respond, she pours one of each into small cups to make the choice more concrete. When Heather and Molly reach for both, they are instructed again to make a choice. The children clamor for second helpings before Teresa completes the round.

Anita quells the uprising with an offer of crackers. Again, there is a choice of two kinds: "Do you want the monkey cracker or the bear? Show me which one you want," Anita says.

Molly shouts out, "More."

"More apple juice or more cranberry juice?"

Molly just repeats "More juice," which suffices, though Teresa is careful to say as she pours, "More apple juice, please." When Doreen points without saying anything, however, she is told, "Use your words, Doreen."

Heather jumps up to get the can herself and creates a ruckus when led back to her seat. She wriggles away from Anita and onto the floor, yelling, "Gimme my juice, I want my juice."

Teresa tells Anita: "I guess Heather isn't ready for juice yet. Maybe she will be more ready after some quiet time," and whisks her off to the timeout chair for a minute. Carl only has to indicate his interest in juice by reaching and he is served. All three adults are kept busy asking questions, responding to requests, cleaning up spills, and reminding children to throw away their paper goods.

As they finish their snacks, the children are invited to "go play." Heather, Doreen at her heels, moves toward the doll corner, but stops when she sees beanbags on a shelf. She grabs several, saying, "I'm Superman, I'm Batman." With a big windup she throws them at nothing in particular. Doreen retrieves one and, clutching it to her chest, wanders off to the doll corner where she deposits it in the baby carriage. Molly, also in the doll corner, gathers up utensils and dumps forks, spoons, and cups into the carriage along with a baby doll.

Heather tries to join but is rejected; so she takes loose objects from the shelves and stuffs them into the oven. She then finds herself a pair of high-heel shoes and a purse. Stomping back to the carriage, she announces: "We go shop now."

As Heather stalks off with the carriage, Molly climbs into the open oven cuddling a doll, and Doreen, after closing the oven door, goes over to the full-length mirror. She lifts up her shirt and inspects her stomach. Bending her body from the waist in a partial bow, she peeks up and says "hi" to her image, repeats this movement a few times, then gets down on her knees and bows from that position.

Larry and Stephen go back to resume their earlier block play, and Austin takes a book over to the window where—it is hard to say—he either looks at the pictures or at light and shadow patterns he makes by tilting the book in front of the blinds. Carl remains at the table with Teresa, who is trying to get him to drink his juice with a straw.

After 5 minutes, Teresa dims the lights and announces, "It's time to clean up and come to circle so we can do our work." There is much to be done. Alice and Anita help the girls put away all the objects in the oven and baby carriage. Doreen and Molly are happy to oblige, but not Heather—she is now "shopping." So as the staff returns the plastic foods that she has removed from the shelves and strewn about in the carriage, on chairs, on the floor, and in her purse, she pulls them out again and shouts: "I need this. Buy this one now."

WORK TIME

By 10:00 the children are assembled and "work" (IEP) time begins. Teresa, with her staff's help, has prepared for this period as carefully as for art. She normally divides the children into two or three groups. Since Austin and Carl are out of the room on Mondays at 10:00 (Austin has language therapy; Carl, physical therapy), she has decided on two groups today.

Teresa assigns Stephen, Larry, and David to Alice. The boys are working on letter and shape identification, form matching, prepositions, and sequencing. Alice picks up a flannel board attached to a metal stand and a plastic box with colored felt objects for mounting. Consistent with the current theme, the teachers have collected turkeys and various foods made of felt. They cut out brown tables with a large enough surface to hold several food items at once. Under Teresa's guidance, Heather has already brought to the table several plastic bins containing parquetry blocks, a set of colorful beads of different shapes, several homemade laminated strips illustrating different bead arrangements, lotto games (matching animals, matching activities, matching objects, and the initial letters that name them), and an alphabet board (letters in upper and lower case engraved on levers which, when pressed, flip up to reveal underneath an object that starts with the corresponding surface letter). (For teaching numbers the process is reversed. At the bottom of the board, each lever has a series of dots—1 through 10—which opens, when pressed, to reveal the corresponding arabic numeral.)

Once the three boys are assembled, Alice starts with the flannel board. She attaches the paper table and, pulling out a few turkeys, asks David: "Can you tell me what this is, David?"

"Rooster. Cock-a-doodle-doo."

"Almost, David. Good try. Larry, do you know what it is?"

"No."

Stephen: "It's a turkey."

"And what sound does a turkey make?" asks Alice.

"Gobble-gobble-gobble," responds David, and he gets up and starts to flap his arms.

"Good, David, but you need to sit down now."

Alice asks Larry to "put the turkey *next to* the table." He puts it *on top of*. She points to *next to*, and he corrects his error. The exercise continues. Different foods are brought out. The boys are asked to identify them by name and color and put them *on, behind, in front of*, and *next to* the turkey; *under* and *on top of* the table; and put *two* apples at one end, *one* apple at the other. They rarely are correct on the prepositions and numbers and miss many of the food items, but for the most part they know their colors. Then Alice lines up a "turkey family" on the flannel board and asks David to pick out the *biggest* turkey. He does so, but the biggest happens also to be the nearest. When then asked to pick the *smallest*, he points to the biggest again.

"David," asks Alice, "isn't this the one you said was the *biggest?*"

"Yes."

"Then it can't be the *smallest*, can it?" A quizzical look from David. "No, David, this is the small one. The *biggest* cannot be the *smallest*, right?"

David assents, "Yes, right."

The boys are restless. Larry starts tipping his chair back and David immediately follows suit. Alice reminds them it is work time and shifts to the next activity. Larry and Stephen each get a set of parquetry blocks. David asks for the letter board but is told by Alice, "First you need to do your beads." The task for David is to thread beads according to the alternating pattern (red round, green square, blue oblong) found on the laminated strip that Alice lays next to the box of beads. He begins to remove beads from the box at random and then comes to a complete stop, preferring to watch the other two boys. Alice suggests, "If you need help, David, ask me. Can you say 'help me, please'?" David repeats, "Help me, please." Alice strings a few beads, explaining as she goes, "You look here up top and see that you need a red circle, so you pull out of the box a red circle and put it on your string. Is that hard, David?"

"Yes."

Alice rejoins, "No, it's not hard for you. I've seen you do it. It's easy, isn't it?"

David: "Yes."

"Good," says Alice, "I'll do one more and then you need to do the rest." When the task is turned over to David, he again strings randomly. Teresa comes to the table and suggests that Alice take a handful of red circles, green squares, and blue oblongs from the box so David won't get confused by the other shapes and colors. This simplifies the task for David, and he proceeds to get many correct, as well as incorrect, sequences. The parquetry blocks are difficult and uninteresting for Larry and Stephen. They work very slowly, sometimes following the guide sheet lining the box they are filling, sometimes not. After this activity, it is time for lotto. Alice holds up one picture after another for the children to find on their cards.

Meanwhile Anita has taken Doreen, Heather, and Molly to a table with an assortment of square and round pegboards, single insert puzzles of objects and shapes, plastic plates color-coordinated with innumerable small monkeys, laminated picture cards of household objects, and an Etch-A-Sketch. She instructs Doreen to complete a pegboard; asks Molly to do the color sorting; and places the Etch-A-Sketch in front of Heather. Moving behind Heather's chair and holding her hands, "together" they start to draw as Anita explains, "Now we're making the line go *down, down, down*, now *up, up, up*. Good drawing, Heather. Let's do it again."

Heather objects, "Me do it. Me do it myself." Anita lets go, and Heather, working both hands simultaneously, produces a cross-quilt of jagged lines while chanting, "*down, down, down, up, up, up*."

Molly has laid out the plates and dumped the monkeys onto the table. Rather than sort them onto the plates, however, she guides them up the sides of the plastic tub and lets them drop, exclaiming, "No bite, monkey."

She repeats this with several monkeys when Anita reminds her: "It's time to put the monkeys on their plates, Molly, like this," and she quickly demonstrates how to match the monkey with its color-coordinated plate.

Doreen gathers up the pegs and starts dropping them into Molly's monkey bin. Anita moves her own chair between Molly and Doreen, separates the monkeys and pegs, and monitors the work of each girl. The pegboard is not difficult for Doreen. Molly searches for the red monkeys to put on the red plate but randomly adds blue and yellow ones. After each error, Anita asks: "Is this *red*?"

Molly: "No red."

"Right," says Anita, "then does it go on this plate?"

"No plate."

"Good," says Anita, "it goes on the *blue* plate here." She points, and Molly follows her lead.

During this time Teresa is working with individual children, marking their performance on "data sheets." David, at long last, gets to do the alphabet board. He can label 10 letters and knows at least one word that starts with each letter. Today Teresa puts a different spin on the exercise. She starts by opening the levers, revealing the pictures underneath—apple, banana, coat—and asks David for the initial letter and sound. No problem. He also gets all the letters correct. Lots of check marks gather on the data sheet. Next, Teresa asks David to find something in the room that begins with "B." He hasn't a notion. She asks: "Does b-b-boy begin with B?"

"Yes, 'boy' gives us B."

"Good. What else begins with B?" No response. Teresa makes a note to work on David's generalization of "B." They then go on to numbers. Although David has some difficulty counting, he reads off all the numerals to 10.

Doreen is called up. Teresa has made an individualized word book for the three girls and Austin. On the front of each is a candid photograph of the child, and inside are pictures of family members, rooms, personal objects, pets—whatever the family supplied. Doreen recognizes and labels "Mommy," "Daddy," "Willy" (the dog), "woof-woof-woof," "me bed," "me doggie" (stuffed animal of a bear), and several other common objects. She calls a comb, "brush," a dish towel, "wash," a refrigerator, "eat," and, after 3 months, still misses pot, pan, bed, rug, coat, dress, hat, mittens, boots. But when Teresa asks, pointing to the dress, "What do you do with this?" Doreen makes a beeline for the doll corner and brings back a ladies' dress, which she steps into backward saying, "Look me, look me."

Pleased, Teresa says: "Good, Doreen. That's a dress. You look very pretty in it. A dress is something we wear. We wear dresses. Now, can you tell me what we do with a dress? Do we wear it?"

"Wear it."

Teresa is satisfied and makes some check marks in Doreen's work book. "Doreen," Teresa continues, "I would like you to take the dress *off* and put it *under* the table, *down under* the table." Doreen starts to climb onto the table. "No, Doreen. Look, we'll take this dress and put it *up on* the table." She demonstrates with an exaggerated lift of the dress and hands it to Doreen who does it correctly this time. "Good job. Now," says Teresa, "let's take it *down* and put it *under* the table." After another dramatic demonstration ("*Down* it comes, and *under* it goes"), Teresa turns the dress over to Doreen, who puts it back *on* the table. Teresa makes a note to repeat the exercise tomorrow.

Teresa summons Heather, saying, "Today we are going to go fishing, Heather, just like we did last week. You need to remember that the fish stay right here in the water" (and she lays out a dyed blue sheet). Heather dives under the sheet and, wriggling her body, shouts, "Me fish." Teresa hauls her up:

"You are the fisherwoman today. You catch the fish. If you have trouble catching the fish, just ask me for help. Use your words and say 'Help me.' OK, Heather?" Not expecting an answer, Teresa dumps a dozen different colored fish with magnetic tails onto the sheet, hands a string rod with a magnetic tip to Heather, and keeps one for herself. After spreading the fish about, she continues, " I'll take the first turn. I think I will find a blue fish to take home." As she moves her rod over the "water, " Teresa asks: "Let's see, is this a blue fish? No, it's a yellow fish, I wonder if there are any blue fish around today? I sure would like to find a blue fish. Do you see a blue fish, Heather?"

Heather exclaims, "Blue fish, blue fish, here blue fish. Me get it," and she swings her pole over the blue fish, but misses.

"Good try, Heather. When it's your turn, you'll have another chance to catch it." But Heather can't wait, and clasping in her hand the magnetic piece attached to the end of her string, she places it on top of the blue fish and, ignoring the string, picks up both the fish and magnet. Teresa, careful not to criticize, demonstrates the correct action while commenting: "Look, Heather, this is the way we catch a blue fish. We move our rod over the fish we want v-e-r-y gently, and then v-e-r-y v-e-r-y carefully we lower the string to the tail of the fish. See? And after we've caught it, we pull the string up v-e-r-y slowly. Remember, the fish is in the water, and we are in a boat so we can't reach in and grab it, can we?" After the fishing game—Heather got check marks for several colors—Heather is sent back to the table.

Molly is working on shapes. In the room are numerous puzzles and sorters for shape recognition. With Molly, Teresa has been using a simple wood box that has a hinged top with five cut-outs for a circle, square, rectangle, triangle, and diamond. Molly starts without instruction. She opens the lid, dumps the pieces, and lays them out around the table. Then she puts a couple back in, reaching under the lid to do so, and shakes the box with both hands, saying "honk-honk-honk" (from "The Wheels on the Bus" song). Teresa reminds her, "It is time to do shapes now. We are going to put them *in* the right hole. Watch me. I take this circle and put it *in* here, then I take it *out*. Now it's your turn"—she hands Molly a circle—"to find where it fits." Molly gets it right immediately. Teresa comments, "Good job. You put it *in* just right. Now take it *out* and try again." Once more Molly succeeds quickly, and Teresa makes a check mark in her workbook. Teresa hands Molly the triangle. Molly knows where it goes but has trouble inserting it. Teresa suggests, "Make it flat, then slide it along the top. That's right; only when you get to the hole, you need to stop and press it in. You almost have it. Move it down just a bit like this" (and she puts her hand over Molly's). "Good, you got it." Next it's the square, which Molly hasn't mastered yet, so Teresa advises: "First, feel the square. Now look at each hole. Does it go here, or here, or here? Look carefully. Feel the square with your fingers" (she rubs Molly's fingers around the piece). "Now feel the holes on the box like this" (she puts Molly's hands over the square hole), and Molly drops it in.

GROSS-MOTOR TIME

By the time Teresa finishes with Molly it is 10:30, and work time is over—she'll get to the other four children tomorrow. While the assistants busy themselves putting the materials away, diapering and toileting, Teresa brings the children to the circle and asks each to select a sticker from an array that she presents as a reward for their good behavior. When Heather makes her choice, she is reminded, "You did pretty well, Heather, much better than last Friday, but you need to pay attention all the time, not just some of the time, OK?" Teresa then explains that since it is a bad day today, rain is threatening—she points to the pictures of cold and cloudy on the wall—they will stay inside. "We are going to do something all of you like a lot. Can you guess what that is?"

Stephen: "Hoops, hoowa-hoops."

David: "Do letter game."

Teresa: "No, we are going to do an obstacle course. First Austin, Heather, Stephen, and Larry will do it with Alice and me, while Molly, Doreen, David, and Carl play in the doll corner with Anita; then we'll shift so everyone has a turn." The higher level boys like this plan. Larry suggests they jump into the beanbag. Stephen wants to jump "from very high up." Teresa, Heather in tow as her "helper," starts to set up the course. When requested, Heather loudly pushes tables and chairs against the wall, knocking over the paint easel as she goes. Stephen helps bring in a small bench from the hallway, which is placed as the starting point in the middle of the windows, one end almost against the wall, the other extending into the room. Next a cloth-covered wire tunnel is taken out of the supply closet and put down at right angles to the bench. Teresa situates the rocking chair and three small chairs, with big spaces between them, in a diagonal line heading back to the center of the room. Here they join the jungle gym with the slide. At the bottom of the slide she pulls over the big beanbag.

With the activity set up and the children sitting on the floor along the wall, Teresa demonstrates how to go through the course. She climbs up onto the bench and begins: "We walk real slowly across the bench like this, one foot in front of the other. Then we jump off and crawl into the tunnel." Teresa gets down on all fours, decides she is too big, and walks by the side of the tunnel. "We don't stop in the middle but come out and take a short rock in the rocking chair. Then we slither like a snake" (and she makes a hissing sound) "zigzagging around the chairs until we get to the climbing structure. You climb up here if you can, or we will help you, then you slide down onto the beanbag and roll off" (this she actually demonstrates to the delight off the children) "and come back to the end of the line. If everyone does it right, we will have time for two turns."

Stephen and Larry are up on their feet, both pushing to be first. Teresa declares: "Stephen, since you got to help set up, we'll let Larry start." The words are no sooner out of her mouth than Larry is up and across the bench. Teresa sees he knows just what to do—she is very pleased with his good watching and recall—but curbs what she perceives as recklessness. "Larry, slower through the tunnel . . . The rocker isn't a swing . . . Gently, Larry, on the rocker . . . Careful when you climb."

At the top of the climbing structure, Larry, ignoring the slide, makes a jump for the beanbag. That gives Teresa a real scare: "No, Larry, you can jump on the beanbag but not off the climbing structure. You could get hurt that way." Stephen is next. "Nice waiting," Teresa notes as she summons him. He takes his turn uneventfully.

Alice, who has been holding Heather on her lap, stays by her side through the obstacle course. She needs lots of "redirection." Her first impulse is to mount the climbing structure. Turned back to the beginning bench ("This is where we start, Heather"), she dives for the tunnel. Teresa takes her aside and, holding Heather's face in her hands so they can look eyeball to eyeball, says calmly and forcefully: "We have to follow the rules, Heather. You need to let Alice help you unless you want quiet time." Her turn then proceeds smoothly, aside from knocked-over chairs.

Austin has left the group to stand by the window. Teresa takes his hand and says, " It's your turn, Austin." He echoes her line but pulls back from her grasp. She applies more pressure, insists he walk across the bench and rock in the rocking chair, after which she lets him go back to the window.

As the rest of the children take their turns on the obstacle course, Anita is supervising the other four in the doll corner. Using one of the tables that had been moved aside, she has put out a large hunk of Play-Doh, rolling pins, cookie cutters, and cookie sheets. Carl is sitting on the floor with an armrest pillow for support. David, Molly, and Doreen all like Play-Doh. The girls start by poking, pulling, and squeezing the individual allotments Anita has given them. As the mounds flatten out, Molly takes small amounts from the hunk, and Doreen copies her. Molly then takes a cookie cutter and bangs it on top of her mound; Doreen picks pieces of

Play-Doh and attaches them to her left arm, saying appreciatively as she does so, "Me pretty."

Anita steps in. "Doreen, let's make some cookies. Here, I'll roll out the dough, and then you can cut cookies out." She flattens the Play-Doh with a rolling pin and hands Doreen a cookie cutter. Doreen makes overlapping imprints. Anita tells her to press down harder and helps her do so. Anita then releases the "cookie" from the surrounding Play-Doh and suggests: "Heather would you like to put your cookie on a tray, then when we get a bunch of them they can be cooked."

"No cook."

Anita acquiesces: "OK, we'll just pretend to eat them."

Meanwhile David has been in continuous action. He started by putting his entire portion of Play-Doh in the oven saying, "Hot, hot." Then, noticing a timer, he counted, "1, 2, 3, 4, 5." On "5," he opened the oven and removed the Play-Doh, brought it back to the table, and began pounding it with a spatula. Then he returned to the oven with the spatula, and his irregular, but flatter, hunk, and counted again. This time he removed the Play-Doh and put it on a tray, brought it back to the table, and immediately returned again to the oven to insert the Play-Doh-on-tray. Observing Anita picking up a nearby doll, he grabbed another one and stuffed it into the oven on top of the tray. He then pulled out the tray, picked up the doll with one hand, Play-Doh with the other, and commanded the baby to "eat." Seemingly surprised by the doll's lack of response, he hurled it, the tray, and the Play-Doh back into the oven and began counting yet again. At this point, Anita comes over to help him sequence his actions more rationally: "David, shall we make cookies for the baby? First, we need to roll out the dough," and she takes him through the steps.

After 10 minutes it is time for this group to try the obstacle course. Anita tells them, "Time to clean up." Doreen, who prefers sponging to just about anything else, runs to get her favorite sponge yelping, "Me help." Molly is always glad to throw materials into a bin without regard for separating Play-Doh bits from cookie cutters and implements. David, however, resists: "I make cookies. Baby hungry. More cookie time."

"You fed your baby very well," comments Anita. "She is all done eating. She will get sick if she eats more" (Anita clutches her stomach and gives a mock groan). "We need to put everything away now. Doreen, that's enough sponging." After a bit more of this back-and-forth, David and Doreen submit.

After the two groups shift, Carl is carried over the bench,

rolled along the tunnel, pushed in the rocker, and held down the slide. Teresa instructs and monitors the other children on each piece of the course. Except for David, they need physical assistance here and there. But even with the supervision, Molly slips through the first bar space of the jungle gym and lies down inside the protected square made by the four sides of the structure. Doreen jumps out of line and crawls in next to her. After trying to persuade the girls to come out—"Mr. Bear is waiting for you on the beanbag. He wants you to slide down and give him a hug"—Teresa, realizing that the morning is swiftly drawing to a close, lets them stay and gives David an additional turn.

DEPARTURE

By the time the obstacle course is dismantled, clean-up completed, and the children brought back to circle, it is 10:50, almost time for the buses to arrive. Alice takes charge of the group, while Teresa and Anita write notes in the children's journals. The lateness of the hour means skipping the final story today. Alice, with a little help from Larry, Stephen, and David sing goodbye to each child, a repeat of the morning hello: "Goodbye, Heather. Goodbye, Heather. Goodbye, Heather, we're so sorry to see you go." Anita helps prepare for dismissal by laying out the jackets. She takes Molly, Doreen, Heather, and David, who are not yet independent dressers, to the top of their jackets so they can put both arms in and flip the garments over their heads. Doreen's and Austin's mothers enter the classroom to pick up their children. Teresa puts Carl in the wagon and asks Doreen to take David's hand.

The procession of teachers and children winds its way down the corridor, as at the beginning of the day. This time Doreen decides to stop at the water fountain, attracted by the broad steps at its feet. She mounts the lowest, exclaiming "Me up!" and starts on the second. Teresa is genuinely delighted: "Good climbing, Doreen. Now it's time to get the buses." Somewhat to Teresa's surprise, Doreen lowers herself and, stomach on the steps, slides down: "Me down!" But as Teresa moves on, Doreen tries to repeat the climb. As in a similar episode at the start of school, Teresa has no time to negotiate; she picks Doreen up and puts her in the wagon with Carl.

After the buses pull away, Teresa talks about her experience as a teacher while she eats her sandwich and tidies the room in preparation for her afternoon class:

"I love being with these kids, their little accomplishments mean so much. I know everyone thinks I'm crazy to do this sort of work, but really you get as much back from them as you give. The first time they say my name, which often isn't until January, or give me a hug, or even pee in the toilet, I'm in the clouds. And when they accomplish a new skill after months and months of work, it's the ultimate satisfaction. They are all so special: funny, needy, excitable, lovable.

"Most of the families are also great to work with. We become a big part of their lives. For instance, Molly's mom has had trouble grocery shopping because she can't get Molly into the cart. Mom tries to keep her next to the cart, but she constantly gets away and climbs onto the shelves. Since I live close by, I've gone with them and shown Mom that if you bring along some food and toys and put Molly in the cart before entering the store, she will behave. When you're building coping skills like this with a parent and child, you know it's forever. They learn management skills they didn't need with their regular children.

"We are close to most families. I write in the children's journals every day even to the parents who never write me. Parents want to know every little detail because the children tell them nothing. If I tell them we made turkeys, they can ask their children more specifically about what happened at preschool. It gives the parents something to talk about, which is important since their conversations are largely one-way affairs. Many of them do write back; just little stuff like how their child slept, ate, something the family did. But when you read this every day, it adds up to a lot of detailed knowledge. And most of the parents who don't write will call on the phone or drop in to ask questions; one way or another they keep me posted on what's going on at home. There are families, though, that frankly are not very involved, and often they are the ones that need help the most.

"I also like the freedom I have. I'm encouraged to take professional development courses, try out new ideas, and pretty much do what I want. The Director of Preschool Special Education used to teach and is, therefore, very understanding. She's always asking us for our 'wish list' of equipment, and much of the time I get what I ask for, like this new computer. However, she is not the person in charge. Officially, I'm under the building principal who has no background in special education. The problem is that those in authority are not experts, and the experts have no authority.

"The therapists, and the other special ed teachers are terrific colleagues. Although it is a small group, we do a lot of joint planning. I've learned from the physical and occupational therapists how to do fine-motor activities like drawing and cutting, how I should position children if they cannot control their own movements, how to do sensory stimulation. The speech therapist comes into class several times a week to consult with me, sees children individually, and runs language groups. She gives me ideas about how to get the kids to talk more and develop concepts.

"I have two big gripes. First is the paperwork. It's absurd. I'm always testing, writing IEPs that run 9–12 pages long, collecting data on children's IEP objectives and updating them every 9 weeks (actually, I don't do much of this, but I'm supposed to), and filling in forms. There's a form for everything: when we call parents, when we see parents, permission slips, survey forms. None of us can get the paperwork done during the day, so I have to work a part of every weekend. Some paperwork is important, but it has gotten out of hand, and I can see it is beginning to create burnout. Lately we've had to take language samples, write down everything a child says, and then analyze it for semantics and pragmatics. This is in addition to the data collection you saw me doing during IEP time. I don't see how this helps the children or parents, and it's not why I became a teacher. It drags me down.

"Second is the lack of integration. I know my children would do better if they had 'typical' children around them from whom to learn, if only there were some little kids in this school. We have tried to do mainstreaming with the kindergarten, and David still goes to one of them for visits. However, their classes are too big and our children end up ignored or else made to be the 'baby' in pretend play. Reverse mainstreaming—the kindergarten children come into my class—is better. But this takes more coordination and cooperation from teachers and parents than we've been getting. I even tried taking our class to a nearby day-care center, the one used by Stephen and David in the afternoon. It didn't work for long because they had a problem with our lower functioning children. I still haven't given up; there must be some way to solve the problem. It's really important to me.

"I don't think most people realize what a hard job this is. You wouldn't think a class of eight children twice a day with two aides was tough, but it is. I'm emotionally and physically wiped out by the end of the week and spend much of Saturday recuperating, that is when I'm not doing paperwork. We really need more time and more staff—more time to see the children, 2½ hours per day is not enough, more time to visit parents, more time to talk with one another when the children are not here, more staff to handle the difficult kids, more staff to do the 'chores' and free me for one-on-one work, and more therapy time, though that is a bit of a problem. It is hard to plan around the therapists' schedules; in fact, it is hard just to keep track of their schedules. Whether they work in the class, do 'pull-outs,' or try to consult with me, it always seems to be disruptive; yet they are very good, and the families are always asking for more therapy.

"I hope I haven't painted too negative a picture. As I've said, the children and their parents make up for all the difficulties. Right now, I never think about switching jobs, certainly not going into administration. I'm not an office person; I don't want all that paperwork, but if a new opportunity outside of teaching knocked on my door, I might consider it."

And with that, Teresa excused herself to pick up the afternoon group of children.

CHAPTER FIVE

Curriculum and Instruction—
Teachers versus Students

All in all, the problem under discussion amounts to this:
should passage from one stage of development be accelerated
or not? To be sure all education, in one way or another, is
just such an acceleration, but it remains to be decided to
what extent it is beneficial. It is not without significance that
it takes man much longer to reach maturity than the other
animals. Consequently, it is highly probable that there is an
optimum rate of development, to exceed or fall behind which
would be equally harmful.

— PIAGET (1976, p. 223)

What one "sees" as characteristic of settings depends naturally
on one's interests and "slots" for storing observations. The school
principal evaluating Midwood concentrates on Teresa's behavior—Does she have good daily lesson plans? Are they carried
out in an orderly and efficient manner?—and scarcely notices the
individual children. A parent may go years without even knowing
there are such things as lesson plans. Doreen's mother looks only
to see if her child is happy and performing up to expectations. A
state supervisor sees neither child nor teacher but counts the
number of children and staff , and inspects IEPs, safety and health
regulations for compliance to state and federal laws. A janitor
looks at the debris on the floor and smudges on the walls. As a
psychologist interested in the development of delayed preschoolers, I looked primarily at the point of contact between teacher and
child. What was the teacher's agenda, what was the child's agenda,
and how did each go about accomplishing her ends?

What I saw were teachers earnestly trying to instill in children a common set of skills and information which they, the teachers, consider key to future academic and social success. The elements in the curriculum, selected largely from a limited number of developmental checklists, are subdivided into goal areas—language, cognitive, fine- and gross-motor, social, and self-help—and treated almost as separate subjects, much like English, math, and history in later school years. The day is parceled out among each of these subjects: circle time is for cognitive goals, snack time for social and language, art time for fine-motor, the obstacle course for gross-motor. But there is also overlap—key instructional objectives are given privileged overriding status and intentionally repeated throughout the day to induce generalization.

Teachers are rarely sidetracked from their serious and earnest pursuit of the curriculum. Despite their difficult charge and charges, they maintain a remarkably unflappable poise, mild-mannered but always in control of the children and their teaching agenda. Above all, they constantly affirm their children, responding even to misbehavior with positive "redirection" (e.g., "I can help you listen") rather than criticism ("stop throwing"). They avoid extremes: do not get angry, raise their voices, and only rarely use direct physical control. When they do so, it is always to restrain, never to hurt. They guide, direct, talk a great deal, do some touching and holding, but are not likely to be either detached or physically exuberant, for example, in chasing, tickling, or rough-housing.

Teachers operate all day within this narrow, sedate, "professional" behavioral range and expect children to do likewise: sit, listen, respond when spoken to ("use your words"), stay "on task." They are expected not to be too silly, noisy, active, or exuberant; not to grab, throw, or hit. There is a steady demand on the children to control their bodies and voices and to maintain a happy emotional state.[1]

The problem is that moderately retarded children have difficulty meeting these expectations—both academic and behavioral. They do not catch on to the preacademics, forget the right answers they may have given the day before, and are restless with the work demands. They are not naturally physically restrained, even-tempered, or emotionally benign. Rather than sitting in chairs at tables, they are inclined to crawl under, and sometimes on top of, the furnishings. Even when seated, their arms and hands are constantly reaching to touch another child's hair and clothes. Paste, paint, and markers may be licked, smelled, smeared, and applied to inappropriate surfaces. By nature the children are noisy, often loudly demanding, sometimes crying and tantruming. By nature they are not interested in preacademics.

Teachers, therefore, must work very hard to accomplish their goals. They cannot, Summerhill style, just put out the materials and let the children loose. The curriculum is broken down into discrete objectives constantly reiterated. Gently, but firmly, the teachers, moment by moment, tamp down unacceptable behavior. They have developed a number of rather subtle techniques that keep the children quiet and calm, even when they grapple with tasks that are beyond them. These include: hiding children's poor performance by "cheating" on their behalf; taking over activities and turning the children into helpers; relying on the higher functioning children to carry the curriculum; disguising immature impulses by distorting the children's intentions; monitoring and controlling behavior through the fast-paced schedule; a high adult–child ratio; constant reinforcement; and few degrees of behavioral freedom. This chapter reviews the content and delivery of the common core curriculum as it rubs up against the nature of moderately retarded preschoolers. The chapter that follows looks at the methods teachers use to maintain the semblance of success. Both content and method fall well within the cultural transmission (behavioral) model.

At one level the enterprise works. Teachers are uniformly kind and good humored, and the days proceed smoothly. They radiate affection and pleasure at the children's accomplishments, however small. Teachers regularly stay after school to talk with, or visit, parents and, from their own small salaries, buy those extra supplies and gifts that school budgets do not provide. They acquire intimate knowledge of the children: their eating, toileting, and sleep habits; their bodies—who is sensitive to diaper rash and requires extra care, who has a scar from a fall or a sore that needs to be watched for infection; their medical and mental history and status. They know the families: the occupants, layout, and furnishings of their homes; hobbies and pets; relatives and friends; religion and values; points of tension and conflict. They understand the trust transferred to them when families open up these most private realms, and they act accordingly. They are much closer to their clients than most professionals but as careful as any in refusing to make judgments.

As we saw at Midwood, Teresa is devoted to the children and their parents, and they to her. She is well-organized, gets through her daily agenda with rather little distress, considering the ages and problems of her students. Children know what is expected and for the most part comply. They are rarely spoken to harshly and never physically mishandled. Family and supervisors are pleased.

But at another, more fundamental, level, early intervention is not working. Teachers are struggling valiantly to impose a body of knowledge and code of behavior but the "take" is slim. The distance between the positions of teachers and children is vast. This applies both to the curricular and behavioral expectations. The curriculum is too daunting and of too little interest for the children to succeed. The children often spend years on the same objectives with barely perceptible progress. Because the content is "academic," remote from experience, it must be forced upon children whose natural inclinations are out of step with most school demands.

The behavioral constraints upon children, while temporarily successful, are at odds with the child's natural habits, as we shall see by looking at children under conditions of instruction and conditions of freedom. Difficult as it is for teachers to maintain their steady emotional poise, it is all the harder for children whose just dawning impulses must be repressed. Teachers react to children's behavioral indiscretions by trying even harder, spiralling the controls upward, never lowering their expectations. That means more use of adult authority, more demands on children, less opportunity for uninhibited exploration and expression.

THE CURRICULUM

For parents whose understanding of young children is limited to recollecting their own childhood, caring for siblings, and babysitting, the introduction to early intervention must be strange and overwhelming. What Molly's parents perceive is a slow 4-year-old—late to walk and still likely to fall, late to talk and still limited in the amount and range of speech, too content to be alone, seemingly unaware of much that goes on around her, unable to play well or long with other kids. The professionals introduce them to a host of other concerns they had never considered. The strands of their little bundle are separated and closely inspected. Discussions are held on the child's fine-motor skills (Can she fold paper, cut in a line, draw a circle?); on her gross-motor skills (Can she walk backward, sideways, stand on one foot?); on her cognitive skills (Can she recognize a triangle, circle, and square, sort objects by category or distinguish few versus many?); on her receptive and expressive language skills (Does she use plurals, articles, compound sentences, can she respond to questions using where, why, and who?); on her personal–social skills (Does she know her sex, recognize herself in photographs, initiate greetings, experience difficulties with transitions, and monitor her own behavior?); and on her self-help skills (Does she undress completely or partially, with or without supervision, blow or just wipe her nose, dry or just wash her hands?).

Common Items on Developmental Inventories

Answers to such questions are determined by the develomental inventories administered as tests to children on, or before, entrance to an early intervention program. The items on all scales are sorted into domains and roughly sequenced by normal age of attainment. From the inventories, teachers determine the current level of a child and what the next attainment should be. The test results, or rather the failed items on the tests, form the core of the educational plan, though they may be supplemented by additional tasks on the basis of teacher observations or parent wishes.

Most of the centers visited rely on one or more of seven different inventories in evaluating and planning for the education of children ages 3 through 5 without special sensory or motor handicaps. The tests most frequently used were: Battelle Developmental Inventory (Newborg, Stock, & Wnek, 1984), Brigance Diagnostic Inventory of Early Development (Brigance, 1978), Early Intervention Developmental Profile (EIDP; Vol. 3 of Developmental Programming for Infants and Young Children; (Schafer & Moersch, 1981), Hawaii Early Learning Profile (HELP; Furuno et al., 1984; only through age 3), HICOMP Preschool Curriculum (Willoughby-Herb & Neisworth, 1983a), Learning Accomplishment Profile (LAP; Sanford & Zelman, 1981), and Portage Guide to Early Education (Bluma, Shearer, Frohman, & Hilliard, 1976). (The Carolina Curriculum for Handicapped Infants and Infants at Risk by Johnson-Martin, Jens, & Attermeier, 1986, was also widely used but not included in this review because until 1990 it did not go beyond age 2.) With the exception of the Battelle, activity guides accompany the diagnostic inventories. Not surprisingly, there is a great deal of overlap among the inventories. A colleague and early intervention teacher, Elizabeth Pollak, charted the overlap by listing every item on every inventory; the following analysis relies heavily upon her work.

In the cognitive area, the inventories stress children's ability to distinguish and/or match shapes (especially circle, triangle, and square), match or sort colors (except Battelle), comprehend quantity (one, two, few, many, first, last), name numerals, count by rote, recognize size differences (big and little), complete puzzles (including form boards), comprehend time distinctions (except HELP, which cuts off at age 3), sequence (by overall size, height, length, number, and pattern, except HELP), and recognize letters (except HELP and EIDP). All but three inventories also include the ability to recognize textural differences (rough–smooth, hard–soft), identify heavy, sort and match objects by conceptual categories (e.g., food), understand the value of money, and read several words.

Of all these, color recognition appears to be the overriding objective in the programs. It is a prime example of a task that crosses divisions of time, teaching modality, and child groupings. It is regularly an IEP goal and so covered in the one-to-one instruction time. A teacher is apt to ask children to identify a color when reading a story (and often selects stories about colors), when talking to them during circle time ("Will the children with red on stand up"), when the children are building, doing a puzzle, or at play. The primary colors with their labels attached decorate the walls and are the principal motif of many games and toys. Teresa had colors on her mind throughout the morning. Colored circles adorn her walls. She has colored the days of the calendar and asks the children to name them. She asks the children to name colors when selecting items from the grab bag, during art, and at IEP time.

In the language area, all the inventories stress extending vocabulary and sentence length (from two to three words), using plurals (except HICOMP), using pronouns (except EIDP), identifying body parts (except Battelle), identifying objects by functional use (e.g., "Show me what we cook on," except Battelle and HICOMP), answering "wh-" questions (what, why, where, who, and when, except Brigance and HELP), following directions (one, two, or three steps) and understanding or using prepositions (except EIDP).

In the fine-motor area, all inventories include: strings beads, folds paper, uses a scissors, holds a writing implement (except Battelle), imitates a horizontal or vertical line, draws (circle, square, or triangle), recognizes letters (except HELP and EIDP), builds a tower or bridge with blocks (except Battelle), inserts or pounds pegs into a board (except Battelle), and independently uses Play-Doh or clay (except Battelle and EIDP).

In the gross-motor domain, the common items are: walks on

tiptoes (except Battelle), walks a straight line (except Portage and EDIP), alternates feet in climbing upstairs or downstairs, walks downstairs using a handrail (except Battelle and LAP), walks a balance beam (except Battelle and LAP), skips (except HELP), runs (except Battelle and LAP), jumps, hops, stands on one leg, throws or catches a ball, kicks a ball (except Battelle), climbs (except Battelle), and pedals a trike (except Battelle).

In self-help, the items of agreement are: uses a cup (except Battelle), spoon, or fork, pours liquid (except Battelle and HICOMP), puts on socks or shoes (except Battelle), dresses independently, buttons or unbuttons, zips or unzips (except Battelle and Portage), washes or dries hands, brushes teeth (except Battelle), uses toilet, and demonstrates caution (except LAP and EIDP).

There is much less overlap among the inventories in the personal–social domain. The most common items measure whether the child engages in dramatic play (except Brigance), plays cooperatively (except Brigance), acknowledges feelings (such as happy, sad, mad, except HELP and Brigance), offers independently to take turns (except HELP and Brigance), and knows first and/or last name. And on all but three: uses pronouns to refer to self (HICOMP and EDIP).

From my observations, those items that crop up on most of the inventories are a good approximation of the core curriculum shared by most early intervention centers. That is, regardless of how programs may otherwise differ, they all instruct children in material close to these core items. For example, although not every program works regularly on big and little (though most seem to), they all teach a variety of antonyms (e.g., heavy–light, hot–cold, happy–sad). More broadly, at least in the language and cognitive domains, the common core curriculum is saturated with discrete bits of knowledge, often quite abstract and remote. Teachers call it "preacademic," a preparation for the "academic" instruction of elementary school.[2]

To verify the impression that the items common to the several inventories are core to instruction, Ms. Pollak reviewed the cognitive objectives for 174 children from 20 programs. Specifically, she tallied how many children had as an objective on their IEP at least one of the five most frequently reappearing items from the inventories for this developmental age range: colors, numbers (1– 10), shapes, three-piece puzzles (usually form boards), and big– little. In this collection of IEPs, 75% listed at least one of the five items. The core items are assigned regardless of mental level. We

were able to estimate that 22 children in the group were functioning at the mildly retarded range (i.e., at approximately two thirds
of their chronological age with developmental levels from 2 to 3½).
Of these, 18 (82%) had one of the five core items on their IEPs.
Another 46 children fell in the moderately retarded range (i.e., at
approximately half their age, with developmental levels of 18
months to 2½ years). Of these, 39 (85%) had one of the five core
items on their IEPs. Finally, 22 children were severely retarded
(i.e., functioning at approximately one third or less of their age,
with developmental levels below 18 months). Of these 22 children, at
the level of a toddler or below, 20 (91%) had one of the five core
items on their IEPs! (We were unable to estimate mental level on
the remaining 84 children because of inadequate information on
functional levels.)

The core content described above is not, of course, the exclusive content in the programs' curricula. Teachers introduce other
material, and there are times during the day when the teaching
agenda is suspended in favor of play, gross-motor activities, and
self-help skills. They also have overriding themes—among them
farm animals, pets, zoo animals, seasons, holidays, community
helpers, safety, food, family, houses, myself, to name just a few—
with field trips, art projects, stories, and games arranged around
the themes. Nonetheless, these items are hallmarks of the programs, the most universally repeated content, and one can predictably count on seeing some of them emerge at every center
every day.

Teaching the Core Curriculum

Instruction in the core curriculum is most commonly done
during circle and "work" time. But it also seeps into art, snack
time, and even free play.

Circle time, which may last anywhere from 10 to 30 minutes
and occurs at least once daily, is remarkably uniform across settings.

> It starts with a song welcoming each child individually by *name*.
> (Items italicized in this description frequently appear on IEPs
> and are seen by teachers as important teaching objectives. They
> are by no means exhaustive but give the flavor of what teachers
> are trying to accomplish.) Sometimes children are asked to ac-
> knowledge their own presence when their name is mentioned, or
> to greet each other in song by name; always they are encouraged

to join the teachers in the song. The song often becomes a roll call. Children select their name cards or photographs from a given location and mount them on the wall. Those absent are noted. (As an aside, it is remarkable, and very satisfying to parents and teachers, that after sufficient daily repetition, even quite retarded 3- to 5-year-olds come to recognize their printed name and often the names of their classmates.) This exercise is supplemented in many instances by asking children for their address, age, and sex.

Then come the calendar and weather. Children are asked to recite the days of the week and *count* up to today's date. Counting is important. Teachers may try to enhance children's interest by having them count *fast* then *slow*, *loudly* then *quietly*, stress alternate numbers, clap while they count, insert the next number when the teacher stops suddenly (e.g., 4, 5, 6, pause). Often the teacher will ask about the day, date or weather from *yesterday*, the date for *tomorrow*

After the greeting, calendar and weather, there is usually a group activity emphasizing *vocabulary*. The teacher may read a story, illustrate a story by placing forms on a felt board, show glossy pictures (often of animals or familiar objects), recount a past or future event, review *dressing* and *body parts* with a doll or the children themselves, bring out a toy or game. In this context, she will ask the children to identify *objects, colors, shapes, size differences*. When they give single-word responses, she will often expand the single word into a two- or three-word sentence and have them repeat it (e.g., Teacher: "Does the horse run *slow* or *fast*?" Child: "Fast." Teacher: "The horse runs fast." And at Midwood, Teresa: "Who is here today?" Larry: "Stephen." Teresa: "Stephen is here today." Larry: "Stephen is here today.").

Songs are traditionally included during circle time. Again and again one hears the same familiar ones repeated across programs (the all-time favorite being "The Wheels on the Bus"). Many of them involve doing actions with different *body parts* (e.g., "Put Your Hands Up in the Air," "Shake Something," "Action Song," "Hokey Pokey," "If You're Happy and You Know It," "Turn Around," often recorded by Hap Palmer and published by Educational Activities, Inc., Freeport, NY).

"Work" time (sometimes called activity or IEP time) is devoted entirely to the sort of items we find on the developmental inventories.

All classrooms have racks of *form boards* and *puzzles* of great variety; multiple assortments of *beads* for stringing, snapping, *matching by color and shape;* a variety of *pegboards, form sorter boxes (round hole for the round form) for shape discrimination;*

lotto games for *matching by object, form, number, letter, color;* blocks in a range of sizes and materials for *stacking*, building, *copying designs* (parquetry), *color sorting and matching.* Many programs have computers with programs largely devoted to *number, colors, letters, sequencing,* and *opposites (fast–slow, big–little, hard–soft, same–different, many–few),* and *prepositions (such as under–over, in–out, front–back).*

Art period is another essential component of early intervention programs usually occurring at least once daily. Because art is a flexible medium and relies on individual imagination, it suits the core curriculum less well than the circle and work periods. That is, the materials of circle and work time tend to restrict a child's options more than the materials of art. If you give a child a three-piece puzzle requiring placement of a circle, square, and triangle, there is not much he can do other than insert the forms.

Teachers use lots of different materials with the children during art (string, cotton balls, sand, rice, starch, shaving cream, Jello, macaroni, paints, brushes, finger paints, crayons, markers, Play-Doh) and sometimes permit them to explore materials without instruction. However, even with free-form material, one regularly sees teachers seizing the opportunity to push the core curriculum. When using finger paint or Play-Doh, for instance, a child will be asked to make a *line, square, or circle.* When stringing pasta shells he will be told to alternate *big and little* shells. When a child is painting or drawing, teachers generally inquire about *colors.* During art time at Midwood Alice, the teacher aide, asks the children for the *shapes, colors, and numbers* of plates and food. Not infrequently the project itself will be to draw particular shapes with particular colors. A prominent IEP objective in early intervention programs is training children in the use of *scissors.* Teachers have on hand a variety of scissors for left- and right-handers, for less and more advanced cutters, and a variety of paper that cuts more and less easily. Cutting ability is subdivided into refined stages: grasping the scissors, slicing, snipping, cuts a straight line, cuts a curved line. To assist beginning cutters, they have developed a range of techniques to stabilize a child's hand or paper. The detailed instruction in scissor use, as contrasted, for instance, with lack of attention to training children in molding clay or constructing block structures, exemplifies how specific items prominent in the inventories become prominent in the curriculum.

The teachers' desire for "nice" productions further inhibits the free use of art materials. Because an art project exemplifies a concerted teacher–child effort and has a life after completion (it goes home or is pinned to the wall), teachers care that the result looks good. As I studied the bright, lively murals that decorate the walls of most programs and the clever projects developed for children, I often thought that art skill must be an entry-level requirement for teachers. But the price of high artistic standards is that frequently teachers dominate the productions with children serving as their assistants. Teachers conceptualize the projects and assemble the necessary components. For example, a teacher will draw and cut out forms, parts to a snowman, monkeys, or trees. The child's task is limited to coloring and pasting. A teacher will plan how to make a lion's face or flower from paper plates and have the child pull yarn through punched holes or glue on cotton balls. Teresa's project to construct Thanksgiving tables had children participate in coloring and/or pasting precut foods. Despite the greater diversity of the art projects than of the work time products, the teacher's role is similar. She may be teaching pasting rather than counting, but she is still trying to get the child to make the correct predetermined right moves (paralleling her effort to get them to give the right answers).

Eating time—usually a snack of juice, crackers, or cereal, but sometimes full meals—is another universal in early intervention. There are teachers who relax instruction slightly during this period, allowing children to concentrate on their food and one another. But eating time is not usually a relaxed or permissive period.

Left to their own devices the children have little to say and likely as not would touch one another or leave the table. Rather than support silence, touching, or leaving, teachers have opted to use snack time for the development of self-help, cognitive, and language skills. Before snack begins, children usually *put away* toys and clean play tables, use the *toilet, wash and dry hands and face;* during snack they *pour,* use a *cup and utensils, spread soft foods.* After snack they again *clean-up* (throw away paper goods, sponge the table), sometimes *brush teeth.* It is also a time for language expansion and instruction in manners (Teresa: "Tell me what you want." Molly: "More." Teresa: "More apple juice or more cranberry juice?" Molly: "More juice." Teresa: "More apple juice, please."). When passing the juice and crackers, teachers characteristically give children alternative choices (Teresa and Anita ask whether the children want apple or cranberry juice, monkey or bear cracker). This popular practice pushes the child to make decisions—for no response means no food—by speaking, signing or pointing. Often the interaction around choice can be extended into a mini-session on *color, quantity, and number* (e.g., "What color juice do you want?" "Do you want more?" "Do you want half a glass?" "Do you want two crackers?"). Snack time is also an opportunity for teachers to work on fine-motor skills and socialization. Children are encouraged to *chew,* use a *straw.* They are urged to wait as the teacher passes the pitcher of juice, *ask for help, take turns* in setting and clearing the table, or pouring, and to *share* the extra food.

The other universal period is play time, which may or may not be distinguishable from work time. Play receives different treatment across early intervention centers and there is a corresponding range of teacher behavior from supervision, to support, to amplification, to direction. Sometimes play is just a traditional recess; children are turned loose to follow their own pursuits, and teachers intervene only to keep them safe. This degree of freedom is generally confined to outdoors. When indoors, with space and materials more restricted and teachers more conscious of who is doing what to whom, there is likely to be more guidance of play (alternatively called "choice," "option," or "center" time). Again, there is a range of teacher involvement. Some teachers take the lead from children during these periods and restrict their own role to facilitation. They move in only if children request help or are in danger; they do not try to shape play. For example, in one classroom I visited during play time, two children wanted to be individually twirled in a Sit-and-Spin. The teacher, with remarkable forbearance, followed their requests for a total of 17 turns, at which point they finally were ready to spin each other! Moving along the continuum, teachers may join children more actively by reflecting verbally on what they are doing.

> For example, a teacher comments to a child named Rachel who is trying to stuff a block in a doll's mouth and then drops both doll and block: "Oh, Rachel, you're feeding the doll. Uh-oh, you dropped the baby." More often a teacher will amplify this sort of incident by taking on a character role: "Oh, Rachel, you're feeding the doll. She likes being fed." The teacher makes slurping eating sounds and then adds: "Uh-oh, you dropped the baby. Ouch! That hurt baby. Wah-wah." Or they may ask questions: "Is the baby hungry?" "Are you the mother?" "What are you feeding baby?"

In these interventions the teacher is supporting the child's actions—although probably reading into the child's acts a false intention to feed the doll—not instructing the child in a specific curriculum objective (except insofar as she has set up the play materials). However, it is only a slim step from amplification to direction. I found that only a few teachers choose to (or are able to) limit themselves to amplification. Most of the children, after all, don't play well. They have few ideas, do the same thing over and over again, lose interest quickly, use materials inappropriately, look bad in their play (because they often have infantile habits of mouthing, smelling, and fingering objects).

> Teresa, noting how bad Austin appeared making saliva marks on the window, directs him to play with a helicopter. When he spins a coke bottle, the aide, Alice, tries to introduce a more social element by requesting food, and in the process alludes to *yellow* and *green*. The aide, Anita, tries to enlarge upon David and Doreen's household play and in the process brings in *big and small*. So it is natural that the teacher with Rachel does not limit herself to reflection and questions but makes suggestions: "Why don't you give baby a bottle, Rachel?" "Oh, the baby was hurt, Rachel, you need to hold her." And when Rachel does not respond, the teacher becomes more assertive: "Rachel, please feed me some lunch. I'm hungry. I'd like *two* eggs on the *red* plate." In this instance we are at least partially back to the core curriculum *(colors, numbers, and following a two-step command)*.

It may be the teacher's intention to use play time as an occasion for reintroducing, and thereby reinforcing, the core curriculum; or it may be that instruction during play is unintentional. The curricular items are, after all, the substance of the teaching, and so they reappear naturally when a teacher wants to activate play in a child who is unproductive or on the verge of quitting.

Moving still further on the continuum of direction, teachers may assign play activities, asking a child, for example, to join in a memory card game, a color lotto game, building a house or a zoo. Gross-motor activities such as Teresa's obstacle course, sometimes conceived of as play, are also highly directed. Teresa makes a conscious effort to teach the children skills such as walking a line, jumping, and following instructions. At this point play and work time merge.[3] Poorly self-directed children are particularly likely to elicit coercion from teachers, as in the following example of doll and housekeeping play during which Marta's teacher, Susan, was determined to keep the child focused.

> Susan sits on the ledge of a small table watching and directing Marta as she moves into the housekeeping corner. When Marta goes to the cabinet, Susan directs: "Marta, let's get the milk and

feed the baby." Marta starts opening the doors of a freezer. "No, not the freezer, right here." Susan points to the refrigerator as Marta goes for the stove. "No, down here. The refrigerator, not the stove. Get it out, get milk, pour it in the cup. Did you give the baby some? Pour the rest back so you don't spill any on the floor, and then put it away." Each of these commands anticipates a move; that is, when Marta gets out the milk (actually an empty imitation carton), she is told to pour it. When she pours it, she is asked, did she give it to the baby? When Marta shows no interest in returning the milk, Susan directs her again to feeding: "Where's baby's cup?" Susan then actually gets it and gives it to Marta. "Put the milk in the cup, Marta. Good girl. Now put it back in the refrigerator." Marta starts to put the cup in the refrigerator. "No, not the *cup*, the *milk*." Again Marta isn't following commands to put the milk back, so Susan again returns to feeding. "Milk, baby wants her milk." Susan holds Marta's hand, and together they feed the baby. "That's the girl. Good. Baby wants her milk. OK, now we have to get the eggs . . ."

We see here the tense struggle between Susan's determination to have Marta perform an appropriate social act and Marta's preference for movement and manipulation, without regard to socially meaningful sequences. Judging from Marta's independent play, if left alone, she probably would have opened and closed doors, and stuffed all the objects she could reach into the cabinets, stove, and refrigerator, at random. The teacher has in mind a series of acts beginning with feeding a baby milk and moving on to other food. Each time Marta pulls away, Susan pulls her back to the doll and milk. In the next scene with eggs, the same struggle is repeated. Susan stops Marta when she abandons the baby in favor of pushing a pot and utensils over the counter surfaces; through a combination of admonitions, demonstrations, and actual hand-over-hand actions, Susan keeps Marta feeding the doll.

The meeting of teacher and child during relatively unstructured periods is a delicate and difficult business, much harder than handling the preplanned circle, work time, art, and snack. Even with normal children, adults need to tread gently and sensitively when they attempt to encourage but not coerce (and thereby risk stifling) play development. It is vastly more difficult with handicapped children whose behavioral patterns are primitive and whose justification for being at school is to catch up with normal peers. Their passivity creates a vacuum for teacher action. Their silence impels teachers to talk; their inappropriate use of materials, to model correct usage; their marginal attention, to keep up a stream of directions; their repetition, to suggest changes; their slowness, to present higher order ("more productive") actions. The result, in play as in the directed work periods, is that the children are pressed into doing what is too hard and goes against their natural interests.

Evidence that life is too difficult for the moderately retarded in early intervention centers comes from at least three sources: first, the contrast between what children do spontaneously (most obvious in play) and what teachers are requesting of them; second, the poor responses of children to teacher direction in formal work time; and third, the discrepancies between the children's mental age and the expected age for learning the material. A discussion of each follows.

THE DISTANCE BETWEEN TEACHERS AND CHILDREN

The Position of Children

The children I targeted for observation were 3- to 5-year-olds functioning at approximately the 18 month to 2½-year level. That means, using Piaget as a guide, they were in the sensorimotor and very early preoperational developmental stage. What occupies such children? Mostly moving themselves and moving things, learning about the nature of objects and their relationship to objects by operating upon them, the beginning of "make believe" expressed through the condensed replay of familiar scenes.

A look at the spontaneous behavior of Doreen, Molly, and Heather, three moderately retarded children from Midwood, gives a more concrete sense of what typifies retarded children in this age range. When left alone, the children's activities are quite simple and repetitive, reducible to just a few themes. A major interest is their bodies.

> The children touch themselves and each other; put on and off hats, ties, necklaces, dresses, jackets, etc. Doreen moves a hat about her head and is fascinated by the changes it produces in her appearance; she attempts to cover herself with a blanket; she, along with Molly and David, touch one another's hair and arms during circle; she and Molly enjoy each other's hands under the water spigot. Molly takes off a sneaker and sock; plays with her skirt and David's belt; enjoys the feel of paste on her hands and fingers. After snack Doreen returns to a mirror, lifts up her shirt and inspects her stomach, and greets herself from various positions; later she covers her arm with Play-Doh.

The children are interested in the relationship of objects to each other—experiences of in–out, on–off.

> Doreen puts an adult hat over a baby doll, pulls a diaper out of a bag; Heather dumps a container of blocks, puts blocks in and out of a sand pail; Molly fills a wagon with blocks from a shelf and—in what must rate as one of the most enjoyable in–out activities—rearranges the contents of children's backpacks. During work time Molly prefers dropping the plastic monkeys into the bin to sorting them onto plates by color. Doreen picks up her pegs and drops them into the monkey bin.

Collecting and depositing, throwing and retrieving are often attached to in–out actions.

> Hurling objects is one of Heather's favorite actions—blocks, sand, plastic foods. After snack time, Heather throws and retrieves beanbags, Doreen retrieves and deposits one in a baby carriage. Molly collects forks, spoons and cups, dumps them into the carriage, and starts to push it. She is interrupted by Heather who, having stuffed assorted objects into the oven, decides to go "shopping" with the carriage. She removes plastic foods from a shelf and redistributes them in her purse, in the carriage, and on chairs.

Moving and climbing are popular activities—the physical enactments of in–out, up–down, under–over.

> Doreen tries to snuggle under a blanket, puts herself *on* the table, rather than a dress *under* (as commanded), wants to repeat climbing up and down the steps by the water fountain. Molly lies down inside the jungle gym, slips under tables, crawls into cubbies, and even into the oven. Heather climbs onto a window ledge, dives under the "water" to swim, moves out of turn to mount the climbing structure, and plunges into the tunnel.

The natural activities of these children can be described as circular rather than linear. In–out, on–off, open–close, and up–down are repetitive rather than sequential. They go nowhere, have no start or completion. Piaget (1952) explains how children, during the first 2 years of life (sensorimotor stage) delight in the endless repetition of an act—batting a mobile, opening and closing a drawer. Through such acts they learn the nature and function of the physical world and how they can be causal agents in the world. This is the essence of early mastery. But to an observer, the behavior appears idle, and unproductive, particularly when the child is 3 or 4 years old. The immaturity tolerated in an 18-month-old looks inappropriate in a bigger body.

The Position of Teachers

Teachers, whose goal is higher-level attainments, have cause for displeasure in children's spontaneous behavior. Heather gets into trouble for almost everything she does. Before our morning visit Teresa had removed a playpen filled with colored balls because Heather threw the balls about the room, and a sandbox was at least temporarily off limits. She gets into trouble for dumping blocks, then for putting the blocks into the wrong container, for diving under the "water" and being a fish (or swimmer?) instead of a fisherwoman. She is admonished for not waiting her turn during juice and gross-motor time.

School demands are opposed to the spontaneous acts of even less rambunctious children. The children are expected to keep hands on lap and are interrupted when they have hands on each other (e.g., circle time at Midwood).

> Molly is brought back to circle when she darts away and is not permitted to nest in cubbies. Doreen's efforts to sponge the table are twice quashed, first, so snack can proceed, and second, so she can have a turn on the obstacle course. Hand washing that becomes water play between Doreen and Molly is interrupted so that snack can proceed.

Teachers also try to improve, make more complex, even the quiet play activities of children.

> Anita wants Doreen to shift from preening in the mirror to feeding a doll. Teresa takes the jar of paste away from Molly, who is gouging it with a crayon and rubbing it on her fingers, so that she will attend to the task—mounting paper food onto a paper table. Anita redirects Molly and Doreen, who are dropping monkeys and pegs into a container, to their work objectives—sorting monkeys by color and inserting pegs into a board.

In theory, Teresa could relax her vigilance and permit Doreen an extended wipe-up time; she could "not notice" Molly's dumping and filling of backpacks. She could even make washing, wiping, and transferring material pedagogical objectives for the children, thereby narrowing the distance between herself and them. In actuality, Teresa would view consenting to, rather than curtailing, these behaviors as retrogressive and not in the children's best interests. She believes "higher" behaviors—looking, listening, and talking—must replace "lower" behaviors—messing in water, moving objects, moving their own bodies—if the children are to progress through the curriculum. Leaving children free to do their own thing would be an abdication of her professional responsibilities, unacceptable to families and to her own work ethic.

Teachers cannot simultaneously be permissive toward the instincts and impulses of Doreens, Heathers, and Mollys, and still serve the curriculum. The children, at the developmental level of a toddler, cannot be counted on, as it were, incidentally, to "pick up" colors, comparisons, and shapes within a few months or even years. Teachers must instill the knowledge, and the installation is conditional upon "mature" behaviors: children must stay on task and keep reasonably quiet, listen and watch rather than move about, follow the routines and schedules. The core curriculum cannot be divorced from its required set of preparatory behaviors any more than an athletic sport, military battle, or classical dance can be separated from its particular personal discipline. As long as Molly plays with her feet she is not learning colors and shapes—or anything else that is respected by the curriculum. Whenever children become disruptive, teachers try to restrain them either physically (e.g., at Midwood, holding Heather during circle) or verbally (e.g., at Midwood: "It is time to listen now." "Molly wants you to help her sit."). The more resistant the child, the more controlling the teacher must become. But increased talk and authority only add to the discomfort of children; teachers then crank up interventions another notch. And so the cycle goes: the restive child receives more restraint, and that restraint may increase the restiveness. In the end the teacher always wins but pays the price of constantly bearing down on the child. Yet teachers, if they are to respect the core curriculum, have no choice but to repress (or sometimes redirect) children's natural impulses.

PROBLEM OF THE "TAKE"

The "Take" in Play

Because of the distance between teachers and children, most teacher interventions, even in children's play, are unsuccessful;

there is no "take." Even when teachers mean only to expand existing play, they almost always lose the child who cannot meet the
increased demands. There is too big a leap between what the child
is doing and what the teachers want. Adults, in their eagerness to
normalize and improve children, misread their play purposes—
usually granting to the child more than was intended. They depart
too radically from what the child has initiated and, when the child
fails to respond, accelerate their input rather than returning to the
point of departure. Consequently, most of the play suggestions at
Midwood fell on uncomprehending ears.

> During free play David, with a baby in his arms and dressed in a
> man's jacket, necktie, and fireman's hat, announces he is going to
> "work." Anita suggests that he take lunch; he rejects the sugges-
> tion, saying he is taking the baby. Anita then urges him to take
> the lunch, too, and drop the baby off at a day-care center. David
> leaves and returns, with baby and no lunch, so that both Anita's
> suggestions are rejected. Anita's effort to have Doreen care for her
> baby rather than preen in the mirror is also rejected. Austin, the
> autistic child, is willing to substitute helicopter twirling for sali-
> va painting but the change is merely cosmetic. Austin did not
> comply with Alice's request for food.

Anita has overinterpreted the degree to which David and Doreen are engaging in symbolic play. What David means by "going
to work" is dressing up and going out with no particular destination in mind, as witness his speedy return. Because he is enacting a
departure–return scene with Doreen, not thinking of another mode
of existence in another place, he sees no need to dispense with the
baby or take along a lunch. Even though David is in many respects
advanced for a child with Down syndrome, he is capable only of
reliving a regularly witnessed scene; he cannot project beyond
what he has observed. Anita, who every morning dresses up, makes
household arrangements for the day, and then departs for work,
has assumed that David, too, is capable of considering the future
(lunch and childcare) in the present.

For Doreen, at a slightly lower level than David, undergoing a
clothing change is not tantamount to undergoing a role change. As
we've seen, she is interested in the physical relationships of objects
to each other and to herself. When she puts on a hat and preens,
she is not pretending to be a mother and, therefore, cannot shift
naturally to feeding the doll. Anita's further suggestion to cover
the doll with a blanket is more responsive to Doreen's psychological state and her preceding move—she has just taken the hat from

her own head and covered the doll with it. But even this is too advanced for Doreen, who prefers to cover herself. Her body, not the doll's, is of primary interest.

Teresa, in recommending that Austin fly a helicopter, over-estimates his ability to symbolize. She may perceive him to be "flying" the helicopter, but he is simply attached to the twirling motion. Repetitive twirling, like repetitive movement from win-dow to beanbag chair, or repetitive grazing of the hands, are typical means that autistic children have for sensory gratification. Austin does not sufficiently understand the workings of the world to put a helicopter through its paces. Similarly, when he rotates a Coke bottle and chants "It's the real thing," he is not pretending to drink or even enacting a commercial. Typical of autistic children, he is combining an object with a rote phrase, the meaning of which he doesn't understand. Alice's later effort to engage him in feeding her is entirely discordant with his psychological state. Because he understands Alice wants something, he produces a pot, but this, like the helicopter flying, is not an interaction likely to be repeated without more instruction, for Austin's engagement is in twirling something, not sharing a meal with Alice.

Teachers often try to extend children's play by developing appropriate sequences. The children, however, are not so much making errors in sequences as stringing together isolated single-step acts.

> David is using Play-Doh in conjunction with an oven and doll. He puts the entire hunk of dough into the oven, counts, opens the oven, returns the cooked dough to the table and begins pounding, then back to the oven, with the dough, back to the table, back to the oven, this time with the addition of a doll who also gets cooked. When the doll refuses his invitation to eat, she, tray and dough go back into the oven for another cooking. Anita comes over to help David make cookies for the baby.

David does not combine a series of acts guided by the overall goal of feeding cookies to a doll. His series of actions are unrelated to each other, there is no plan. He construes the Play-Doh in relationship to the oven or banging or feeding; the doll in relation-ship to the oven or feeding. His play, while somewhat more sym-bolic than the girls', is still limited to a back-and-forth, two-step sequence, dominated by his trips to and from the oven. The plea-sure and interest in this play probably come from the in–out movements—the doll goes in and out of the oven, food gets cooked and recooked, shaped and reshaped—not from the rendition of a pretend cookie preparation routine. Anita might, if she wishes, get David to plan ahead a bit more, perhaps have the doll wait while he cooks, or put only molded Play-Doh into the oven. But she is unlikely to get him to think through the series of steps—molding the Play-Doh, putting it on a cooking tray, taking it to the oven, setting a timer, cooking, preparing the doll, feeding the doll— necessary to carry out a proper cooking–feeding scene. Before assuming he wants to prepare cookies for the baby, it would be a good idea to find out what his intentions are.

Not infrequently a teacher will be tuned in to a child's mental state, but becomes restless when the child keeps doing a simple act over and over again, finding the repetition tedious and a waste of time for the child. As we see in the following vignettes, under conditions of repetitive play teachers are likely to intervene with suggestions for higher level play, often resorting to the familiar mandates of the curriculum. The child loses interest, and either the play episode ends, or it becomes teacher's play.

Melanie is a 3½-year-old child with Down syndrome. When alone she plays *open–close* — doors in the room, toilet covers, doors to a Fisher-Price barn. And she plays *in–out* — inserts a small doll into a long tube and tilts it so that the doll comes out the other end, laughs and repeats, picks up a plastic cow and puts it on a chair, climbs in and out of the chair herself repeatedly. And she plays *up–down* — pushes the cow off the chair, replaces it, and pushes it down again. The teacher, Margaret, sits down, and Melanie approaches her with the cow (it is not clear what Mela- nie has in mind). Margaret, not wanting a cow in her face, com- ments, "Nice cow. I'll give it a kiss. Now you give it a kiss." Instead, Melanie follows what was apparently her original inten- tion and puts the cow on the teacher's head (part of her up–down, object relationship interests). The teacher accommodates. She tilts her head so that the cow falls to the floor. Melanie is de- lighted and says, "More." Margaret asks: "You want it to fall down?" Melanie nods and Margaret obliges. Melanie again gig- gles with pleasure and says, "More." Margaret responds, "Last time," and, despite Melanie's importuning, "More, more," shifts gear by asking: "Where does the cow live?" No response. "In a house or in a barn?" No response. Then both teacher and child separate.

Pedro is 5 years old with a mental age of 2. Outdoors he reveals his true collecting–depositing interests. Oblivious to others, he wanders over to a set of pine trees and begins to pick up cones. He brings a few over to a bench, deposits them, goes off for more, dumps and scavenges again. This time, rather than dumping the cones onto the bench, he inserts each one into the spaces made by the slats of the bench. Having lined up four, he is about to set off again when he notices the puddle of cones from his prior forays. He begins to pick them up and stick them one at a time between the slats, making two rows of pine cones. Teacher Pat, who has had her eye on him all the time, comes over, stopping on the way to pick up some cones. She hands Pedro a cone. He smiles and starts a new row with it. She continues handing over cones, and he continues creating rows. Pedro is obviously more engaged by this activity than Pat, who asks him: "Which one is longer, Pedro?" No response. "Let's count and find out." She begins by counting and pointing. Pedro joins her up to number 5, which is as far as he can go. Pat then suggests they arrange the cones in a circle. Pedro starts to leave for another cone foray but is called back to help the teacher. He is now asked to hand the cones to the teacher while she makes a circle and then other formations.

Pat, sensitive to Pedro's disinterest, suggests that he might like to "drive" a push car (feet move on the ground rather than on pedals). Pedro does so briefly, then stops to watch a group of children playing. Pat tries to reengage him by coming to the front of the car. She opens her arms and says: "Stop, I'm a cop. Let me see your driver's license." When he doesn't produce one, she says he is under arrest. Then she pretends to find the license and waves him on, telling him to be sure to stop at the red lights. He looks confused, but "drives" the car a bit further. She reappears in front of him again and, with arms extended, tells him: "Stop. Red light," at which point she is summoned to another child.

Both Margaret and Pat sensitively "tune in" to what the child is doing — up–down, collecting–depositing–lining up. But they quickly grow restless with behavior that seems to be simplistic and going nowhere. They do not so much expand on existing play, as shift it. A horizontal expansion of Melanie's up–down play would be to drop the cow from the arms and legs of both teacher and child, drop the cow off other surfaces beyond one's body, drop different objects, drop several objects at a time and then find them all, do other kinds of up–down movements; a vertical expansion might be to go from up–down to acting out related concepts achieved at roughly the same developmental period such as give–return, in–out, and open–close. When Melanie approaches Margaret with a cow, Margaret suggests giving it a kiss; a little later she asks where the cow lives (or she might have asked, as is commonly done, what sound the cow makes). In each instance she treats the cow as an object with complex characteristics—capable of receiving affection, residing in particular places, making unique sounds. But for Melanie the object is something that she can drop—*cowness*, if recognized, is not of interest. When Margaret begins to talk about kissing cows and barns, she is not on Melanie's wavelength.

Pat knows what Pedro is doing, no question here of symbolic play. She loses Pedro not through any misinterpretation but by moving too far from his interests. Had Pat stayed with Pedro's activity she might have extended the play by joining him in collecting other objects, using a pail in conjunction with the objects (in–out), stacking the objects (up–down). If, in gathering, sorting, or sequencing various objects, he showed even an inkling of pattern, she could elaborate upon it. But, as so often happens when an industrious teacher observes what she perceives to be static behavior, Pat reaches for the core curriculum (comparison of length, counting, shapes), and Pedro rejects it. Pat sees she has floundered in her effort to have Pedro sort cones by shape, but rather than going back to Pedro's lining-up play and simplifying her intervention, she keeps increasing the demands—from making shapes, to driving a car, to acting out a highly *symbolic* traffic scene. It has become her game, not his.

We all make mistakes all the time in "reading" children's behavior. When Melanie picks up a cow, we take for granted she is pretending it is a cow and wants to play cow, just as when Doreen puts on a hat it is natural to think she is pretending to be a mother. But misinterpretations can be corrected by careful observation of a child's play and her response to adult suggestions. The repetitive nature of Melanie's raising–dropping actions strongly suggests that she could be using any object—a piece of chalk or pine cones would do as well; her failure to respond to the kiss-the-cow suggestion, or where-does-the-cow-live inquiry, confirms this. Pedro rejects the idea of making shapes with the cones. No response usually means one took a wrong turn; the solution is to go back and try an elaboration closer to the observed behavior. Even when a child complies with an intervention, as Pedro did briefly in driving the car, there may not have been a good "take." A suggestion that "takes" and is permanently incorporated into a child's behavioral repertoire, rather than existing as a moment of rote compliance, will reappear on another day and in another context.

Following are more examples of typical incidents that illustrate the distance between teachers and children:

A child in a sandbox is filling a shovel with sand and watching it spill out. The teacher suggests building a roadway for cars. The teacher leaves and the child returns to former play. *Analysis:* The leap from pouring sand to constructing a roadway is too big, as the child indicates by returning, when permitted, to his prior activity. Better to model or suggest pouring sand through one's fingers, pouring sand into a bucket, using a funnel—if indeed any change is required.

A child is removing animals and blocks from a shelf. The teacher suggests building a zoo with the blocks and animals. The child, interested in removing and lining up, cannot participate in the zoo construction. The teacher picks up an animal, pokes it in the child's stomach, and says: "Monkey is going to get you." The child giggles. The teacher then tries to retain the child's attention by constructing cages with the blocks and putting an animal in each. *Analysis:* Teachers often try to reengage a child who is not joining in play by becoming more physical, dramatic, and interactive. The problem is that the teacher has diverted the child from what was purposeful, if limited, activity and placed her in a passive position, a receiver of entertainment.

A child spontaneously moves a car back and forth without releasing it from his hands. The teacher, having successfully gotten the child to roll cars to her, asks: "Will you send me the big car or the little one?" No response. "The small car or the police car?" *Analysis:* By staying with the child's interest and his back-and-forth movements, the teacher has helped this child transform a simple self-contained act into a social game. The new achievement needs to be practiced and enjoyed. Bringing in abstract, remote irrelevancies (big–little) is more discouraging than reinforcing.

A child randomly throws and retrieves a beanbag. The teacher puts out (as a target) an upright clown face with holes for the eyes, nose and mouth. She asks the child to throw the beanbags at the face. The child continues, throwing randomly around the room. The teacher then says: "First, we'll throw the beanbag in the green eyes; next, in the red mouth. We'll take turns. I'll start." *Analysis:* The child is throwing and retrieving, not throwing to an object. Getting her to throw at the clown's face is already a large expansion; when that fails the teacher should retreat, not further expand her demand to throw by facial feature and color.

A child makes a pot whistle by pushing down on the lever. He repeats and repeats the action. A teacher comments: "Oh, you're making coffee. Just what I wanted," and instructs him to get the cups and saucers. He continues making the pot whistle, and she becomes more insistent, finally bringing the equipment to the table and, her hand over his, pours. *Analysis:* The child is riveted on his ability to create a noise; the attachment of whistle to pot is entirely incidental. The teacher misinterprets the act as a symbolic enactment. His refusal to "cook" prompts her to take over the activity so that the play can be successfully concluded.

The "Take" at Work

The distance between teachers and children is even more striking during the bulk of the day dedicated to accomplishing particular goals—circle, art, work time. During these periods the teacher is "instructing," not "joining," the child's self-selected activity; she has less room to adjust her agenda to the child's receptivity. Evidence that the curriculum is too hard for the children comes from low participation and high failure rates. The consequence of persistent failure is often a widening gap between children and teachers: children stop attending and respond to questions by random guessing; teachers then tighten their oversight by further controlling every detail of a child's response. Let us look at the instruction–response gap during lesson periods at Midwood and elsewhere.

The single most universal activity in the preschools I visited across the country is circle time, and almost invariably the same routine prevails: a greeting followed by calendar and weather. Yet without exception I found that children participate widely only in the greeting routine. The calendar and weather are beyond nearly all the children; teachers get through the exercise only by giving repeated and broad hints, filling in many blanks themselves.

> At Midwood participation in the circle is dominated by Larry and Stephen. No one else goes through the entire "Who came to school today?" routine without error. Molly, Doreen, and of course Carl, cannot manage to repeat the sentence, "I came to school today," even after hearing it repeatedly recited by the other boys and Teresa. Austin, quite willing to repeat any sentence anytime, cannot answer the question, "Are you here today?" and Heather opts out altogether. No one can manage the calendar and weather. Even Larry is confused, substituting season (winter) and holiday (Thanksgiving) for month (November). None of the children correctly labels the date or day of the week. Although weather appears to go better—Heather gets "cloudy" and Larry,

"cold"—because Teresa poses the question with only two options, it is hardly a fair test of their knowledge.

The children's capacity to participate in music—almost as conventional a part of circle time as greetings, calendar, and weather—is also limited. Children like the rhythms, the chance to move and gesture, and the teachers' enthusiasm, but they rarely know more than a small part of each song, if that. The rapid-fire commands, as seen in the following hit songs, are extremely difficult:

In "Put Your Hands Up in the Air" the child, in sequence, is supposed to: put hands on nose, hands in the air, touch toes, turn around, jump up and down, right hand in the air, right hand on hips, left hand in the air, both hands on hips, turn around, jump up and down, back to seat, hands in lap, bow head, and take a nap.

In the "Action Song" the child is asked to close and open eyes, turn around, close and open mouth, wriggle nose, touch ears, scratch back, rub stomach, stamp feet loudly, stamp feet softly, clap hands loudly, clap hands softly, bend legs, bend waist, etc.

In "Hokey Pokey" the child is supposed to put the right hand in, then out, then in; do the same with the left hand, right foot, left foot, right elbow, left elbow, right hip, left hip, head, back side, and whole self.

When they do participate, and a good many always do not, the children are more likely to join in the actions than the singing, which is left to the adults. Because the children usually get their clues, not by listening to the verbal instructions on the congo, but by watching the teacher's movements, and because they have trouble shifting from one gesture to another, they are always out of synchrony with the singer. A teacher may go through half a dozen movements while the child is still repeating the first one. Doreen sticks with the honk-honk gesture and sound for "The Wheels on the Bus" but misses all the other verses; she stays about two gestures behind the verse in "Hokey Pokey," shaking her leg when she should be waving her arms, jumping when she should be turning. During music, unlike work time, teachers accept errors and poor participation. They do not, for example, repeat the songs, simplify, or scale down the number of gestures. Once a song is completed, teachers proceed to the next, equally difficult, one, typically going through five songs in 10–12 minutes.

Games played at early intervention also demand more than these children can deliver. Hiding and chasing games such as "Duck Duck Goose," and "Doggie, Doggie, Where's My Bone?" are particularly popular. Retarded children, with approximate mental levels of 18 months to 2½ years, understand and delight in disappearance–reappearance activities like jack-in-the-box, but transforming this simple, informal play into formal, complex, rule-driven games is a different matter. Here is what occurs:

> "Duck Duck Goose" is a variation on "tisket-a-tasket." Children sit or stand in a circle. The child who is "it" moves around the back of the circle, touching the others sequentially and saying "duck" until he selects his "goose"—indicated by "it" tapping a child on the shoulder while he says "goose" (usually "it" is instructed to pick someone who has not been previously selected). The "goose" is then supposed to chase the "it" around the circle while "it" tries to get into the exact space left vacant by the "goose." Assuming the "it" reaches his destination without being caught by the "goose" (and from my observation whether or not he is caught), the new "goose" is now the "it." Common mistakes made in this game are: the "it" does not understand he is to run fast to escape the touch of the "goose," the "it" does not understand his destination, the "goose" does not understand he needs to tag "it" before "it" reaches his destination at which point he is safe, the "it" fails to tap a new child not previously selected, the "it" does not equate "duck" with no chase and "goose" with chase, so that children run whenever they are tapped regardless of whether "it" says "duck" or "goose." Because of all these errors, the teacher must constantly direct and redirect the "it," the "goose," and the sedentary children.
>
> "Doggie, Doggie, Where's My Bone?" is a variant on "hide-and-seek." The "it" (pretending to be a doggie) is sent out of the room while the teacher hides the bone (usually under a child's rear or tucked into his clothes) and tells the children to keep the secret. Regularly, neither the "it" nor the children understand their respective roles. When "it" returns he does not know what to do. Even when told to find the bone, he does not know where to look for something he cannot see. One can safely bet that when the teacher asks: "Where is the bone?" the possessor will jump up and say "Here it is," although sometimes he, too, will fall victim to the out-of-sight-out-of-mind condition. The children do not see the point of the game—that there is a hider and seeker, that the hiders have a secret from the "it," and that the fun comes from not revealing their special knowledge. Because the game is usually up before it begins, I never saw the "it" go through a systematic

search or the teacher able to offer useful clues. At best, after one wrong guess by "it," whoever has the bone reveals his secret.

Art time, like music, gives the children an opportunity to be somewhat active, but here, too, the failure and correction rate is sky high. The overall problem is that moderately retarded pre-school children are more interested in the process, teachers more focused on the product. The children enjoy the feel of different materials—finger paint, shaving cream, Play-Doh, etc. They like stroking with a paintbrush or crayon, smearing, rubbing, pound-ing, tearing, smelling, and mouthing. But they do not easily take on the discipline of confining their movements to the teacher's specifications—coloring within boundaries, cutting out a form, pasting only a small piece of paper. Therefore, when teachers want a product, they must heavily monitor and constantly correct the children's actions. Problems with paste illustrate well the distance between teacher and child.

> Teresa, it will be recalled, has the children paste paper food (the more advanced children are supposed to paste food onto plates, plates onto cut-out tables, a table onto a big piece of construction paper; the slower children are to paste the food directly onto the cut-out tables). For Molly and Doreen paste is something that feels good on their hands, they savor the sticky sensation by rubbing their fingers together. As a somewhat novel medium with a thick consistency, it is fun to smell, lick, spread, and gouge with a crayon. The children do not understand that paste is used for adhesion. The quality of stickiness that they find compelling does not translate into binding one object to another. So Teresa does the actual pasting and has the children pound on the ob-jects, but they do not understand that their pounding is part of a gluing process.

In center after center I noted that paste, though very appealing to the children as a novel texture, is always used "inappropriately" and requires heavy adult supervision. For the same reasons—interest in the material, not the product—painting is also problem-atic, as the following incident illustrates.

> Six children are given small brushes, a box of watercolors, a cup of water, and a big piece of paper. The teacher explains and illustrates the procedures to be used: first, the brush is dipped into water, then in a single color, then applied to the paper, then dipped again into water so that it is clean for the next paint application. Out of the group, only one understands the pro-

cedure, and even she, when the paints are removed, rubs her hand on the wet colorful paper, looks at her hand admiringly, and licks her fingers. The other children do lots of wrong things: They may get the sequence confused—brush goes into paint, then into water, and then often into the mouth. They forget to dunk the brush into the water, so that all the paints, as well as the picture, begin to turn brown. They do not confine paint to paper but apply it to their fingers and, liking the appearance, proceed to their hand, thence to other parts of their body and clothing. The teacher, enlisting the help of an aide, stops these responses and, her hand over a child's hand, walks each through the right sequence. After having them make a few proper strokes, she hurriedly removes the paper to a drying rack.

Not all teachers select such an ambitious project, but even when it is paint on an easel or crayoning a paper, the children and adults are in different places.

Duane, a hyperactive–distractible 4-year-old, accepts an invitation to paint at an easel (having refused coloring and cutting). There is something about the opportunity—thick paint, big brush, bright color, large paper, standing position?—that attracts him. He begins stroking with the blue paint (the only color made available to him). There is a lot of action in the room, and he is slightly diverted. He turns and takes a step toward a group of children, notices the brush in his hand, and goes back to his more or less up–down strokes. Soon he is off the paper and onto the easel. The teacher reminds him to stay on the paper. He pays no attention. She comes over and introduces red paint, suggesting he fill in the blank spaces with red. He takes the new paint and "misuses" it as he did the old paint, so that the teacher decides it is time for another child to do some painting.

Again, it is the medium and the movement that attract Duane. Although this teacher is not demanding a particular outcome, her limits—the paper edge—are not relevant to Duane. When he fails to discipline his movements, she, like so many others, increases rather than decreases the demands. Instead of suggesting use of another color, she might simply have attached a larger sheet of paper to a larger surface so that Duane would not be limited by paper boundaries. Teachers, however, want to advance children, and this might look to them like retreat. So when a task is not going well, they prod children to do more, not less. All too often the effort results in additional failure.

Children's high failure rate is most apparent during conditions of explicit questioning like work time, even though, as we shall see, teachers try hard to elicit the right answer. As a general observation, whenever teachers bring up the staples of the curriculum—counting, colors, shapes, letters, verbal labels, antonyms (e.g., big–little, happy–sad)—children make frequent mistakes. The low ratio of right to wrong responses at Midwood is typical.

> We have already reviewed the difficulties children had with the calendar. While still at circle, Teresa asks David to identify which is bigger, an apple or table. Heather responds: "Big apple, big, very big apple." Her answer indicates that, beyond making an error, she has not understood the question. Heather is using "big" as an absolute, rather than relative, quality. She can conceive of apples as big (though it could be confused with good) but cannot compare the size of apples and tables. That would mean disregarding all the ways tables and apples differ and focusing only on size, too abstract a task for Heather. Teresa, as is true of most teachers, skips over Heather's problem with the question and, instead, dramatizes the right answer. Molly, Doreen, and Heather get about half the labels right during the grab-bag game. In their small IEP group, Heather makes jagged rather than vertical lines; Molly does not sort the animals by color; Doreen succeeds with the pegboard.
>
> At individual time Doreen misses at least half the objects in her personal book, though she has been drilled in them for months. When asked to put a dress under the table, she begins to climb on top of the table. Again, she has not merely confused under and on but misconstrued the question as a request to do something with her body, not her garment. As usual, Teresa, rather than taking the lead from Doreen and shifting to a game of climbing on and under, keeps the objective intact (placing something on and under) and demonstrates the right answers; Doreen copies her, correctly once, incorrectly once. Molly can insert the circle into the form board but requires hand-over-hand assistance for the triangle and square.

Authorities may argue about just how many wrong answers are right for good teaching. However, at a time when errorless learning is widely acclaimed, a persistent error rate of over 50%, on tasks that are hardly new, must be of concern. Further indications that the uptake must be low come from the repetition of objectives over multiple IEPs, and rough norms indicating the age at which children are expected to accomplish the tasks. We turn now to this evidence.

TOO HARD

Repetition of Items

One line of support for the "too tough" argument is the repetition of objectives over time. It is bad enough for a child to be wrong over half the time in November, even worse to be confused by the same questions in June and have to face them again the next fall.

In each of the 20 centers I collected two IEPs, separated by 8–12 months, for at least two children. It is clear from a review of these documents that objectives are repeated again and again, although exactly how often is hard to judge because areas are dropped and added without explanation. Following are typical examples of the same or similar objectives repeated over time.

Juanita, a child with Down syndrome, was 5 years 1 month when I visited her program, and functioning at approximately 2½ years. Her first evaluation was completed 4/88 when she was 3 years 11 months; her second, 5/89 when she was 5 years old. Juanita's 1988 objectives:

A. Juanita will rote count 1 to 10 in four out of five trials.

B. Juanita will put objects in one-to-one correspondence in four out of five trials.

C. Juanita will take apart and put together a five- to seven-piece puzzle with adjacent pieces, in four out of five trials.

D. Juanita will remain seated for 10 minutes when given instructions to do so during an activity or in a waiting situation in four out of five trials.

One year later, Juanita's IEP was an exact repetition of objectives A through D.

Victor was 4½ when observed and functioning at approximately the 2½ year level. His first IEP was completed 5/88 when he was 3 years 5 months; his second, 1/89 when he was 4 years 1 month. Victor's 1988 objectives:

A. Victor will build a three-block train using cubes.

B. Victor will grasp a pencil between thumb and forefinger.

C. Victor will understand the concept of 1.

D. Victor will point to big and little on request.

E. Victor will draw a vertical line.

Eight months later, Victor's IEP goals were an exact repetition of A through D, and with one addition:

E. Victor will draw a circle.

Nina was 4 years old and functioning at the 18–24 month level when I visited her program. Here are items from her first IEP, written on 11/87 when she was 2 years 4 months; and her second IEP, written on 10/88 when she was 3 years 3 months. Nina's 1987 objectives:

A. Will match two identical objects when one like object and one distractor are placed on the table and Nina is handed the other like object. She will do this with four different objects.

B. Nina will demonstrate object combinations in play (e.g., put the baby to bed and cover the baby) in three different routines.

C. Nina will stack four 1-inch cubes in a tower when given a model to copy on three out of four trials.

Nina's 1988 objectives:

A. Nina will match four objects with 100% accuracy.

B. Nina will combine two to three steps in her play with common objects with 80% accuracy four times during a 2-week period.

C. Nina will stack four 1-inch blocks in three out of three trials.

The repetition of these exercises for 2 years indicates, at the very least, that they were initially too hard. One might retort that because retarded children make slow progress it is appropriate to give them very similar objectives, even over 2 years. Perhaps the teacher was overambitious in suggesting that Nina learn to stack four blocks in 1 year, but an objective of two blocks the first year and four the second or, for Juanita, counting to 5 the first year and 10 the second, would have been suitable. The problem with this position is that it mistakenly equates the length (amount) of a task with its complexity, and supposes that by reducing the former, you will always reduce the latter. Although counting to 5 may be marginally easier than counting to 10, a genuine simplification would postpone counting until the child demonstrates competency in prerequisite tasks, such as lining up, sorting, and matching. When a child has reached the developmental threshold for talking, reading, counting, or stacking blocks, progress is rapid, though somewhat slower, in a retarded child. Think how quickly a 2-year-old compared to a 1-year-old picks up new words. According to estimates, normal children between 1 and 6 learn five to eight words a day (Chapman, 1981; de Villiers & de Villiers, 1978). That means a moderately retarded child who is ready should learn close to 900 words a year, not the half-dozen targeted on the IEP.[4]

The moderately retarded child, once developmentally ready, should not take more than twice the time of an ordinary child to learn a given objective. If a year of instruction in block stacking or counting is too long for the nonhandicapped child, then 2 years on the same task is too long for a retarded one. By assigning virtually the same objective for 2 years, the teacher subjects herself—and the child—to monotonous and oppressive drilling. Teachers impose these drills out of the utmost good will. Several told me with obvious commitment and resolve that it was time to stop "underestimating" the potential of these children. What they have not considered is the psychological cost of year-in, year-out repetition. Although we do not have good research data on the academic outcome of moderately retarded children with long preschool histories (and it is always possible to reverse previous predictions), current information suggests that most children with Down syndrome never attain even a first-grade level in reading or math.[5]

The infinitely slow progress, repetitious preacademic drill, and distance between student and teacher have, as previously mentioned, an analogue in oral instruction for the deaf—an analogue that may help illuminate the shortcomings of early intervention instruction. From the 1880s to the 1960s the goals of deaf education in this country were speech and speechreading (Sacks, 1989). At both residential and day schools deaf children managed to express themselves naturally only behind teachers' backs, in the bathrooms, hallways and dormitories. Student failure—only 25% left school reading as high as the fourth-grade level (Sacks, 1989), 30% were functionally illiterate (Jacobs, 1989)—did not deter schools from persisting in the official oral-only policy. But academic failure was just a small part of the damage incurred.

> Spontaneous outbursts of laughter in the classroom were often stilled by scornful reprimands from our fifth-grade teacher . . . because he said they sounded disgustingly unpleasant or irritating—even animalistic . . . We were forced to undergo various exercises like breathing through the nose only—breathing through the mouth only—either with sound or without—doing these repeatedly with our hands on our stomachs or heads. Compliments were often lavished upon those who came up with forced but perfectly controlled laughter—and glares were given to those who failed to laugh "properly" or didn't sound like a "normal" person . . . Some of us have since then forgotten how to laugh the way we had been taught. And there are two or three

from our group who have chosen to laugh silently for the rest of their lives. (Gannon, 1981, p. 355)

Only in recent years, with increased respect for the wishes of the deaf community and for sign language, has "total communication" replaced oralism (a combination of American Sign Language, signed English, finger spelling, and speech). Today, "there seems to be unanimous consensus that the young deaf child exposed to the difficult spoken English environment is extremely impoverished" (Meadow, 1980, p. 27). The switch in language instruction has brought about a shift in the teacher's role. As noted by Hans Furth (1973), an eminent scholar of intellectual development in the deaf:

> Language drill, speech drill, and lipreading drill are the main activities of the young deaf child in a traditional classroom; under oralism the deaf child regurgitates the linguistic patterns that the teacher imposes on him . . . In contrast, total communication emphasizes the *spontaneous expressions* of the child . . . However, the point is not to teach sign language but rather to use the spontaneous communication of signing to encourage a two-language communicative exchange. For this purpose the teacher reflects the child's own expressions to provide informal occasions for spontaneously improving these expressions; he will sign back to the child in a more adequate manner, and he will accompany all signing by English speech . . . The school atmosphere is not centered on language but on the child's communicative *interest;* language per se is considered too narrow an education goal. This is really the only psychologically sound way to acquire a language, particularly a first language. (p. 41, italics added)

In both deaf education and early intervention, the ambition of normalizing the handicapped—in the one case through speech, in the other, through preacademics (including speech)—is hard to fault (although, as portrayed in *Children of a Lesser God* [Medoff, 1980], some in the deaf community have a principled objection to speech instruction). But in both instances adults decide without adequately considering the child's receptivity; the result has been little "take." Hour after hour, day after day, and year after year children passively endure what they cannot readily absorb. Meanwhile, programs disallow the children's more natural expressions—sign language in the deaf, toddler-like behavior in the retarded—that may, in fact, be paths to more fulfilled lives.

Predicted Attainment for Objectives

There is no set age at which normal children learn colors, numbers, shapes, particular games, and songs. However, one can safely assume that material developed and routinely used with normal 3- to 5-year-olds is by and large too difficult for children functioning at 18 months to 2½ years. Some equipment— household objects, Play-Doh, finger paint, large cardboard boxes— is sufficiently supple that children of very different abilities can use it well. But books, games, and songs are less flexible.

Stories provide a good illustration of the "too hard" theme, as every teacher reads regularly to her students. The classrooms always have a diversity of books: some that identify animals, numbers, and colors; some about seasons, holidays, and community helpers; some that tell traditional and modern stories. A very popular one is *Harry the Dirty Dog*, found also in preschools for normal 3- to 5-year-olds. I heard it read to groups of handicapped children in several centers; as far as I could see, no one ever understood it adequately, and the moderately retarded children were at a total loss. The dust jacket advertises the book for children ages 4 to 8.

> In the story Harry the dog—who buries a scrub brush in the back yard because he does not like to be bathed—runs away from home and undergoes a series of adventures that transform him from a white dog with black spots into a black dog with white spots. When he returns home, tired and hungry, his family does not recognize him, despite the familiar tricks he performs, until he unearths the scrub brush, jumps into the tub, and is bathed by the children. To understand this story a child needs to know the relation of physical appearance to social recognition, why an animal would want to run away from home (dislikes baths), and then want to return (hunger, fatigue, concern that his family believes he has truly run away), and must recollect the buried scrub brush. That identifying these transformations and motivations is way beyond the capacities of moderately retarded preschoolers can be seen by responses in one classroom.

> The teacher is reading to six children and conscientiously asking questions. As is so often the case, only two are responding. When she asks, "Who is Harry?" one comments, "Harry the dog," the other, "Harry is the dirty dog." When the teacher asks, "Why did he leave home?" the only response is, "Gets dirty," and "Dog gone." Teacher: "What happened when he ran home?" Child: "Ran back home." Teacher: "Did the children know him?" Child:

"Dirty dog." Teacher: "That's right they didn't know him because he was dirty." Teacher: "What happens after the bath?" Child questioningly: "Dog gone?"

Another popular instructional tool is the *Peabody Early Experiences Kit* (PEEK; Dunn et al., 1976). It consists of 250 lessons aimed at developing "basic cognitive skills" (p. 43) that are easily incorporated into circle time. Each activity is introduced by Mr. Pazoo, an appealing puppet with his own theme song. Because the activities, with their accompanying attractive materials (records, drawstring bags, photographs, cards, posters, beads and ropes, assorted small objects, etc.), include a major focus on shapes, colors, body parts, and vocabulary development, they are a convenient way to implement IEP objectives. But "primarily PEEK is designed for three-year-old children . . . PEEK is especially suited for the broad 85 percent of average children" (p. 37).

The authors are explicit on what they conceive to be 3-year-old attainments. Cognitively, normal children "are beginning to express imagination by playing roles . . . are curious about their immediate environment as expressed through frequent questions . . . are beginning to spot the absurdity of such questions as 'Do tables play?' . . . understand and retell simple stories expressed in narrative form" (p. 22). Linguistically, normal children "speak in a mixture of complete and incomplete sentences and phrases averaging five utterances in length . . . have a receptive vocabulary of about 800 words . . . have an expressive vocabulary of about 500 words which is sufficient for labeling and describing a wide array of objects, actions and thoughts . . . are embarking on the period of most rapid language acquisition" (p. 22). "Rapid language acquisition" is also made explicit: within a year (i.e., by their fourth birthday), it is anticipated that the children will "have a receptive vocabulary approaching 2,500 words . . . have an expressive vocabulary of nearly 1,250 words" (p. 23). Most of the moderately retarded children I observed do not have the competencies described as typical of a 3-year-old and certainly do not make the annual gains projected by the authors of PEEK.

IEP Items

The preacademic items selected from the developmental inventories for the children's IEPs are often unreasonably difficult. Take Doreen, who has a chronological age of 38 months and, according to a standardized developmental test, an overall mental age of 21 months.* Included in the cognitive goals for her are: identifying big versus little, in–on–under, and three colors; and matching three shapes (circle, triangle, square). Yet according to the Battelle—of the seven frequently used developmental inventories the only one that is standardized—identification of big and small shapes occurs at the 36- to 47-month level; matching shapes, at 24–35 months; and demonstrates understanding of prepositions, at 25–35 months. The Battelle does not have color items, but five of the inventories do, and their youngest age for color identification ranges from 30 to 36 months. Even without tests to document age expectations, simple observation of normal children at preschool is proof enough that Doreen is in over her head. Normal 3-year-olds in mainstreamed classes struggle with colors and simple counting; 4- to 5-year-olds, with days and months (often confusing the two), and one-to-one correspondence.

There is a great range among the eight developmental inventories on where they place "core curriculum" items (to be expected, given that they are not standardized). But even the wide band of posted ranges put the tasks beyond the comfortable reach of moderately retarded 3- to 5-year-olds. Here are a few examples:

> *Distinguishes square, triangle, and circle:* Range is 36 to 60 months of age.
> *Sorts by shape and color:* Range is 24 months (only the Carolina) to 59 months.
> *Differentiates colors:* Range is 30 to 60 months (commonly 36 to 48 months).
> *Completes simple puzzle:* Range is 24 to 71 months (commonly 36 to 48 months for three to five pieces).
> *Counts by rote:* Range is 36 to 72 months, but at 36 months, counts only 1 to 3.

As we saw in reviewing the IEPs from 20 programs, 91% of the severely mentally retarded children—functioning at or below 18 months—had as an objective the learning of color, numbers, shapes, three-piece puzzle, or big–little.

SUMMING UP

Early intervention programs have taken on a very tough task. They have accepted as their mandate instructing children in a

---

*Although Doreen is a composite, the mental levels and IEP objectives are from an actual child.

"preacademic" curriculum that might well be rejected by non-handicapped preschoolers. The core curriculum is derived from frequently used developmental inventories. Moderately retarded children in the 3- to 5-year range are expected to learn something about colors, forms, numbers, size, sequence, opposites, puzzles, time, and letters. Learning this material, which is not the natural habitat of small children, requires a strict teacher-directed behavioral regimen (cultural transmission model). As part of their professionalism, teachers maintain a poised, controlled presence with children. Like Teresa, no matter how much unexpected commotion erupts—tantrums, toilet accidents, spills after clean-up—they stay calm, unflappable, modulated. With one hand they right the disruption, with the other push forward the agenda. To carry out their work teachers need children to be quiet, listen attentively, talk (or point), respond to questions, maintain—as the adults do—an even-tempered, positive, and patient attitude.

I have argued that both the academic and behavioral requirements are too difficult. The actual world of these toddler-like children is planets away from the artificial world imposed by the teacher. We can see this by the discrepancy between what children do naturally and what teachers want. When unsupervised, children are in motion, not in talk. They move objects, dump objects, replace objects (usually to a spot where they don't belong), get to know their bodies and space by touching and moving. They live prepositions (in, out, on, under, behind, in front of), but do not verbally identify them. They prefer circular movements to sequential ones, repeating over and over an act—for example, pushing a button to make a noise—in which they are effective agents. They are interested in making and doing, not in right answers. Their ability for delayed symbolic play is primitive. They may literally put themselves into the shoes of another person, but they cannot live out any substantial part of another person's life. They are very unlikely to string together a series of actions or to enact scenes in which they have not participated. Behaviorally they are egocentric, they are beginning to perceive their own wants but are unaware of the wants of others. They are ruled by inner, not outer, clocks. Sometimes this means long absorption, sometimes fitful. They are emotionally labile, moving so swiftly and unpredictably from one extreme to another that often one cannot be certain if their excitement signals joy or distress.

Early intervention programs are trying to turn toddlers into students. We ask children who are naturally in motion to do a great deal of sitting; children who talk little, to listen and respond with words; children who know by doing, to deal with abstractions; children who are interested in the process, to turn out a product; children who are impatient to express themselves, to be patient, considerate, wait their turn, abide by group standards; children who are driven by their own interests, to subordinate those interests to a swiftly moving time schedule; children who are exuberant and emotionally reactive, to be "nice," restrained, calm.

Because of the distance between children and teachers, there is a great deal of failure. Children are not responding to teacher suggestions in play, and they are not, for the most part, "taking" the instruction although they may give the appearance of learning. David, for example, is a master at preacademics, but it is a rote knowledge that he cannot use. Witness, his failure when given the task of threading beads by a color–shape pattern or finding something in the room beginning with "B" (even though he has told Teresa, "Boy begins with B"). In the face of student failure, teachers press on rather than joining the children at a less demanding level. Objectives get repeated year after year with only slight modification. Programs are making too little allowance for the retardation, expecting the handicapped to work with the same materials, ideas, and knowledge as do their nonhandicapped peers.

Admittedly, there are achievements; they are hard come by and rightly to be treasured. When a retarded child masters a task after long labor, the pride of accomplishment for all involved is deep and abiding. But, at early intervention the minuscule progress is vastly overshadowed by the mammoth amount of failure. And that failure is particularly onerous coming, as it does, from tasks imposed by adults, rather than objectives sought by the children themselves. The cost of so much failure on the children's aspirations and selfhood—perhaps because invisible and slowly cumulative—seems not to be a matter of concern to early interventionists.

One might ask, if the distance between teachers and children is as great as I claim, why don't children rebel? How do teachers maintain not just order, but a peaceful atmosphere in the classroom? To keep children working on tasks that are not to their liking with a minimum of protest, and to hide the degree and nature of their retardation, teachers have adopted a number of specific techniques. We turn to them in the next chapter.

CHAPTER SIX

Managing Children— Masking Retardation

> We like children who are a little afraid of us, docile,
> deferential children, though not, of course, if they are so
> obviously afraid that they threaten our image of ourselves as
> kind, lovable people whom there is no reason to fear. We
> find the ideal the kind of "good" children who are just
> enough afraid of us to do everything we want, without
> making us feel that fear of us is what is making them do it
> . . . You can do this [create docile children] in the
> old-fashioned way, openly and avowedly, with the threat of
> harsh words, infringement of liberty, or physical punishment.
> Or you can do it in the modern way, subtly, smoothly,
> quietly, by withholding the acceptance and approval which
> you and others have trained the children to depend on.
>   —HOLT (1964, pp. 168, 179–180)

Teachers try to be—and, for the most part, succeed in being—kind, gentle, and patient with children. They offer unstinting praise and rarely criticize. But alongside the gentleness, teachers are operating very tight ships very authoritatively. Their use of authority is subtle but pervasive and required to bridge the expectation–performance gap. One rarely sees naked use of power through force or even verbal coercion. Children are not called "bad" or threatened with "punishment" (although one might interpret "Do you want timeout?" as a threat). But most of the time children are submitting to teacher authority and inhibiting natural inclinations. The techniques to be discussed—teachers compensating for children through excessive cueing and assistance, teachers dominating activities, teachers enlisting the more competent students as proxies for the class, teachers distorting children's true intentions, teachers adhering to a rigid regimen, high adult–child ratios, constant reinforcement, and a narrow range of permissible behavior—all restrict a child's freedom. When a teacher offers only two options to a question, the child cannot give a third. When a teacher takes over an activity, the child cannot invent a response. When only some children know the answers, others must remain silent. A child cannot contradict the teacher who tells him how he feels. When it is "time to," the child must submit to the routine. High adult–child ratios make it possible to monitor every move a child makes and even to anticipate those he is about to make. The steady stream of reinforcement leaves a child without opportunities to learn from mistakes, and narrowly channeling the permissible deprives him of experiencing the possible. In their totality these techniques succeed not just in controlling and subduing children but in producing a *seemingly* high level of student attainment, veiling the retardation.

DISGUISING RETARDATION

"Cheating" for Children

Teachers, because they are so thoroughly on the side of children, do what we all do in relationships of affection—they seek to avoid seeing the children fail. In practice this means "cheating" on the child's behalf by excessively shaping responses. Favorite means of doing this are to limit the number of possible answers to two, to extract the right response from children's familiar rote recitations, to monitor children's responses closely and guide them physically when necessary, and sometimes simply to supply the right answer. As a result, the children appear to be doing better than they really are. Parents, of course, are pleased and can hardly be expected to complain about the deception. But there are some pernicious consequences. Children become oriented to teacher-pleasing. Often, with no notion of the right answer, they guess wildly or search the teacher for hints rather than think independently. Teacher-pleasing, or teacher-appeasing, and wild guessing work against personal autonomy, integrity, self-reliance, independence—core values of all educators.

Asking questions in the alternative is a common strategy. Not only does this give the child at least a 50% hit rate, but it permits the teacher many additional ways to guide the child's answer without giving it to him outright. Often a teacher will use extreme alternatives to get the right answer: "Is the child happy or sad?" "Are you a girl or a boy?" "Is it applesauce or peanut butter?" She may offer ridiculous alternatives as a hint: "Are chairs or toilets in the living room?" "Is it a house or dinosaur?" This is a bit risky, for when the child errs he reveals his total lack of understanding. A teacher may further increase the odds by underscoring the right answer with her voice. Or she may pick up on children's habitual ways of responding. For example, in an object discrimination problem, the teacher may consistently place the correct alternative to the left side of a child if he consistently reaches with his left hand; in a verbal question she may always present the right option last if the child habitually selects the last alternative. Teresa uses an either–or format in much of her questioning.

> With Heather: "Is it cloudy or sunny?" Heather correctly says cloudy but it seems she was merely guessing. Her first response to Teresa's weather inquiry was to open the window, suggesting she may not have understood the question. Even after getting the right answer, she wants to attach both the cloudy and sunny faces to the calendar. Teresa rescues her from error by accepting only the cloudy face.

> Teresa asks the class if winter is "cold or hot?" Larry gets "cold," but is uncertain whether a shivering or sweating child correctly represents cold. He looks to Teresa for a hint. She nods and smiles as he starts reaching toward the right choice.

> David is asked if an apple is round or square. He responds, "Apple gives us A," and Austin chimes in, "Apple juice is good for you." Neither child has absorbed the question. On repetition, David says, "Square." This failure is a clue for Stephen, so that whether or not he knows the right answer, he offers the remaining alternative.

> Teresa holds up two apples, then an apple and banana and asks for each twosome, "are they the same or different?" A bit later she asks, "Which is bigger, an apple or a table?"

Sometimes Teresa asks a question in which the child's response is restricted to a yes–no option.

> To David: "Does b-b-boy begin with B?" To Doreen: "Can you tell me what we do with a dress? Do we wear it?" To Austin: "Are you here today?" To Heather: "What are you pasting? Is it an apple?"

Another way teachers "cheat" for children is to extract a correct response from their rote memory bank.

Teresa asks Austin what the day is. He begins to recite the days of the week starting with Saturday. When he reaches Monday, Teresa interrupts and tells him, "That's right, today is Monday." When no one knows the date, she has the class start counting from 1, stops them at 11, asks for the next number and, when David gets "12," says, "That's right, today is November 12th."

Not infrequently teachers give the answer straight out.

When Austin does not answer Teresa's question: "Are you here today?" she tells him to say, "I am here today." Although he complies, and superficially that may look better than silence, there is no reason to believe he has done more than parrot some words. An echolalic autistic child, Austin frequently just repeats what he has heard.

When Larry answers a question on the month with "winter" and Stephen, with "Thanksgiving," Teresa responds: "This is November. Can you say November?" He, too, complies, but is he more knowledgeable about months than before he gave the "correct" answer?

Teresa helps Stephen to find something orange in the room by staring at a pumpkin.

At work time, Alice asks Larry to put the turkey next to the table. When he puts it on top of the table, she points out "next to." David correctly picks the biggest turkey on command, but apparently it was just luck, for when asked to find the smallest, he points to the same big turkey—perhaps reasoning that if Alice liked what he did the first time, he should do it again. Quite clearly David does not understand this antonym, but Alice persists, saying: "No, David, here is the small one. The biggest cannot be the smallest, right?"

Dominating Activities

When children do poorly a teacher has several options: she can withdraw her efforts, simplify the objective, or give more help. Teachers, eager to increase children's performances, react to failure by trying to "help" more. They are not inclined to give up, reduce demands, or even search for a child's comfort level. The only way teachers can further help the inattentive, error-ridden child who has not responded to coaching or answer-shaping, is to dominate the action. We have seen already that in many art activities there is a role reversal, with teachers planning and carrying out the bulk of the project while children serve as helpers. The children's job is to do a bit of pasting, cutting, or coloring on forms that the teachers have prepared and will mount. We have seen also that what sometimes starts out as "child help" turns into "teacher play," as when Pat transforms Pedro's cone gathering into cop play. There is no getting around the fact that for an imaginative, energetic teacher the play of these children is tedious, and it must be very tempting for anyone with a bit of inventiveness to make it more interesting. I found teacher play particularly prominent with unstructured materials such as Play-Doh and blocks, where the gap between a creative teacher and simple child is so glaringly apparent. The problem of teacher play is that when there is no "take," there is also no continuity; the children look impressive only while the teacher dominates the play. When the teacher quits, so does the child. The following examples from programs are illustrative.

> It is first thing in the morning, and a teacher invites a few children to play with her until the others arrive. She constructs a roadway that goes under a tunnel as it approaches the airport. She has one child zoom an airplane overhead, a second one move a car along the road. Then she has them crash. A third child is instructed to bring the ambulance and take the car passengers quickly to the hospital. The children play out their roles with lots of coaching, and the teacher is animated and enthusiastic; but when she leaves, all the children disperse.

This is not to imply teacher suggestions never work. Sometimes children do continue with, elaborate upon, or simplify a teacher's idea. The following task was sufficiently open-ended that children of very different levels could all find it absorbing.

> At circle time a teacher has introduced the concept of sink and float by filling a plastic pool with water and dropping in assorted items she has strewn about a table—wood spools, paper clips, balls, pebbles, plastic tub animals, soap bars, plastic flowers, and food. As each child prepares for her chance to experiment with an object, the teacher asks everyone to guess before dropping the object whether it will sink or float. Even those who won't guess,

or can't because they have no notion of sinking or floating, enjoy tossing something into the water and keep their eyes riveted on the object's movement. The teacher does not object when the children spontaneously leave their seats and gather around the pool. After circle, several of the children choose to continue experimenting during their free play time. Since the teacher has not imposed any complex set of sequences the children must follow— sorting the objects by buoyancy, material, size, color—they are able to continue with minimal supervision.

Taking over also means using a steady stream of directives to move children through a project.

The instructions flow from Alice during art at Midwood: "OK, boys, I want you to find the cut-out table. Good, you found it. Now put paste on one side. That's right, very good. Now paste the table onto your paper . . . Now you need to find the plates. Each of you is to take two plates and paste them at each end of your table. David, look at what you are doing," etc.

At work time Molly is sorting colored monkeys onto a red and blue plate. She has a general idea but makes lots of errors. Each time she makes a mistake Anita says: "Is this red? . . . Does it go on this plate? Then does it go on this plate? . . . It goes on the blue plate," and she shows Molly the proper match.

Teachers go so far as to control a child's movements in order to elicit the correct responses.

To "help" Doreen make cookies, Anita flattens the Play-Doh with a rolling pin, gives Doreen a cookie cutter, and presses down on the cutter with Doreen to make the imprint. To get Doreen's paper food pasted onto paper, Teresa turns the food over, sticky side to paper, and picking up Doreen's hand, presses it on top of the cut-outs. Before snack she completes the art projects for Molly and Doreen. Teresa verbally and motorically guides Molly as she inserts a triangle and square into a form box.

As Heather goes through the obstacle course, Alice does not move from Heather's side. Anita takes Heather's hand in hers as "together" they pick up and replace blocks and again "together" draw vertical lines.

It is quite usual for teachers to guide children's hands during cutting and drawing activities. Typically, the teacher sits behind or next to the child, places her hand over the child's hand, and "together" they cut or draw. It can certainly be maintained that this is a good way for teachers to give children the feel of a new objective or to assist when they are stuck. However, the frequency of hand-over-hand helping suggests it is more than an initial introduction or strategy of last resort.

Yet another way teachers try to engage children and heighten their performance is through the dramatization of activities. Teachers, in an effort to gain a child's attention, or having failed to get a question answered, resort to theatrics. The teacher building a zoo, for a child more interested in removing and replacing blocks, reaches for the child through dramatization.

> "Look, we'll put the monkeys here in this pretend cage," she says. Then she lopes about scratching under her arms, making monkey noises while pleading, "I want a banana. Please give me a banana." The teacher gets flat on the floor, wriggles her arm between two blocks, and pleads again, "A banana please, just one banana." No banana is given. The teacher begins to whimper. Still no banana. Then she gives the child a banana, moves the child's hand (with the banana) to her (teacher's) mouth, pretends to chomp on the food, and jumps about exclaiming, "Oh, delicious. Thank-you *so* much."

While one cannot but admire the energy, originality, and job investment reflected in teacher theatrics, the dramatizations keep children looking, listening, and riveted on the teacher's performance—a passive position. The more the teacher becomes the actor, the more the child becomes the stilled, compliant audience.

Using the Competent

During small and large group instruction, teachers cope with the wide spread of children in their classrooms (from a Carl to a Stephen) by relying on the most competent. Although teachers earnestly try to adapt tasks to individual levels, they depend upon the more mature children to keep the answers flowing. Gearing instruction to the higher children is a successful device for maintaining a tough—too tough—curriculum. Teresa, for example, would not have done weather and calendar with a class of only Doreens, Mollys, and Carls who do not count, even by rote, and know nothing of days and dates. But, thanks to the responsiveness of the higher children, she can ignore the slower ones and maintain a rather normal preschool curriculum. Similarly, with *Harry the*

Dirty Dog: Heather, Molly, and Doreen can only point to the dog and go "bow-wow." Without Stephen, Larry, and David, who have a marginal understanding of the story line, Teresa would not have read it, but with their participation she can rationalize that the reading supports the slower children's "listening skills," while stretching the higher children's comprehension, and everyone benefits from the group experience. The higher functioning children, even if they number but one or two, provide a rationale for moving ahead, even if a large number of children are left far behind.

Teachers do modify tasks for slower children when possible. With the grab bag, Teresa asks the more advanced children to identify objects without first looking, while the slower children are permitted to look first and then label. In the art project, the more advanced children are required to paste the objects on plates, the slower ones directly on the paper table. But alterations of this sort are often not enough. If a child has no comprehension of colors, it does little good to require him to match or point, rather than label. There is no way the slower children can be helped to do the calendar or follow what is, for them, a complex story plot. If the objective for the slower children is animal identification, then *Harry the Dirty Dog* is a poor choice. As a general rule, I noted, a lesson is continued (and repeated on subsequent days) as long as *some* children respond. The slower children always have their turn, but usually they are the beneficiaries of substantial teacher "cheating."

The problem of leaning on the more competent is particularly acute in programs that combine handicapped and nonhandicapped children of the same age. If a majority of the children are participating well, the teacher does not (perhaps cannot) make substantial modifications for the few very slow children. This leaves the latter thoroughly lost and frequently scolded by the teacher and other children.

Ricky is 3½, functioning at 18 to 24 months in an integrated classroom with normal children ages 3 to 4. I observed him, when left alone, raise and lower a telephone receiver, pull an alarm switch up and down, try to eat and then toss away plastic fruit, open and close a cash register, arrange chairs around a table, remove and replace rings on a stick, wander, and use the words "hi" and "bye." Meanwhile his chronological age peers cluster around a train and track, play "campfire," karate kid, and the big bad wolf, and talk about birthday parties and water safety. During circle time, the teacher asks the children to identify different aspects of dressing. They think of zipping, buttoning, snapping, and tying. She adds buckling. They talk of what clothes go over, what clothes go under. The teacher gives everyone a flat cardboard cut-out shoe with punched holes to lace. Ricky steps on the "shoe" and tries to walk, surprised that it fails to accompany him. A child raises his hand and asks to "go potty." Ricky gets up imitatively to follow him, but is told to stay. He nonetheless says "bye-bye" and starts to pull his pants down, revealing his diapers. The children giggle. After being seated, Ricky starts rubbing his neighbor's arm and hair. The neighbor backs away. Ricky rubs his own fingers and then touches the girl on his other side, who complains, "Ricky pulled my hair again." The teacher reprimands Ricky and then asks the children a variety of questions concerning what they would like for snack. Ricky, not understanding the questions and slavishly imitating the other children, raises his hand in response to each question. The teacher has children count their crackers. Ricky at first is silent. But when he sees his neighbor touch each cracker while counting, he reaches over and touches a few of her crackers as well. Ricky eats his crackers oddly. The children laugh. Ricky, not understanding the ridicule, joins the laughter. The teacher throws a beanbag to a child. It is the signal for the child to name what he will play with during center time. When the bag comes to Ricky, he misses the catch, picks it up, and throws it aimlessly. The teacher suggests: "How about playing in housekeeping?"

Ricky, like other retarded children, has techniques for handling a set of too-hard demands. He follows the visual rather than the verbal cues, which he cannot grasp, just as children imitate visual gestures rather than listen to recorded gestures in action songs. He imitates rather than understands, gets up when another child stands, raises his hand when the others do. Often he is silent, watching—perhaps vicariously enjoying—the activities of others, or sometimes drifting off. He narrows his range, focuses on only one other child, watches the crackers as they are passed about, studies the floor. He is holding onto fragments. To an observer it may look like marginal participation, but it is hardly even that, for his hand raising is not a response to a question and his pointing to crackers is not counting. Finally, when he cannot grasp what's going on, he turns inward to his own body, as did Molly at Midwood.

Distorting Children's Intentions

Teachers disguise the motor restlessness, negativism, and failures that are part of a retarded child's immaturity by subtly distorting children's feelings. This is a curious phenomenon, for teachers also have a habit of "reflecting" emotions by verbalizing children's ongoing experiences. Frequently one hears a teacher remark, "I know you are angry now, but it is time to go inside," or "I know you want Jacob's ball, but he got it first and you will get it later." At the same time, they often put words of agreement in the mouth of a child who, in fact, wants to disagree. The denial of children's true intentions makes programs look more harmonious and collaborative than they truly are.

> Teresa says to Doreen, who is playing in the corridor with an excavated diaper, "Can I help you put away your diaper?"

> When Molly leaves circle during "weather," crawls under a table, and removes her sneaker, Teresa says to Anita, "Molly wants you to help her sit."

As Teresa knows full well, Doreen does not want help to return a diaper she is enjoying, she wants to play with it more; and Molly wants to be freed from, not helped in, sitting.

> When Molly takes Larry's candy, Anita comments, "She is sorry, aren't you, Molly?"

Molly is only sorry that she cannot have the candy.

> When Heather, because of a throwing incident, is denied sand, Anita says cheerfully, "I know soon you will stop throwing sand because you want to follow the rules."

Nothing Heather does suggests such a desire; it's sand she wants, not rules.

> When Heather "falls out" because Anita stops her from grabbing juice, she yells, "Gimme my juice. I want my juice." Teresa replies, "I guess Heather isn't ready for juice yet. Maybe she will be more ready after some quiet time."

Of course, Heather is ready for juice; she is just not ready to wait her turn.

> And when Heather is too boisterous on the obstacle course, Teresa tells her to follow the rules unless she "wants quiet time."

Heather, of course, has no desire for quiet time.

> When David has difficulty with imitating bead patterns, Alice asks, "Is that hard, David?" To his "yes," Alice rebuts, "No, it's not hard for you. I've seen you do it. It's easy, isn't it?"

David is making a lot of errors—clearly it is hard for him.

These incidents have in common the projection of teachers' wishes upon children. It is the teachers who want the children to follow the rules—sit in the circle, walk down the corridor, not throw the sand, wait for juice, go slowly in the obstacle course, find bead stringing easy. It is the teachers who want to timeout the child if she does not behave. Why do the teachers intentionally misconstrue children's intentions? Perhaps because they do not wish to appear to themselves and others as authoritative, controlling, and threatening. Teachers want to (and do) "make nice" with children; adopt a gentle, not heavy approach; avoid head-on confrontations, disagreement, and dissension; and establish an atmosphere of friendliness and harmony. Acting positively affirms a child's sense of well-being; acting negatively denies it. Perhaps, too, teachers believe that attributing better intentions to children will become self-fulfilling. That would be consistent with their efforts to instruct by giving information.

Praise, discussed more fully later as a major technique to control behavior, also distorts children's feelings—the approval is often a command. "Good sitting" means "keep sitting, do not get up, you must sit." It may be delivered after a child has been bad (i.e., not sitting), so that the child hears praise in the context of a reprimand. Similarly, when a child is told "good trying" after doing poorly, the praise conflicts with his own disappointment, which often is not acknowledged. Teachers would never say, "That coloring job wasn't too good, was it?" They are so reluctant to be negative that many inhibit dispensing simple orders such as, "You must sit, you must not run" and replace it with "I can help you sit" and "Good walking."

The distortions may seem harmless—after all, they represent a manner of talking that adults use with children all the time. But before shrugging them off, think of the message. If a teacher says, "You must sit, like it or not," she is bluntly exercising adult authority and leaves the child free to oppose the demand, to be angry, sulky, and resistant. The child knows the teacher disapproves and can nurse his wounds or resentment. Failure, disappointment, and disapproval are part of life. Every child and adult experiences them regularly. To "protect" children from negative feelings and reactions distorts their reality and, conceivably, makes coping with the inevitable negatives in life more difficult. When teachers mask their superior authority by complimenting a child for his unwilling submission ("that's nice sitting now") or distorting his intentions ("you want help sitting"), they are in fact saying, "You don't really feel what you feel, you will feel what I tell you to feel." Denying a child the authenticity of his own drives seems a particularly bad form of brainwashing. It is respectful and honest to set limits, rules, and structure, and to enforce them with approval *and disapproval;* it is disrespectful and dishonest to tell children they *want* to follow the rules when they do not, or that they are good and doing well, when they are bad and doing poorly. The distortion is particularly hard to defend when directed at children who are weak, powerless, and rather easy to manipulate.

CONTROLLING BEHAVIOR

The above techniques—"cheating" for children, dominating activities, using the competent, distorting intentions—obscure the low functioning and immaturities of retarded preschoolers. They cast a patina of near normalcy on the children who, in their responses to questions and use of materials, seem to be acting very much like nonretarded children. Never mind the slippage that would occur if the teachers stepped out of the room; what shows up on the tests, in the reports to parents and administrators, and in the teachers' own internal ledgers, are the accomplishments, however marginal. These techniques are double-edged. At the same time they bring out high-level performance, they also inhibit spontaneous, albeit low-level, behavior. It could be argued that the following techniques—tight scheduling, high adult–child ratios, heavy positive reinforcement, restricting the permissible—also have the same dual function, but I have organized them separately because they seem more explicitly methods of control.

Control through Schedules

The daily schedule is a powerful tool for teachers to modulate and regulate children's behavior. Frequent prescribed changes of activity keep children's behavior from exceeding carefully constructed boundaries.

Every early intervention program I visited is broken into a series of scheduled time blocks. On paper, periods extend from 15 to 30 minutes, but in actuality they are shorter because of transitions. In a 2½-hour program there are, typically, six to eight scheduled periods: toileting, free play, circle, food, work time, gross- and/or fine-motor. Found less universally, not always held every day, and sometimes inserted into the more traditional set, are periods for language, story, art, music, and sensory integration. Schedules are complicated further by the children's standard therapies (most commonly, occupational, physical, and language). Therapists work through "pull-outs," with individuals or small groups in the classroom, and, occasionally, with the entire group. They also give teachers activities to carry out, and consult with parents. Although every program I visited offers some specialized therapy to each class, who receives it, and how frequently, depends on the school's resources and the child's needs. This makes scheduling quite complex. The therapies, seen by teachers and families as essential components of early intervention, add another layer of order and control upon the flow of events. The therapists have a large number of clients and minimal flexibility. When Doreen is due for physical therapy, she will have to stop her mirror play.

Schedules serve many purposes. Most obviously, they give teachers a framework for insuring that activities they want covered will be covered—songs will be sung at circle time, IEP objectives covered at work time, etc. Schedules enable teachers to guarantee children a variety to each day—a chance to play, a chance to work, a large group time, an individual time. Schedules create predictability for teachers and children, a routine gets established that many children internalize—everyone knows after juice comes quiet time, so they need not be reminded to get a book after throwing away their cups. Consistency, structured expectations, and familiarity increase the security of children. Boundaries and frameworks provide safe spaces that can encourage children to be more expressive than an unregulated unpredictable environment.

But as schedules become tighter and more rigid, they also restrict behavior. They strictly define an established order to which everyone must conform. Children and teachers alike rush to complete a project before a scheduled time period has elapsed.

A firm schedule can seriously limit children's freedom while getting the teacher off the hook. It is the schedule, not the teacher, that must be obeyed—"it is *time* to sit," not, "*I want* you to sit, *I want* you to clean up."

Periodic mandatory shifts break up any difficulty a teacher may be having with a child, keep the teacher in firm control, and keep children quiescent. They serve to dam overflowing behavior, while preserving the calm steady rhythms of the day. If Molly cannot tolerate circle and darts away, no matter, after a few incidents the start of another activity will curtail this behavior. If Heather is creating a disturbance during free play with her banging and dumping, Teresa can take heart that soon she will be pacified by work time. Children's excitement with their block play is limited by the need to clean up and move on after a few minutes. To stop the children, Teresa does not have to denounce them or even give orders. She merely states, "It is time to . . ."

Transition routines that book-end each individual activity put a further brake on children. These requirements—laying out materials, putting away materials, sponging tables, toileting—occupy a significant amount of time and are an effective means of keeping children obedient to external demands. Teachers may consume 10 minutes out of a 20- to 30-minute period with these tasks, if there has been a messy activity and children participate in the wipe-up, if teachers have the children collect and properly replace all the bits and pieces of their toys and puzzles, if there is a lot of toileting to be done—even when children cooperate and teachers are efficient. Then, after clean-up, teachers consume more minutes moving children from one part of the room to another, getting out new materials and giving out new instructions. For activities scheduled in another room (e.g., bathroom, gross-motor, art, music), there must be a line-up or assembling by the door and a prescribed procedure for how to move the group, often encumbered by wagons and wheelchairs. And usually there are laggards or break-away children who protract the transition even more. A child takes advantage of an unsupervised moment to go after a coveted object, another spills an entire cannister of blocks on his way to the shelf. During the transitions, children are either complying with instructions or waiting for others to do so. Waiting occupies a lot of time: they wait for activities to begin, they wait while activities are finished, they wait while disruptions are handled, and they wait for their turn during a teacher-led activity.

Teachers tighten their control over children even more by breaking up a single short activity into numerous, still smaller, subactivities. It seems there is always more to do than can be done in the allotted time frame. The rush to complete, very characteristic of the programs I visited, combined with the complex sequence of steps within each activity, creates a powerful pressure to keep children at the imposed task.

> A creative teacher has children sit and watch while she sets up a gross-motor activity. First, they are to step through a series of hula-hoops, then jump in and out, label the colors of the hoops, and finally throw beanbags at animals she has placed inside the hoops. Of course the children cannot remember the sequence, so the teacher continually reminds them: "Now step in . . . now jump . . . what's this animal . . . hit the bear with the beanbag . . . ," etc.

> Teresa, during art, in the course of just a very few minutes, asks the children to paste a precut table onto construction paper, paste plates onto the table, cut out and color paper food, and paste the food onto the plates—and all the while she questions them about what shape, what color, and how many. By snack time, the art project is still incomplete, and the teachers must hurriedly finish it themselves. The steady stream of commands and the quick pace have helped to keep the children on task and on time.

Short time periods, punctuated with set-up and clean-up rituals, and numerous small tasks to be accomplished within each period, also hide children's incompetence. The teacher must continuously direct the child. If a child starts to have trouble, the teacher must assist; there is no time to let him flounder or spiral downward. The fast-paced schedule provides a momentum that suppresses all off-course behaviors.

At Midwood the schedule is omnipresent. Nothing lasts long. Free play is sandwiched into 5- or 10-minute slots—after arrival and before circle, after snack and before work.

> The children arrive at 8:30, enter the room at 8:35, take off jackets and have toileting. When done, they have free play. But at 8:50 Teresa interrupts to tell them it is almost time to clean up and at 8:55 she dims the lights to indicate now it is time to clean up. Circle time, which lasts from 9:00 to 9:20, has multiple subcomponents—greeting, calendar, weather, six songs, a grab bag. Teresa directs each of these, while the children sit and wait for their turn. Art goes from 9:20 to 9:40, but it, too, is shortened by the need to herd children to their preassigned groups, bring out material, return material, and clean up. From 9:40 until 10:00

children get their snack, clean up and have free play. From 10:00 to 10:30 there is individual and small group work time and another clean-up. From 10:30 to 10:50 the group is divided in two, and each half has the obstacle course, a Play-Doh opportunity, and another clean-up time.

In this scenario there is not much opportunity for trouble to develop, but there is also not much time for a child to probe her own capacities and interests as they intersect with outside opportunities. Children are not usually finished with what they are doing when the lights flicker to indicate a period is ending. At Midwood, for example, Doreen was not satiated with mirror play when first period ended. She would have liked to linger, admiring herself in the glass. Molly, too, gave no indication that she was through moving blocks from shelf to truck, to floor, to shelf. Both girls needed reminding to be "all done now," and come to circle. David was deep into cookie-making and Doreen into sponging when Anita insisted they attend the obstacle course. The teachers' common practice of issuing warnings that a period is soon to end, is a likely result of the children's reluctance to make the switches. The teachers' warnings support my own observations that children's activities are often prematurely terminated. The justification for demanding the frequent shifts is that these children tend to get involved in "nonproductive" (i.e., low-level) activities and, for their advancement, need the stimulation of the next planned curricular period. Yet it is curious that in a population where "attention deficit" is a widely cited problem, the teacher so often interrupts the engrossed, attentive child.

Adult–Child Ratios

Teachers exercise control indirectly by observing tight schedules and, more directly, through the close monitoring afforded by high teacher–pupil ratios. Teacher–pupil ratios are formally set by state law and vary somewhat according to the particular state and level of the children. However, due to high levels of absenteeism in this young population, the official ratio is rarely the actual. I calculated the adult–child ratios in 27 classrooms (a few were omitted because atypical circumstances on the days I visited would have increased the average even further). The lowest ratio, observed in two classrooms, was one adult to four children. This was balanced by a ratio of 1 : 1, also in two classrooms. *The average ratio was one adult to every 2.2 children.* A few of the adults were volunteers, foster grandparents, or retarded young adults; but the usual pattern was a teacher, two aides, and six or seven children (of perhaps nine actually enrolled). Such ratios allow for a high level of adult supervision and monitoring. We have seen at Midwood, with eight children and three adults, how rarely the children are free of tight oversight. At circle, two adults are seated behind the eight children. But since Carl cannot move, Stephen, Larry, and David do not care to move, and Austin is always oblivious, two adults can hover behind the three moderately retarded children who are likely to be disruptive—Heather, Doreen, and Molly—while Teresa tries to control the group from the front. The only time a child can make an unobserved move is when the adults concentrate on a single child or get busy setting up and cleaning up.

Conscientious teachers like Teresa know every move a child makes and anticipate the next move that each is likely to make. They believe their professionalism obligates them to intrude at the slightest indication that a child is deviating from course. They want to head off trouble and keep the child accomplishing tasks. Many children, on the other hand, crave privacy and freedom. One sees them hoarding a batch of materials, retreating to a corner, looking over their shoulders to see if they have gotten away without being noticed. It is tough on these children to be constantly under adult oversight.

Because teachers are asking children to produce beyond their capacities and interests, and there is a real risk that the children will relapse into toddler-like pursuits, teachers must remain hypervigilant at all times. They cannot, following a more usual instructional pattern, introduce an activity and then take a back seat, or intrude early in the year but less and less over time.[1] It is impossible, given their mission, to leave children to their own devices and simply come when summoned, as is done in many regular day-care programs. We have already seen the many forms of this hypervigilance. Teachers maintain a close physical presence, sometimes holding children in their laps or on small chairs. Teachers demonstrate what they want children to do and lead them through the tasks. Mostly, teachers regale children with verbal suggestions, directives, questions, and explanations. While directed to elicit correct, high-level responses, the nonstop talk also holds a child in check. At snack time, for example, a teacher in one program prevented children from getting silly, messy, grabby, and touching each other by asking in quick succession: "What do we drink with? . . . What do we eat with? . . . What do we need for the applesauce? . . . Which cracker do you want? . . . What color is it? . . . Is it a cookie or an elephant? . . . Which is bigger, the cup or the can? . . . Do you want more cracker or more juice? . . . Is the juice cold or hot? . . . Do you like it hot or cold? . . . Is the table wet or dry? . . . What should we do if it is wet? . . . Where are the crackers, in the cupboard or in the sink?" etc. To increase the likelihood of a response, teachers embroider the talk with animation and drama; laced through it all is a pattern of repeated praise that further reins in children.

Positive Reinforcement

Without doubt the most widely used technique to control children is positive reinforcement. Going down a school hallway, one can always identify the special ed preschool room by the phrases "good sitting," "good using your words," "good helping" coming through the door. Everyone does it, knowing that approval is fundamental to a child's sense of self-worth. Children seek it, and so praise becomes a potent means of manipulating them. But teachers heap so much praise on children in early intervention programs that, like excessive chocolate, the sweetness may lose its power to gratify.[2]

Praising children is a tricky business. To understand its use in early intervention centers, we need to distinguish between praise that rewards a child's achievement and reinforces his pleasure in it, and praise, without achievement, that disguises a command. A child comes to his mother flushed with satisfaction and presents her with a clay sculpture. He is pleased with his product and pleased to present a gift. Her "Wow, that's wonderful," acknowledges and resonates with his own pleasure and perceived competence. She certainly reinforces his action—and can expect more gifts as a result—but because her remark concludes a long chain of events, it leaves intact his pride of accomplishment. Very different from this shared rejoicing is praise prior to any accomplishment—for instance, at the initial point in the chain of events ("good looking at the pictures"), or before the chain has started ("good sitting," "good listening"). Heaping praise on a child when he is not feeling pleased or even looking for an adult judgment, undermines that child's personal authenticity. It only thinly masks the true message: "Do what you're told, don't be disobedient." In early intervention, teachers praise children for each step in a task, for the steps leading up to a task, and for not being out of step. They praise children for poor work and overpraise them for ordinary work. They give them bits of food and stickers, stamp their hands, and add links on a chain just for not misbehaving.

> Cessation of naughtiness gets rewarded: "I like the way you've stopped hitting . . ." "That's good not kicking back . . ." "You're a good boy for not crying anymore."

> Simple compliance gets rewarded: "I like the way you're waiting your turn . . ." "I like the way you're being quiet . . ." "You're sitting nicely. Good keeping your hands in your lap . . ." "I like the way you're using your listening ears."

> Any effort to respond, right or wrong, gets rewarded: "Good try . . ." "Good pointing . . ." "Good coming up to the board . . ." "Almost right . . ." "Good trying to remember."

> Effusive praise often accompanies a correct or near correct response: "I'm so proud of you . . ." "You're so smart, you're almost ready for college . . ." "I don't believe how great you are . . ." "Nice pouring. Great pouring . . ." "Beautiful, gorgeous cutting."

At a certain threshold, the constant outpouring of praise works against what it is designed to promote—self-worth. The child is not given a chance to evaluate his own efforts, to move on from experiences of disappointment and discouragement, to differentiate on his own a good from an inferior production. Teacher approval becomes a substitute for child effectiveness. Praise inflation, like grade inflation, equalizes all efforts and discourages initiative. Too much external praise saps a child of his native motivation. In this atmosphere of excessive, nondiscriminating evaluation, the child is deprived of neutral space to work or play as he is inclined, without the direction of adult commentary. It is as if the teacher is saying, "Since you cannot do much, I'll praise your effort and compliance" (which explains why there appears to be so much less positive reinforcement in classrooms for nonhandicapped children, who accomplish more). When constant praise works, the child becomes addicted, looking to the teacher for approval after each subcomponent of an action and waiting for approval before making the next move.

Narrow Realm of the Permissible

Much of what toddlers do naturally, and do regularly in their homes, is either forbidden or confined to special times and places in school. By limiting what is allowable at school, teachers have yet another device to minimize disruptions. Basically children are supposed to act a lot like teachers: curb their emotional and physical responses; maintain a positive, calm, patient manner; keep to the assigned task; abide by the rules of collective living with consideration and patience.

There are physical restraints: Children are not allowed to climb, kick, and run (except in gross-motor or outdoor play); crawl under furnishings or into spaces (ovens, doll carriages, cradles, cubbies); climb on top of furnishings (tables, bureaus, chairs, shelves); touch themselves or one another; throw material (except balls and other objects made for throwing, and then only at certain times); wander without purpose; leave (circle, work, the room); shift objects from one place to another, particularly if they are removed to another section of the room (from fine-motor to gross-motor enclosures); mouth or smell (except when it is snack time or there is a lesson in smells); yell, cry, or tantrum. Even sitting on the floor, rather than in chairs, is prohibited in many centers.

There are behavioral restraints: Make no mess (e.g., mix up toys, dump puzzles, spill). Do not grab. Use words rather than hands. Respect the property rights of others—no taking another child's toy, no interrupting another child's play. Always be mindful of adults, listen and follow their commands until the adult releases your attention. Sit and wait—for your turn at circle, for the group to leave the room, for a teacher to help. Follow the daily routine and postpone preferred play. Clean up after each 20–30 minute period. When playing, do so appropriately and with the toys specified. Sometimes the materials children like best—sand (rice, beans, water, whatever is in the tub), jungle gyms, slides, rocking boats, trampolines—will not be present or, if present, not available. The toys that are plentiful—toys with small pieces that stack, sort, nest, fit together, and are designed to help children learn colors, shapes, sequences, part–whole relationships—may require adult supervision. Art material such as paint, crayons, paste, Play-Doh, and, to a lesser extent, housekeeping material, also may require heavy adult supervision. In the context of all the rules, both explicit and informal, the "choices" children are given—during option time they get to select in which of the open centers they care to participate—are very restricted. There is not a whole lot of elbowroom.

There are input restraints: The curriculum is very repetitious. It is not just the recursive schedule but the very same lesson material that is gone over day after day. I have described the privileged status of such items as colors, shapes, numbers, three-piece puzzles, and a small set of verbal antonyms. What makes this material so tedious is that, despite teachers' ingenuity, it does not admit of much variation. Teaching colors is not like teaching sand play. The child either knows or does not know the color. Despite the inventiveness of teachers—associating red with fire while dramatizing heat and sweat, or blue with cold while dramatizing shivering, etc.—the thing is either red or not; it is a thin bit of learning.

SUMMING UP

No one could pass through early intervention programs like Midwood without being struck by the atmosphere of good will and kindness. It is a rare teacher or aide, whether experienced grandparent or recent graduate, who is not conscientious, generous, and caring. Early intervention teachers are either a self-selected lot, or the tender ages and disabilities of the children bring out their kinder selves. There cannot be a group of more earnest professionals. Yet I have described a rather grim environment lurking just under the surface of smooth, orderly functioning and good will, unnatural and strained, where children are unduly repressed and teachers unduly authoritarian. Teachers, from my observations, are trapped by a curriculum that is both too tough and too remote for the children, who inevitably resist it. Caught between the conflicting demands of curriculum and of children, teachers have put in place a range of techniques that, while wrapped in cotton batting, severely curtail the natural, spontaneous desires of children. The techniques manage to keep the operation going smoothly in the face of inappropriate demands; they make children with retardation look more proficient and keep their behavior in check. But it is no gift to children when we deny and distort who they are, what they feel, and what they can do.

I have identified eight different techniques—and the list is not meant to be exhaustive—that teachers use to elevate performance and control behavior. The division between performance and control is somewhat arbitrary, for each technique, to some extent, serves both. But the first four techniques seem more performance-related, and the last four, more control-oriented.

1. Teachers cheat for children by structuring questions so as to get the right answers. By offering just two choices, by facial expressions, by leaving only one word out of an answer for a child

to supply, teachers make it hard for children not to be right. But the "right" answer under these circumstances does not necessarily mean any genuine learning has occurred. The cheating turns many learning episodes into a sort of game where the challenge for children is to pick up on their teacher's hints. This becomes embarrassingly evident when the teacher gives an absurd choice—"Is it ice cream or an elephant?"—and the child picks the wrong one.

2. When heavy coaching is unsuccessful, teachers will take over the task themselves and use the children as aides. They thereby shift the normal relationship from teachers supporting children, to children supporting teachers, and place the children in a more passive position.

3. In pursuit of their too difficult curriculum, teachers turn regularly to the more competent children. They, at least, partially answer the questions and serve as proxies for the entire class. The slower children may try to hang on by watching quietly, imitating movements when they cannot understand language, narrowing their focus to a close neighbor, close object, or their own bodies. Others will misbehave during sessions in which they grasp little. They, then, are managed by teachers, while the more advanced children are instructed.

4. When children disrupt the routines, teachers often cast the best light on the meaning of their behavior by reinterpreting their motives. Thus a child who is fed up and wants to do something else is told, "You want (or need) help in sitting." The teacher is saying, in effect, "You must not feel uncooperative, you must not feel like running." Such distortions may make life look sweeter on the surface, but they deny children the authenticity of their subjective feelings.

5. Teachers harness children's potential run-away actions by organizing the day into a tight fast-paced schedule. Frequent transition times, with the required cleaning up and getting out materials, act as barricades against out-of-line behavior. The interruptions also prevent children from pushing an activity and themselves to a natural point of completion or satiation.

6. Teachers maintain their high level of vigilance over the children through extremely high teacher–child ratios. It is hard for a child to misbehave when he may share the supervision of a teacher with only one other child. The ratios permit a great deal of attention to children, but they prohibit much chance for privacy and freedom.

7. By raining reinforcement on the children—not just for

works completed, but for the first moves in a task, or for simply not misbehaving—teachers exact conformity to the curricular demands. But they also cultivate an investment in teacher-pleasing and answer-guessing rather than in work and self-evaluation. Children turn outward for appraisal rather than inward for ideas. This is especially problematic for a population known to be passive and low in ideation.

8. Finally, teachers keep control by cordoning off the permissible to a narrow set of school-acceptable behaviors. Much of what children do spontaneously and out of school is banned.

This all adds up to a lot of control, but is it too much? No child can ever adapt to a civilized world without a great deal of restraint, shaping and, yes, manipulation. The debatable question is how much restraint at what ages is good for which children, and the further question—what is it we mean by "good"? If restraint leads to more colors learned but less curiosity displayed, is that "good"? If restraint leads to more obedience to school demands but also more passivity and lassitude, is that "good"? Is there too much restraint for a group of children known to be at high risk for attention failures, for low initiative, for a low sense of worth, and for impoverished ideation? What is the trade-off between social conformity and self-expression? We return to these difficult questions in Chapters Ten and Eleven. The point of this chapter was to describe the kind and degree of controls required by teachers when they transform retarded preschoolers into toddler–students.

Assuming teachers are bearing down on children excessively, we are still left with a fundamental question: Why would conscientious professionals develop an unnatural authoritarian superstructure to support an inappropriate curriculum? Part of the answer to this admittedly perplexing matter is that teachers have a lot less instructional choice than one might assume. Their day-to-day lives are controlled by a number of forces that have as a common denominator the press to accelerate children's progress, to make them look smarter, more normal. These pressures, described in Chapters Seven and Eight, force them to introduce items that are beyond the children's comfort level. A second explanation, discussed in Chapter Nine, is that teachers and administrators operate under some questionable psychological premises about mental retardation, learning, and development. Together the pressures and premises are responsible for creating programs in which teachers dominate and students fail.

CHAPTER SEVEN

External Pressures
for Acceleration and
Cultural Transmission

> As policies are more and more centrally determined, abstract
> and salutary goals are reduced and trivialized, and only
> those goals which can be measured are implemented . . . In
> the drive to make educational institutions accountable, goals
> have become narrow, selective, and minimal . . .
> Reductionism is also caused by efforts to give operational
> meaning to words which appear in legal documents . . . The
> exigencies of the policymaking process, together with the
> limited technology for making policies, cause policymakers to
> adopt a narrow view. Their personal goals for the elementary
> schools may be not only to teach basic skills but to instill
> the desire to learn and to develop the potential of the child
> . . . In the real world of policymaking, however, these larger
> goals are not integral to the process.
> —WISE (1979, pp. 58–59, 61)

Teresa and her colleagues have not sat down, like modern
platonic philosopher kings, to devise ideal programs from the
universe of beliefs about how handicapped children grow and
prosper. The balance they have struck—toward restraint and away
from freedom in preschool special education—may be more the
result of external pressures and embedded traditions than of rational deliberation, for in early intervention all the pressures flow
in the same direction, swaying teachers toward controlling rather
than liberating children. Their behavior is under powerful influences including social expectations for children's improvement
made specific in Public Law 99-457, highly specific requirements

for writing "objective" IEPs, demands imposed by schools and administrators, expectations of families with whom teachers develop close alliances, general traditions of teaching and specific traditions of special education. Personal beliefs and educational principles, along with other factors—such as personality, energy, aesthetics—naturally influence programs and contribute to their variety, but teachers also adjust their beliefs to the external forces and to the historical practices of the profession. No one can stand for long the discomfort of not believing in the enterprise, particularly when the work is difficult, tiresome, and poorly rewarded. For some, the task of reconciling beliefs and required practice is easy; what they have to do they believe in doing. For others it is awkward. They manage by the usual tricks we all employ to avoid psychological dissonance: holding onto vague popular slogans that mask our own uncertainties, blending ideologies that are fundamentally incompatible, ignoring the distance between theory and practice, and not inspecting too closely the unspoken rationales underpinning our behavior.

In this chapter I consider the more distant pressures on programs—expectations of the law, the IEP, the pressure to prepare children for integration, the rules of school buildings that bind programs even when their students are "special" (younger, slower). In the next chapter I review the nearer pressures—the hopes of parents who look to the teacher for encouragement and release from the pain of raising a handicapped child, the close parent–teacher working relationship, the special education tradition, and the beliefs teachers hold of their students.

What emerges from these pressures, as we have seen, are didactic classrooms devoted to accelerating progress through a cultural transmission model. Notwithstanding their sincere verbal allegiance to a "developmental model," to "self-esteem" and "fun," teachers, pushed to speed up growth, dominate classes (though always pleasant and praising) and enforce child compliance, adopt narrow preacademic goals and a behavioral technology. Children are held on a tight leash, programmed to perform very specific tasks. Anger, and even exaltation, are muted, the spontaneous is suppressed, not necessarily because teachers want it this way—though many have rationalized their practices as appropriate to the "needs of the retarded"—but because a larger set of forces is controlling their practices. The range of child and teacher expression is inevitably curtailed probably well beyond what is tolerated outside school in a family setting where external constraints are fewer. The picture is by no means uniform; there is a spirit of change in the field. Some teachers are complaining about the expectations, others are actively experimenting with new approaches and goals. But always teachers see the movement toward a less controlled, less accelerated, accomplishment-based curriculum as swimming against the stream of existing practices.

THE LAWS

It is quite clear that the public supports early intervention because of its promise to accelerate progress in handicapped youngsters. This is why in 1986 Congress generously granted an educational entitlement to young handicapped children (Public Law 99-457) that it has denied to normal preschoolers. It is one thing to insist that the disabled and nondisabled receive an *equal* education, as the federal government did in 1975 (Public Law 94-142), quite another to decide that the handicapped qualify for *more* (and more costly) education than others, as the federal government did in 1986 when it declared that the policy of the United States government is to give financial assistance to the states so that they may "develop and implement a statewide, comprehensive, coordinated, multidisciplinary, interagency program of early intervention services for handicapped infants and toddlers and their families" (Part H, Title I Handicapped Infants and Toddlers, Public Law 99-457, p. 3455). To justify this special funding, Congress found that

> there is an urgent and substantial need—(1) to enhance the development of handicapped infants and toddlers and to minimize their potential for developmental delay, (2) to reduce the educational costs to our society, including our Nation's schools, by minimizing the need for special education and related services after handicapped infants and toddlers reach school age, (3) to minimize the likelihood of institutionalization of handicapped individuals and maximize the potential for their independent living in society, and (4) to enhance the capacity of families to meet the special needs of their infants and toddlers with handicaps. (p. 3455)

This is the language of acceleration. Aside from the last provision, to support families, each "urgent and substantial need" refers to removing, insofar as possible, the deficits in these children. It is not the sort of rationale used for public day-care or even Head Start. The further one descends in ability, it seems, the heavier the obligation to accelerate. The purpose of day-care is merely to provide safe nurturing environments for children while their parents work. It is a mandate to protect. The purpose of Head Start is to enable disadvantaged children to achieve social competence. According to the regulations:

> The overall goal of the Head Start program is to bring about a greater degree of social competence in children of low income families . . . To the accomplishment of this goal, Head Start objectives and performance standards provide for: (1) The improvement of the child's health and physical abilities . . . (2) The encouragement of self-confidence, spontaneity, curiosity and self-discipline which will assist in the development of the child's social and emotional health. (3) The enhancement of the child's mental processes and skills with particular attention to conceptual and communications skills. (4) The establishment of patterns and expectations of success for the child, which will create a climate of confidence for present and future learning efforts and overall development. (5) An increase in the ability of the child and the family to relate to each other and to others. (6) The enhancement of the sense of dignity and self-worth within the child and his family. (Chapter XIII—Office of Human Development Services, Department of Health and Human Services, 1989, §1304, 1–3, p. 132)

Even given provision (3), the thrust of this mandate is to expose and enrich, not to correct.

By contrast, the purposes of early intervention are to reduce delay, reduce the need for later special education, reduce the probability of institutionalization and (clearly implied) save the taxpayer expenditures. The largesse of the legislators creates a heavy burden for early intervention.

Congress was willing to impose these standards and hold teachers accountable because they believed that research on early intervention supported their expectations. The 1985 Seventh Annual Report of Congress boldly declares:

> Studies of the effectiveness of preschool education for the handicapped have demonstrated *beyond doubt* the economic and educational benefits of programs for young handicapped children. In addition, the studies have shown that the earlier intervention is started, the greater is the ultimate dollar savings and the higher is the rate of educational attainment by these handicapped children. (Senate Report, 1985, 99-315, 99th Congress, 2d Session, p. 4, italics added)

Unfortunately the research evidence is by no means "beyond doubt." As James Gallagher, a long-time advocate for the handicapped, has stated:

> Keep in mind that these purposes—to enhance the development of the child, reduce educational cost to society, minimize institutionalization, and build the capacity of families to cope with their special problems—are only hypotheses. We have not yet demonstrated that any of these hypotheses are correct. (1989, p. 388)

The only long-term studies available to Congress are with *disadvantaged* children from Head Start or similar programs, not with the *handicapped*. Even with these "at risk" children the results are less than overwhelming. Sandra Scarr and Jeffrey Arnett (1987) summarized the literature on efforts to raise intelligence with disadvantaged children:

> The consistent result across the studies was that, although virtually all of the children were reported to have had IQ gains immediately following the intervention, in almost all cases this result was followed by a steady decline. Thus, in 1975, 3 or 4 years after the termination of the intervention, the IQs did not differ between the experimental and comparison groups. (p. 74)

In the same vein, a review of 210 research reports on the effects of Head Start programs by the U.S. Department of Health and Human Services (McKey et al., 1985) concluded:

> In the long run, cognitive and socioemotional test scores of former Head Start students do *not* remain superior to those disadvantaged children who did not attend Head Start. However, a small subset of studies find that former Head Starters are more likely to be promoted to the next grade and are less likely to be assigned to special education classes. (p. 1, italics added)

The accomplishments of Head Start are not inconsequential even if limited to a "small subset of studies." Better programs can be exemplars for weaker programs; researchers may find equal or more important benefits in the social and health areas that are tougher to document than IQ and achievement; it is unrealistic to expect that the benefits of a good year before first grade will not "fade out" over time (see Zigler & Seitz, 1980). But whatever Head Start may have accomplished, the findings do not put "beyond doubt the economic and educational benefits of programs for young handicapped children."[1]

Early intervention programs themselves have not yet generated any long-term studies; the endeavor is too new. We do know that, as with Head Start, short-term gains are common, but here too, it is entirely possible that the hike in test results will be diluted over time. An increase in how much children *know* at the end of preschool does not indicate changes in their *ability* to learn. This is particularly true in early intervention, where it is common practice for programs to teach to the test. When a child masters specific items (e.g., identifies three shapes) that have been taught, the child's improvement may be limited to those specifically instructed items. Once item instruction stops (or more general tests replace the curriculum-specific tests) other children, not beneficiaries of early intervention, will catch up. Retarded children followed over time with general tests of intelligence (albeit not necessarily beneficiaries of early intervention) generally maintain their level (IQ scores remain constant); that is, they develop at a retarded pace. (For a summary of this literature, see Goodman, 1990.)

Despite our uncertainty about the possibility and actuality of speeding up growth, early intervention professionals have joined ranks with the optimists in Congress. The name of the game is acceleration. Their goal is to give handicapped children the skills, behaviors, ways of coping and thinking, that are needed in the next, hopefully less restrictive, setting; to mold children so that they fit future environments rather than mold environments to fit children (e.g., Anastasiow, 1978; Bailey & Wolery, 1984; Salisbury & Vincent, 1990).

The eagerness of teachers to accelerate their students' progress translates quite naturally into a regime of prescribed instruction. A permissive, play-oriented atmosphere would obviously be irksome for staff intent on preparing children for kindergarten. Even if the handicapped do learn through exploration of their environment (and we shall see that most teachers believe they do not), the compulsion to increase the rate of learning along specific dimensions dictates highly planned instructional activities. Sand and water won't get the job done.

In addition to general statements in the law emphasizing acceleration of mental development—so that youngsters remain out of institutions, special education classes, and treatment by therapists—there are specific requirements to provide every child a written educational program and to educate children in "the least restrictive environment." These requirements further increase the pressure on teachers for skill development.

THE INDIVIDUAL EDUCATIONAL PROGRAM

Of all the strictures to be discussed in this chapter and the next, the IEP most obviously curtails the teacher's freedom to do what she wants in her classroom. It is a universal requirement—no program I visited failed to have one on file for every child. In the IEP, teachers must detail an individual program for each child of just what will be done by when. It is written and reviewed annually; signed by parents as well as school authorities; and should include (among other provisions) a statement of present levels (in each goal area), long-term annual goals, and "short-term instructional objectives," along with "appropriate objective criteria and evaluation procedures and schedules for determining, on at least an annual basis, whether instructional objectives are being achieved" (Public Law 94-142, p. 4).

Those who created the IEP had only the best intentions. They were professionals frustrated with the inadequacy of special education. Leaders in the field found—before the 1975 legislation—that children were labelled and shifted from one educational stream to another without academic benefit. Through the IEP they hoped to develop a means of making teachers accountable for their actions, instructional systems more finely attuned to individual children, the handicapped included in the lives of the nonhandicapped, parents involved in educational planning, and procedural safeguards guaranteed to families.[2] The IEP was the instrument to accomplish these reforms. It would make teachers responsible for what they taught.

The IEP was "not intended to be a detailed instructional plan" (Code of Federal Regulations, 1986, p. 87) nor a mandate for behavioral teaching. It has, however, turned out to be both. Through two key provisions—the requirement to state short-term objectives and evaluate them at least annually with appropriate objective procedures (Public Law 94-142), Congress unwittingly legislated "mandatory behaviorism" (Heshusius, 1986, p. 26). The insistence on establishing objectives that can be reliably *measured* forces teachers to concentrate on fairly narrow accomplishments that lend themselves to behavioral instruction. The requirement to write down in September what you want a child to accomplish by June, and to do so in a way that permits objective measurement, gives teachers little room to watch children and respond to their lead. Thus, although intended to measure progress and impose accountability from well outside the classroom, the IEP drives both curriculum and method of teaching.[3]

Were it permissible to write an IEP with nonspecific broad goals and subjective evaluation procedures, teachers would be freer to develop a range of instructional formats. A program committed to supporting and following children's interests, for example, might elect as a goal improved play patterns. Without the requirement to specify an exact outcome, teachers could watch what evolved over a year and make retrospective judgments. However, "increasing play" does not very readily satisfy the IEP requirement for "objective criteria and evaluation procedures" of "short-term instructional objectives." It is impossible to anticipate in advance just what behaviors will change. A child may increase his skill with a particular subset of toys such as blocks, display more interest in exploring unfamiliar toys on a shelf, become involved in pretend play, or make play overtures to other children. A developmentally oriented teacher who believes in the importance of individual initiative would support any of the emerging initiatives, since each of them represents progress, rather than project a particular area of gain. Because such a teacher would not know at the outset what direction the child's play might take, she would have trouble setting up her IEP objective and deciding upon "objective criteria and evaluation procedures" to determine achievement.

One rather awkward way to preserve an open-ended outcome is to compare extensive samples of behavior videotaped at the start and completion of an IEP period. But it is unrealistic to expect that teachers will have the time and skill required to code enough videotape play samples so that, for comparative purposes, they capture the same behavior twice. Quite naturally, then, even in the play domain, teachers select narrow objectives—using one of several toys, playing in the housekeeping center with the dishes, putting two toys together, etc.—and then plug away at them to demonstrate progress by the IEP expiration date.

Most teachers, faithful to the objective evaluation components of the IEP, predict behavior with unhesitating precision, as for example: "When exposed to a housekeeping setting, Johnny will pretend to feed the doll on two out of three occasions." Some waffle by stating inexactly the expected behaviors and measure progress in terms of *time* spent in an activity, as for example: "When exposed to a housekeeping setting, Johnny will play for 5 minutes."

This form of evaluation may pass muster with a local administrator but not an IEP czar. "Play" is too inexact and nonspecific a behavior, with probable low agreement between observers, to be a good "short-term instructional objective" capable of objective evaluation. Is Molly "playing" when she takes off her shoes and socks, pulls out the contents of her classmates' backpack, or touches David's arms? Perhaps, it is because of these definitional and measurement difficulties that even when play is important to a teacher it is likely to be a low IEP priority, taking a back seat to language and cognitive goals that are clearly specifiable and easily drawn from the developmental inventory used in assessing the child.[4]

Developmental inventories provide the ideal building blocks for constructing IEPs, given the obligation to establish long-term goals and short-term objectives that are a "logical breakdown of the major components of the annual goals" (Code of Federal Regulations, 1986, p. 84). For easy adaptation to the conventional IEP, authors of the inventories conveniently list, more or less by level of difficulty (there is no true ordinal sequence that all children follow; see Garwood, 1982), specific behaviors that are observable, measurable, and organized by domains (cognitive, language, motor, social–behavioral). Because each item is assigned an expected age range for mastery, the manuals suggest establishing a developmental level from the items passed, and a set of IEP objectives from the items failed.[5] Teachers find it convenient to follow this advice, though often they will supplement the inventories with objectives drawn from their own observations and from parent requests. In the following random examples, drawn from the expressive language sections of the inventories, the reader will note that objectives are narrow and highly prescriptive, teaching is didactic—the inevitable outcome of a requirement to prove success.

Portage Guide: "Repeats sounds made by others" (Bluma et al., 1976, Instructional Card I).

> (1) Make sounds that go with game or physical activity (i.e., while using pop beads, say "p/p/p"). (2) Say a sound like "ah" and tell the child, "say ah." Say it with the child and reward him with a goodie or praise—"good ah." . . . (3) Say various vowel sounds to child. Say each one several times and allow child time to repeat. Initially reinforce any approximation of the sound, etc.

Learning Accomplishment Profile: "Names three pictures of common objects" (Sanford & Zelman, 1981, p. 69).

Place page of pictures in front of child. Point to each picture in turn and ask, "What is this?"

Early Intervention Developmental Profile: "Child will combine two words" (Schafer & Moersch, 1981, Vol. 3, p. 70).

When a child says a noun, such as baby, change his statement to a question by asking him where the baby is, or if baby is crying.

HICOMP: "Can answer questions in the form 'What's _____ doing?' " (Willoughby-Herb & Neisworth, 1983b, p. 15).

[Adult begins] by asking about very concrete, observable verbs. Examples are:
    dog barking, "What's Barney doing?"
    playmate running, "What's Billy doing?"
If child does not answer with the *ing* form, model it and ask again. For example, to the first question, child says, "Barney barks." Caregiver says, "Yes, Barney is *barking*. He is *barking* and *barking*. What is he doing?" Reward the imitation of the *ing* form. (italics in original)

Brigance: Picture vocabulary (Brigance, 1978, p. 136). The following is a test item. If failed it becomes, without change, an IEP objective. No instructional advice is given.

The child is presented with drawings of 18 objects (e.g., dog, cat, key, girl, boy, airplane, apple, etc.) and the IEP suggestion is that the child will acquire _____ many words by a specific date.

The common practice of using the inventories both to generate IEP objectives and measure developmental level, contributes to acceleration pressures by inflating children's accomplishments. On an intelligence or aptitude test designed to assess ability (or functional level), individual items are selected opportunistically because they differentiate children by age, not because of their intrinsic importance or pedagogical value (Bailey & Wolery, 1984; Dunst, 1981; Garwood, 1982; Mahoney et al., 1989; Willoughby-Herb, 1983). The argument against teaching to them is that, although they are markers and even predictors of progress, they are in no way essential to progress; learning the items does not enlarge intelligence or competence. As Kohlberg points out: "Unless a predictor of later achievement or adjustment is also a causal determinant of it, it cannot [i.e., should not] be used to define educational objectives" (Kohlberg et al., 1987, p. 73). This is also true of the developmental inventories.

For example, there is no reason to believe that stacking blocks is an important ingredient of intelligence, as opposed to a proxy for intelligence. That is, although 2-year-olds can generally stack six blocks and 1-year-olds cannot, teaching the skill to a 1-year-old does not make him more 2-ish. By the same token, it may be that most 4-year-olds can name four friends, that most 8-year-olds can name four cars, that most 12-year-olds can name four beers and that most 16-year-olds can name four drugs. A child who has *incidentally* acquired this knowledge may be "smarter" than one who has not, but *teaching* the information will not make him smarter.

Developers of aptitude tests try to keep items secret, for when they leak out, and students learn the specific answer (without increasing their aptitude), the test is "ruined." A child who has learned a list of specific vocabulary words under a teacher's regimen, is not the equal of a child who picks up the same words in the course of everyday life, just as a high school student who studies the vocabulary list from the Scholastic Aptitude Test is not equal to the student who receives an identical score drawn from general knowledge. In the former instance, the test evaluates the success of specific teaching; in the latter, it samples attainments from a wide foundation of knowledge. When teachers and parents take as evidence of general "catching up" the mastery of specific skills drawn from developmental inventories—as happens when the inventories are both curriculum objectives and indicators of developmental status—they are likely to overestimate the child's capacities and will inevitably apply still more pressure on the child.

Teachers do some grumbling about the IEP and developmental inventories, but on the whole they have reached a qualified acceptance of both, despite the burdensome time demands these impose.[6] Even those teachers and administrators who advocate a developmental approach to learning—moving away from preacademic content (colors, shapes, letters, numbers)— struggle to make their beliefs fit the IEP requirement. There are a few radical critics who denounce it altogether because it forces them into a stilted, archly academic, overly precise, and uniform format. One teacher went so far as to say she believes in open-ended activities, not "results," and therefore would like truly global objectives such as "improvement in play skills." Other critics would settle for a modification of the current approach by making objectives a bit broader or less preacademic. For example, a teacher who believes more in socialization than preacademics suggests teaching children to say "hello" rather than colors; another wants to avoid teaching specific colors and substitute a general appreciation of color. Still, the complaints are mild. Only a few are ready to repudiate the IEP totally. The prevailing opinion is that it works to ensure accountability, helps keep parents and teachers on the same wavelength (though some teachers doubt the meaningfulness to parents, and most believe parents basically rubber-stamp), and provides a focus for planning, even when much of the classroom activity is outside the IEP. The dispute is less likely to be about whether the IEP makes for good education than whether it is better to teach objectives head-on during "work time" or nest them in classroom activities—for example, point out in passing the color or length of an object that a child is using. Here, in their own words, is the range of opinion*:

The resenters:

"I hate them [IEPs]. For us it's just a formality. We use computerized programs, but even so it takes 3 hours to do one. I don't teach to them. They have no place for the emotions. They just go into the file." . . . "I resent it, rarely look at it, find it artificial. Our objectives shouldn't be color learning, sorting, matching, but social things, like stand in circle, and say hello to a friend. They make parents nervous. It takes me seven hours to do one. They're a big pain in the neck." . . . "They encourage splinter skills like rote counting. We're now looking at more global objectives, less specific words and concepts. We'd like to substitute something like 'will improve in preacademics' instead of specific colors and numbers. Maybe add five additional colors but try not to corner ourselves as to which one. We avoid one on one, it's too stilted, and teach in groups so children will learn from each other."

And, at the other end of the spectrum:

"They are extremely important. All my instruction is based on the IEP. I check it weekly for planning and do data on objectives daily." . . . "I follow them very closely and don't do well without them. It's the centerpiece." . . . "We keep them front and central. I would like it for regular kids. It helps get parents to buy into activities and do them at home. The IEP is better than a report card. It makes us accountable."

*Here and elsewhere the ellipses separate comments of different respondents.

But the typical view is that they are a necessary, though burdensome, part of the job:

"It's a headache, but a necessary headache. It makes you sit with parents and plan. I do my small group planning around the IEP. Lots of functional skills—like lining up, manners—are not on the IEP, and we teach them, too. The problem is the paper work. We're burning out on paper work. The school should computerize the IEP." . . . "It gives me and parents an idea where the child is developmentally, for example, in matching colors, and forces parents and school to agree on priorities. It takes 3 hours to write one, but it's worth it." . . . "We need to be accountable to parents and there is no other way to do it." . . . "It's a tremendous burden, the paper work is horrendous, it takes 4 to 10 hours to do one, but it helps planning. We should eliminate the data recording and monthly progress reports." . . . "I incorporate objectives into activities so that there will be generalization, not splinter skills. I want the principle of stacking, for example, not the accomplishment of stacking three 1-inch cubes so we have the children do lots of things with blocks and learn to stack other materials. I don't want it to become rote, that is, a child sees a 1-inch cube and automatically stacks because that is what he has been taught. There's a danger in teaching to the test. We're moving from training to educating." . . . "We need a measure of what's going on, though colors are overrated. I use many of the usual objectives like matching, sorting, pointing. I don't necessarily teach to them, but I am aware of them. It might be good to have sequencing, like baby and blanket, and causality as goals. I could live without it, but it's a good record-keeper."

Parents, too, like the IEP. It gives them substance around which to communicate with the school, an opportunity to feel that they are participating, and an important symbol of the teacher's interest and concern. Although a few parents find it irrelevant and a waste of resources, theirs is decidedly the minority view.

The dissenters:

"I think people wear themselves out over the IEP. You can ruin programs with data collection—how many times he chokes or drools. There are mountains of paper work. The teachers can't even take the kids out to see the flowers." . . . "It's a lot more important to the teachers than to me. I never review it after our first meeting. I don't really care if he can stack 10 blocks. My daughter at 5 has trouble doing some of the puzzles they expect her to do." . . . "It's only useful for poor teachers. Good ones don't need it. It's not written for parents, too much technical language like 'maintain balance in rotational position.' "

The consensus viewpoint:

"The IEP helps in telling us what our expectations should be. I respect the professionalism of the staff and usually defer to them, but I know they are always open if I disagree with them." . . . "I don't know on a regular basis what happens at school. The IEP gives good information on what he can do and what we can do with him at home." . . . "Every 3 months I talk to them about progress. Every month I get a sheet of objectives, they constantly tell me how he is doing, like right now if he is tolerating different textures in his food." . . . "They go over him from head to toe. They push me to let him do more and not to give in to him. Some goals are unrealistic, like counting objects, but he meets many of them. I can always ask for what I want." . . . "I like the one-step-at-a-time approach, the way they systematically cover all the little steps before walking. In another program they tried to do everything. Here they narrow it down, and that's good. They always ask what's important to me." . . . "The IEP makes people look at her and forces me to look at some things I usually don't. It's necessary and keeps the staff accountable." . . . "I'm glad to have the goals written down, though it's not a bible. The school goes with the child, not just the IEP, and I trust them. But for accountability, I'm glad it's in writing." . . . "I like the process. Aside from the tasks, they take the trouble to know her personal characteristics. They give me something real to shoot for. It helps with other family members. They take it easy on her and stay patient when I tell them she's just at a certain level. It's good professional documentation." . . . "It's excellent. Everyone gets together and voices opinions. I wish we had formal meetings every 8 weeks to review goals. I like the format. It's a way of keeping my child challenged."

The IEP, deeply embedded in early intervention, has to all intents and purposes legislated behavioral instruction and a fairly uniform curriculum derived from a limited number of nationally accepted developmental inventories. The consumers do some complaining, but there is no revolution brewing. It gives teachers and parents a certain reassurance that children are headed in the right direction, accomplishing what they need to know for the next challenge. Checking off objectives that everyone perceives to be signs of developmental progress moves the child closer to the ultimate goal: successful integration with normal children.

MAINSTREAMING

Mainstreaming (also called integration or normalization) the handicapped is both the means through which acceleration is achieved and a demonstration of its success. Virtually everyone favors it.[7] Federal laws require that children be placed in the "least restrictive environment." Researchers in the field, state departments of education, parents, and teachers all approve. The argument is that isolating children in special classes has not been successful; the stigmatization has been greater than any dubious academic benefits. Separate education for the handicapped, as for any other minority group, is inherently unjust. Integration removes the stigmatization, provides handicapped children with good models to imitate, and increases mutual acceptance by exposing normal children to the delayed. A major effort to prove the effectiveness of mainstreaming, called the Regular Education Initiative (e.g., Reynolds, Wang, & Walberg, 1987; Wang, Reynolds, & Walberg, 1988) has attracted considerable attention and was enthusiastically endorsed by Madeleine Will (1986), former Assistant Secretary of Education and Director of the Office of Special Education and Rehabilitative Services. Although there is some controversy about the REI and integration generally (Kauffman, 1989), public policy is increasingly favoring it. Good or bad, mainstreaming provides still more momentum to transform handicapped into normal children quickly, so that they can adjust to more demanding environments.

Most of the parents I spoke with are strong supporters of mainstreaming. It could hardly be otherwise. For parents, integration is the path to normalcy. There are parents, even with severely handicapped children, who want their child entirely mainstreamed, others who want at least partial mainstreaming—a bit of both worlds. Some parents are ambivalent: they want it but have their doubts that it will work. Mainstreaming represents to them the promised miracle of a cure. They and their child will emerge whole and accepted. On the other hand, they worry that their child will be lost, isolated and underprotected. Here are their comments.

The enthusiasts:

"I like mainstreaming. It's wonderful to see the other children interacting with mine. They kiss her and love her. She enjoys it even if she just watches." . . . "I want him to be fully mainstreamed, that way he'll learn to talk, and that's his big problem.

If he goes into the mainstream I think he'll outgrow his difficulty, and no one will ever know he had a learning problem." [This child at 4 was functioning at the 18-month to 2-year level.] . . . "I want him mainstreamed, although maybe partially at first. I have a vision of college and marriage [a nonverbal 5-year-old autistic child]. Mainstreaming prepares our children for the real world. Normal children develop acceptance. Some day they will be hiring our kids, and they should be aware of them. They become friends. It degrades our children to put them in special class. People may make fun of them, but that's life."

Mixed feelings:

"I want my child mainstreamed, even if he just claps and laughs at the children. I want to see normal kids around him. I know he learns from them because I see how he jumps around when he sees his sister and my nephew and nieces. But he also needs a protected environment; in the mainstream I fear he may be forgotten. Even at our table he gets lost when the conversation gets going." . . . "I want as much mainstreaming as she can handle. I know it helps. She watches kids and then does what they do. But in a regular class she can't be a cheerleader or go to the dances. She won't be included in social activities outside of school. She needs half-and-half." . . . "It all depends on how well she's doing at kindergarten age. I don't want her falling further and further behind, at the bottom of the barrel. If she can hang in with the others, fine, but she needs to be successful. I know she can't keep up with her age-mates. I'd rather see her successful in special education than fail in regular education. I also don't want her teased by others. Even now, children ask, 'How come you can't talk?' and grab her toys. If it doesn't hurt her, fine." . . . "Integration is our goal, but you can have integration and no learning. Material must be adapted or everything goes by him. He behaves better in normal settings, but he doesn't learn as much. He should learn normal social skills through integration. Now he growls at kids. Some of them accept him and some don't. I expect him to have friends with and without special needs."

A small dissenting minority:

"I don't want her to be at the bottom of the barrel. She needs special education for security." . . . "I want him in a protected environment. Children in public school can be cruel." . . . "Better to have smaller classes with more structure."

Teachers, too, want mainstreaming because they believe it will accelerate children's progress and, at the heart of the matter, because they want the handicapped to receive the respect and be granted the dignity accorded all other people. However, they recognize, more than parents, that integration will not be effective without careful planning and monitoring. Almost every teacher that I interviewed gave qualified support for integration, preferring it for the higher functioning children, for part of the week, with careful supports, adequate staffing, and in the reversed format—normals coming into their programs. A very few were against it because the handicapped are isolated in a mainstream setting and receive less individual attention. In their own words:

"It's important to be with normal children as long as the special kids can handle it, but I wouldn't want to see a physically handicapped child put in a regular gym class." . . . "Some mainstreaming is important for everyone, even the severe and profound, who may just sit out in the sunshine with the normal children, but our children also need some separation to work on their skills." . . . "I would like normals around all day during these preschool years. Children are accepting and loving of each other when they are young. Our children should have less individualization and more experience of the real world. They might as well start getting along together now because they will be together forever." . . . "We need to have much more mainstreaming, but unfortunately the kindergarten teachers don't want it. However, in my own class I have a big range, which is good for the low children." . . . "I'm an advocate for mainstreaming in preschool but it is best for the mildly delayed. I love the compassion I see developing." . . . "Normal children are good role models for our children. With my really low children it may not be appropriate, but it would be worth trying a couple of days a week." . . . "Heterogeneous grouping is good, but you need to be careful. Sometimes I've seen the lower kids take a tumble. They get isolated if mainstreamed into a high-functioning group or treated like a doll. Janet always was the patient in our integrated class, but I intervened, and now the normal children ask her if she wants to be the doctor. I also had to help the other children be patient with Janet. I've seen changes in them, too. But you can't just dump. You have to place those children with a chance of making it gradually and selectively." . . . "Normal children are great role models. When I say, 'It's time to go out,' the normals get up and the retarded follow. Language is enriched. When I ask, 'What did you do yesterday?' the retarded children grunt and groan, but the normals speak up." . . . "The class is much worse when you don't have reverse mainstreaming. Normals spontaneously help the handicapped. They are effective as role models, especially in bringing up play levels. They are much better in the creative areas than teachers, and the retarded children will imitate them. The problem is in regular classes—there is not enough staffing to help the integration work."

A minority is more doubtful:

"I've seen integration fail. The Down's children just run about, the role models go off and play by themselves." . . . "Lower children are ignored or require constant facilitation. Every time the retarded child puts a coat on the rest of the class has to wait, or the teacher does it for him." . . . "I'm not sure what our children are learning from the others. They are in the same room but are not really mainstreamed." . . . "I'm nervous about mainstreaming because it waters down what we do."

Great efforts are made in early intervention centers to create mainstream experiences. Every day across the country, school buses are taking handicapped preschoolers to consenting day-care centers, or even to regular kindergarten classes, for part of the day. Some school districts have created reverse mainstreaming opportunities, such as buying slots for normal preschool children in special education classes; others have placed the special needs program on the same premises as a day-care center with frequent opportunities for mixing and separation; still others bring older nonhandicapped children from the regular classrooms into the special preschool program or send the retarded children into the regular kindergarten. Arranging what should be an easy matter— mixing together different kinds of children—becomes enormously cumbersome, expensive, time-consuming, and heavily bureaucratic, because it all occurs under public school auspices.

PUBLIC SCHOOL

Most of the programs I observed were run by departments of education and located in public school buildings.[8] This will be increasingly true as early intervention becomes an entitlement across the country. At the time of this study, 7 of the 10 states visited had mandated early intervention services for handicapped children ages 3 to 5; all of them were administered by education departments. Eleven of the 14 programs in these mandated states were located in schools. Generally, the schools like Midwood had both handicapped and regular elementary classes. The 3 states temporarily without a mandate for 3- to 5-year-olds used community centers and churches for their programs. Transportation was provided for all but two programs (nonmandated states). The most common solution to housing early intervention—also the simplest, least expensive, and most "normalizing" one—is to use vacant classrooms in elementary school buildings and transport the children in buses.

Although this format is probably the trend for the future, and therefore the educational implications need to be closely considered, a good deal of experimentation—and a good bit of bumping programs about—is now occurring as educational administrations struggle over where to place their early intervention classes. No consensus has yet emerged, even at the theoretical level. A building constructed for the exclusive use of preschool handicapped children, while fitting their precise developmental needs (no long corridors or distant bathrooms, plentiful appropriate equipment), isolates them. Placing them in a regular elementary school usually means mixing the mentally retarded preschoolers with kindergarten children (unless, through the waiving of fees, younger normal children are recruited). The special needs children located in these schools become the youngest, as well as the lowest functioning, pupils in the building, a deterrence to natural socializing. Administrators are trying a variety of creative resolutions to the twin problems of isolation and mismatching of children, but no one claims to have figured out a "best practice" plan. Regardless of the setting provided, each imposes its own behavioral requirements. Let us inspect the school setting constraints for Teresa's children at Midwood.

We start with the bus ride, a constant of almost all early intervention programs. In a bus children must sit and keep still. Physical restraint, forbidden in most settings, is required in a bus. A teacher will think long and hard before belting a child into a chair during the school day, but the bus matron has no such hesitation. However much one may believe in the young child's need for physical "freedom" and personal "self-expression," buses are not the place for their exhibition. When a child resists the safety requirements of the bus by moving or yelling too much, more restraints are added, often in the form of another paid adult. Here, as so often in these programs, the "needs" of the setting take precedence over any hypothetical "needs" of the child. An extended bus ride is often the only way to get to school, however "inappropriate" it may be for small handicapped children.

Once off the bus, new hazards await. Teresa has to get the children to class safely with a minimum amount of disruption to the surrounding rooms. In the corridor allowable behaviors, and options to control them, are limited. For example, when Doreen stages a "sit-down" in the hallway, Teresa may believe she should ignore Doreen and continue down the hall with her group, betting that as she withdraws her attention, the child's powerful needs for companionship will drive her to her feet in hot pursuit. But a noisy child pulling apart a diaper cannot be left alone in a school corridor, so Teresa begins her verbal cajoling—"Can I help you put away your diaper, Doreen? It's time to walk now. Floors are for walking on, Doreen. We can play in our room"—all to no avail. When talking fails to do the trick, Teresa has no choice but to forcibly put Doreen into the wagon and pull her along. Both the cajoling and physical handling are unnatural to Teresa. If moving from one room to another at home, she would tell Doreen, "Come when you are ready. I have to go now," thereby turning over to Doreen the initiative and control while avoiding a confrontation won through superior force. At Midwood she does not have the option.

Teresa also knows that Austin, preoccupied with sliding his hands along the grainy surface of the walls, is not taking in his social surroundings. It has occurred to her that if the doors they passed were vividly differentiated and the interior classroom activities made more obvious, Austin might begin to decipher the geography of the building. Yet she can hardly start painting doorways different colors and applying various textures, or opening up classrooms to Austin's inspection. Sometimes she has the impulse to take Austin by the hand and run quickly down the corridor with him, stopping abruptly at a door to dramatize the concepts of passage and arrival. But of course this would be an unacceptable breech of decorum. So with him, also, she is reduced to ineffective admonitions: "It is time to get to class now. We need to keep moving. Alice wants to see us. Hands belong by one's side." She has little choice. Principals need corridors that are quiet, safe, and adequately supervised, not places where children have temper tantrums and teachers run about. They also need classrooms that are neat, orderly, and reasonably quiet.

Even within her own room the school constraints continue to dictate codes of restraint over freedom. Teresa must minimize noise and movement levels so as not to disturb neighboring classes. The atmosphere in the classrooms I saw was subdued, restrained. Again, in a home setting Teresa might not object to Heather's banging and messy style of play—she is, after all, a clumsy child—but neat, orderly behavior is a long-standing school tradition. The room is crowded with materials that have many pieces and parts. These are easily mixed up or destroyed by a

Heather, leading to frustrating searches under cabinets and in boxes for missing pegs and color forms. If Heather is allowed to "act up," the seven other children in the room might imitate her banging and crashing. Teresa fears that if she relaxed the boundaries of the permissible for Heather, she would release a contagion of noise and mess that would soon bring complaints from other teachers and the principal, not to mention the janitor. So each time Heather spills the blocks out of the container, she must replace them; if she spills too much, if she continues to break the "rules," there is the timeout chair and removal of the toy. A child like Stephen who wants to plow through a tunnel quickly and jump from the top of the climbing structure to the beanbag, rather than descend via the slide, is cautioned to go slow, to be calm. The value is on safety, not risk-taking, on restraint and conformity, not spontaneous expressiveness. The school atmosphere affords little opportunity for letting the child's impulses play out, or for using more subtle methods to change behavior (e.g., having fewer toys with fewer pieces available to Heather, or providing a messy area that does not infringe on other children's activities).

Clearly, as evidenced by the constant need for teacher monitoring and redirection, the regime is hard for preschoolers with mental levels in the toddler range, and even tougher for those with noisy habits like Heather. Principals do not lose sleep over the requirement that a group of 3- to 4-year-olds, many functioning at half those ages, conform to rules established for 6- to 12-year-olds. Order and decorum are not negotiable issues. Even if self-determination and autonomy are highly valued, they must be carefully curtailed. Control over the major and minor events of the day is vested in the teacher and constantly exercised.

The larger environment in which Teresa works also forces conformity to rigorous time schedules. The handicapped preschoolers at Midwood and elsewhere share space and routines with the rest of the school. They have scheduled access to the gym, music and art rooms, playground, library, and cafeteria (if the children do not eat in their own rooms). Therapists with large caseloads have schedules they must keep with the children. Snacks and hot lunches may be distributed school-wide on a regular schedule. And, of course, the buses come and go at prescribed times, often with only 2½ hours between delivery and pickup. If Doreen and David have just started a game of putting each other to bed with blankets and dolls when it is time to clean up for snack, their play, however fresh and novel, must be interrupted. The distribution and consumption of snacks is an opportunity for language and social growth; other children already assembled cannot wait too long, the ordered sequence of daily events must keep on flowing. This means that, once again, Teresa will be pressing against children's initiative and self-regulation by ordering them, in her kindly way, to stop—"It's time to clean up now. It's time to get ready for lunch. That was nice playing you've been doing." School does not give children the unscheduled hours for improvised self-selected play and flexible meal scheduling provided by parents at home. Whether or not one thinks it is "good" to organize the activities of young handicapped children into 20-minute or half-hour time blocks, external pressures push programs in that direction.

SUMMING UP

The public support for early intervention, while very generous, is not disinterested. The commitment comes with an explicit expectation, written into the enabling legislation, that intervention will quicken the children's pace of development and prevent (or minimize) their becoming a future burden to society. Even though there is not much theory or evidence to justify that expectation, professionals and parents seem to have accepted the mandate. To ensure children's progress, Congress legislated the IEP requirement: for every child, teachers must write out an annual program that specifies exact learning targets and evaluation methods. By being task-oriented and specific, rigorous, objective, and data-minded, accountable and responsible, teachers supposedly will bring these children up to snuff. For all concerned, mainstreaming the handicapped by age 5 or 6 is the broad overall goal. Meanwhile, programs live in school buildings and must conform to school expectations (set, of course, for older and higher functioning children).

The pressures not to have children become a "future burden to society," to get them prepared for the mainstream, and to survive in an educational institution, all quite obviously push programs into an acceleration mode. Somewhat more subtly so, too, does the IEP. Because teachers, on advice of experts, lift instructional objectives from the tests that spell out a child's developmental level, small accomplishments are perceived, wrongly, as indicators of general growth—adding fuel to the acceleration fire. The programs' achievement and "readiness" emphases, as well as the need to prove progress, favor a behavioral model. Waiting upon children's interests and preferences, zigzagging with them and in response to them, staying on their level rather than elevating them to the expected levels—all are luxuries Teresa cannot afford. But the demands are not alien to her; she has incorporated them into her own professional mission. We turn now to the more internal pressures that come from the early intervention players themselves.

CHAPTER EIGHT

Internal Pressures
for Acceleration and
Cultural Transmission

I have seen Children at a Table, who, whatever was there,
never ask'd for any Thing, but contentedly took what was
given them: And at another Place, I have seen others cry for
every thing they saw; must be serv'd out of every Dish, and
that first too. What made this vast difference but this? that
one was accustom'd to have what they call'd or cry'd for, the
other to go without it. The *younger* they are, the less I think
their unruly and disorderly Appetites to be comply'd with;
and the less Reason they have of their own, the more are
they to be under the absolute Power and Restraint of those
in whose Hands they are . . . The *sooner* this Way is begun
with Children, the easier it will be for them and their
Governors too.

— LOCKE (1693/1927, p. 26, italics in original)

Pressures external and internal to programs nourish each
other in a seamless loop. Perceptions of the public that find their
way into laws are determined by, as well as determinative of,
parental and professional opinion. Teresa is a product of a special
education tradition that molds, and is molded by, the contemporary reformist spirit. Through Teresa that spirit is caught by
parents; they then reinforce (and make demands of) teachers. The
pressures to be covered now are those dictated by the expectations
of parents and teachers, the alliance forged between parents and
teachers, the special education traditions of didactic and group
instruction in the context of extreme child diversity, and the

beliefs of teachers about the nature of mental retardation and how to remediate it.

PARENT AND TEACHER EXPECTATIONS

Parents and teachers substantially agree on their goals for early intervention. Both place more emphasis on adjustment goals (independence, getting along with others) than on preacademics, which is not as close to their hearts as practice suggests. For parents, while preacademics make you look normal to school professionals, it is independence and appropriate social behavior that normalize you for the wider world. Parents, of course, yearn to see their children progress, particularly in language (almost always interpreted as speech). Talking is an entry-level requirement for normality. If you do not talk, you are out of the running; the problem cannot be hidden. Even parents who stress across-the-board improvement and acceleration, isolate language as their primary concern (referred to by teachers as the "number one concern of parents," and "the big thing"). But even more important than language or preacademics for parents are independence and social behavior. Notice, however, that the goals of doing for yourself and making it with others often translate into following the rules, and being obedient; not into having more freedom to learn from experience. The personal and social goals are consistent, for these parents, with behaviorism and acceleration:

> "I want Jimmy to be self-sufficient when I'm not here, to be independent, and that is what they are making him. I see him some day in a half-way house. He could stay with me, but I'd rather he do for himself. I know he will." . . . "What matters to parents are independence and self-sufficiency so we won't have to worry. We'll know our child can have a job and be self-sufficient. It's a tedious procedure, teaching him to do things for himself like picking up toys and hanging up a coat, but after a while if the teachers work with us, he gets in the habit." . . . "The goals are practical, and I like that. He will respond when his name is called, will say 'hello,' waits his turn without tantrums, comes when called." . . . "This year my goal is to teach him to be happy playing independently. I leave the preacademics to school. If they want to do them, that's OK, but I care more about daily living skills." . . . "We put our priority on social skills. Betty goes everywhere with us, but she couldn't if they hadn't helped her play with other children and get along with people." . . . "I care

about language and independence. At school they are sent to do errands, carry their own tray in the cafeteria, cooperate with others. That all helps a lot." . . . "Peter is good at letters, learned them at 3, but for me they are an unimportant splinter skill. Nonacademics, like not taking off and not having a tantrum at every transition, are more important." . . . "The cognitive is not a major goal. Actually, you can't teach him much because it requires too much repetition, but that's not a big concern." . . . "I want speech and socialization, especially socialization so that she will work and play well with others. Both are more important than preacademics (colors, shapes, letters, numbers)." . . . "Her progress is amazing. The doctors said she'd probably be a vegetable. She had 21 seizures a day for a week. Now she carries her backpack, follows commands like 'put your diaper in the trash,' even tries to help with her dressing. She's come a long way. I say 'Look at my baby' to everyone." . . . "I've seen progress. They taught him table manners and how to spoon out food." . . . "His attention span has improved. He can complete a task. They got him to obey and to look at books." . . . "We want him to be as functional and independent as possible. The school is always saying, 'Do it yourself, you can do it.' We want that, too. My top priority is walking. It's their priority, too."

The minority view supports across-the-board improvement, or places equal emphasis on preacademics and speech:

"I want her up to par for kindergarten. I don't want her to have learning disabilities all her life. She needs to learn speech and letters and numbers." . . . "I want to see more vocabulary development and more preacademics. Keep working on speech; push a little harder; but also do more academics like numbers and letters. Introduce her to the sounds of letters." . . . "I want him to relate to other people, communicate, and get him into things a 5-year-old would do better, like colors." . . . "My major goal is prekindergarten skills. She needs to do circles, know colors, count to 15, and stack blocks."

Teachers are quite focused on giving children the skills they need for mainstreaming. Getting a child into the mainstream is a personal triumph for the teacher, not to mention the thrill it gives the parent. *Pre*school, almost by definition, is preparatory to kindergarten, and kindergarten preparatory to first grade, so positioning them well at the start is critical to ascending the normal ladder. Being ready for kindergarten and first grade means, according to teachers, strengthening preacademic skills, and more importantly, personal (or "functional") independence, and social skills.[1]

> "I want to get them ready for a transition class and then for a regular class." . . . "Teach them the skills they need in the next environment. Even if a child cannot draw, he can make a mark on a paper; that's what's expected when he gets work sheets, and he better not eat the paper." . . . "I want them to be successful in kindergarten." . . . "I look toward the next environment and know they need to be more compliant, stay in their seats, count, take turns, and improve in speech, even if it is only single-word utterances." . . . "I want my children to survive in regular class—follow directions, listen, respond to limits, cooperate, share, be as normal as possible, learn words like over, under, behind, above, etc., because they are basic to reading."

Given the salience of the cognitive in the daily schedule, it was unexpected that teachers would rank preacademics well below other goals. Over and over, however, almost to a person, they, like parents, spontaneously told me that independence and appropriate social behavior are more important to the children's future success than cognitive skills. For teachers, too, independence and socialization are compatible with behavioral instruction. As they expressed it:

> "What's important is independence and social skills, which they get through reverse mainstreaming. I used to do more skill [preacademic] training and data collection, but there was no generalization." . . . "What matters are social skills. If children can answer questions, listen and follow directions, and react appropriately, it normalizes their whole life. We shouldn't worry so much about counting and A,B,C. If they can be polite, they have more opportunities than if they don't come when called, or run wild." . . . "I try to build up their social skills so they can fit into a regular class later. This means attending, sitting at a table, participating in some kind of language activity, sharing, and cooperating with others." . . . "I really stress independence. Attending is the big thing—sitting in a chair and paying attention, staying seated, and completing a task." . . . "I want the children to be independent. When they put their bags on a hook, express a need, make choices, find something for themselves to do, clean up, wipe their hands, they are achieving independence." . . . "I don't care what skills kids have. I want them to be functional. I don't care about pegs and little skills at 60% accuracy. I want them to be able to dress, potty, identify their name and colors, feed themselves, communicate, not string beads." . . . "We need to

develop functional skills—manners, lining up, saying the pledge, fixing a lunch tray, self-help. I'm not real big on academics." . . . "Our objectives should be functional; teach the child what he needs to function in the environment. We are at the point of a *paradigm shift*. Everyone is tired of teaching skills."

Unlike parents, however, teachers repeatedly mentioned as important the enhancement of self-esteem. That teachers underscore self-esteem as a conscious objective, rather than a derivative (like happiness) of good experiences, may explain why they do so much praising. In their own words:

"What's important is for kids to feel good about themselves and be independent and make social connections. There is plenty of time for [preacademic] skills later." . . . "I believe in self-esteem, though that conflicts with my behavioral theory." . . . "I think self-esteem is more important than the cognitive. The ability to sit, interact with peers, and be independent is more important than colors and numbers." . . . "I want them to have self-esteem, so I give lots of praise whenever that is appropriate. They feel better about themselves if you say, 'I don't like what you're doing,' not 'I don't like you.' "

Generally, teachers who discounted the importance of academic goals did not perceive any discrepancy between their practice and principles. Adjustment goals, not easily written into IEPs, can be attended to outside the IEP. A few, however, noted a tension between their beliefs and the demands of the IEP:

"I want these children to function in the community; that means getting along with others, being generous, kind, caring. Academics are less important than being content with yourself. Social goals, though, don't get on the IEP if you're not disturbed; the cognitive always does." . . . "It's fine with me if we do water and sand, but not in this community, not in these homes." . . . "I would like the children to have fun and feel good about themselves, but when the principal walks in, I better be teaching the IEP—that means red and blue."

Although teachers are remarkably unified in disclaiming academics as their primary goal, even while caring about mainstreaming, the "paradigm shift" may be more apparent than real. When specifying the route to their goals—self-esteem, appropriate social behavior, independence, or "functional" skills—teachers, here again like parents, regularly bring up compliant behaviors:

sitting still, following directions, standing in line, coming when called, manners, listening, waiting your turn, and especially attending. As seen in the above quotes, these virtues are sprinkled through their remarks. Obedience gets you ready for the next environment and is integral to independence, socialization, and self-esteem. This makes sense. A child who can sit still is more highly valued by others, requires less supervision, is more reliable and, in that way, more independent. A child who does what he is told will get along better with other children and adults, will receive more approval, and thus will acquire more self-esteem. But if compliance is the route to the teacher's objectives, no basic shift in teaching will occur. Instead, there will only be a shift in which end of the instructional seesaw gets stressed—sitting still and listening during color and number sessions, rather than actually learning the colors and numbers. A paradigm shift in the Kohlberg sense would come about only if teachers were to decide that the route to self-esteem, independence, and social competence is through more self-determination and freedom, with teachers, metaphorically, shifting from the front to the back of the room. If this happened, the widespread belief that preacademics are not of major importance might presage a change in practice. But such a change will be hard to pull off given the pressures described in this chapter.

THE PARENT–TEACHER ALLIANCE

Parents and teachers have forged an intimacy that goes beyond agreement on matters of procedure and conduct. Of course there are tensions. Parents cannot understand the IEPs that teachers write; teachers find parents unrealistic. But the discord is minimal, the closeness remarkable. Parents are deeply grateful to, and dependent upon, the early intervention staff. It is natural that teachers—all of whom have very low enrollments, responsibility for everything from toileting and feeding to language, and often the same children in their classes for several years—establish much more intimate relationships with both parents and children than is usual in schools. The ties are deepened by the helplessness and vulnerability of the children, their pariah social status, and the teachers' sincere commitments to the inherent worth of the handicapped. Objectivity and realism are discarded on both sides as parents overload teachers with their hopes and prayers, and teachers all but stand on their heads to bring about accomplishments.

Parents are thrilled with early intervention. Its importance in their lives is altogether of a different order from the importance of day-care to families. They see it as a life-saver, the first reprieve from the overwhelming sorrow, pain, stigmatization, loneliness, and terrible sense of responsibility that accompanies the birth of an abnormal child. That most parents eventually adjust and courageously, even cheerfully, go about their lives is a testament to the heroic potential in ordinary people. As much as any person who puts her life on the line to save another, they deserve society's admiration and tributes. But in the beginning, when the going is rough and cheer in short supply, it is the teachers and therapists who lend a hand by telling parents, in word and deed, "I like you, I like your child, I want to help."

This very strong tie creates obligations. Teachers earnestly want to make the lives of parents easier. They spend a lot of time calling, visiting and writing to them. They are nourished by the appreciation of parents and do not want to see them disappointed by a child's poor progress. Sometimes teachers very gingerly try to dampen an obviously impossible expectation, but usually they press hard to accomplish what the parents want, exaggerate the triumphs, and minimize the failures. The intimacy between them is yet another subtle pressure on teachers to accelerate children's development and to endorse the parents' inflationary thinking about their progress.[2] Let us look at what parents have to say about teachers:

"When you bring someone into the world who is imperfect, you feel guilt and pain, you feel ashamed; it's hard for me to believe that anyone can love my child. Years ago they'd have put these children in closets. Now they accept them." ... "My child can't do anything, but the teachers think he is a somebody. He waves his arms around, and they think he is trying to talk. I know he is not, but I'm impressed that they're working with him. It makes me feel so good when they greet him, when they get excited over some small something." ... "I was going nuts before I got into this program. I didn't know how much to stress him or not stress him. One thing was certain, I was all stressed out. Jill has given me reassurance and guidance and relieved my guilt." ... "They know my child really well. They know everything he does at home and at school. We write to each other every day. The feedback is fantastic. I know what he ate, when he pottied, who he played with. His father was impressed by how well they knew him." ... "The first day my child walked on his own, everyone at school called me. The whole staff was involved, even the bus driver was pulling for him. They all lined up outside school until I drove up. It's more than just a job for them. They celebrate his accomplishments as much as I do." . . . "Teachers of early intervention are like family. They come to our home. They take our kids into their home. This is so much more than a job. They love my child. It's like he has another parent." . . . "Now I'm not the only person responsible for my child and in the dark. I can enjoy being her mother for the first time in my life; I don't have to be her occupational therapist, physical therapist, speech therapist, and I don't have to lay awake at night and think I'm not doing enough." . . . "I'm astounded by what we've received. I get overwhelmed with everything you have to do with my child. I don't want to be tied down to the handicap every minute. The physical therapist does the exercises regularly, and that's a relief for me. They are so upbeat. They take one day at a time and tell me everything that happens." . . . "These teachers are the best. They make us feel so welcome. There's nothing they wouldn't do. We're here today because of them, not because of your book."

Parents appreciate the instruction they have received:

"They gave me cards with printed words to review, recipes for Play-Doh, tips on what toys to use, how to read books so that he is involved, how to let him struggle with a puzzle piece and not do it for him." . . . "They showed me how I was contributing to her problem by not making motor demands. They also gave us the list of signs they are using in school." . . . "I know I wouldn't have been able to handle my child without the program. I've never been around a special child. She has a bad temper. They taught me how to handle it. I don't know where I'd be without the program. It helps my whole life, period." . . . "They've taught me to see things through my child's eyes and to be more patient. They've made me a better person. Before, I would put cartoons on and leave the children. Now I color, write, cook, and pull weeds with them. Everything they do, I do, and if I don't get to cook, clean and sew, so what." . . . "The teachers are constantly giving me insights. Last year they sent home a list of toys, how much they cost, and where to get them. That's how I did birthday and Christmas shopping. I don't know what I'd do without them."

Parental optimism is infectious. Doreen's mother is typical. At first she dreamed of making her Down's child the "smartest, cutest, highest functioning one ever born." She gave up this dream but "we still have high hopes." The early intense efforts she and professionals are making, the newness of educating handicapped preschoolers, and changing social attitudes make the horizons a lot brighter. One parent of a Down's child told me: "I expect him to go to college, even get a driving license and a professional job. I see he picks things up so fast." Molly's mother at Midwood dwells on her good memory and believes that, in going through the backpacks, she was intentionally searching for Larry's candy.

All this adulation and these high expectations make it nearly impossible for teachers to tell parents the whole truth and nothing but the truth. Rather, parents and teachers have entered into an unspoken agreement to keep the optimism alive by not discussing the diagnosis, the future, the rate of progress, and to dwell instead on the accomplishments that feed the pride of both teachers and parents. Teachers pull the shades down over the future and focus narrowly on day-to-day behavior, on the small positive changes that tend to obscure the chronicity of the condition. Labels are out, obfuscation is in. Not "telling" produces high expectations and, again, more pressures to succeed. Parents report:

> "I know they used to call children like Andrew mentally retarded, but now they don't use those words. They call them 'developmentally delayed' instead." . . . "I'm not comfortable with the words, 'mentally retarded,' more so with the word 'Down's.' " . . . "We say 'delayed,' not 'retarded.' We don't consider her retarded. She looks younger than 3, but not retarded. We try not to look too far ahead. You can't predict her." . . . "I'm not sure she is retarded [a Down syndrome child]. She's developmentally delayed, or maybe she has a mental disability. I think maybe she'll end up as a child with learning disabilities because she can do some letters and numbers." . . . "We try not to think of the future. We use the word 'delay' mostly. Sometimes we use the word 'retarded' so our other child will understand, but it is not a word that comes out easily." . . . "I'm down on labels and IQ scores. They are not meaningful, and I don't care about them. The program docs not use labels."

Because teachers do not really know the probable rate of the children's progress, estimated by intelligence tests, their obfuscation of retardation is made easy. Despite their intimate knowledge of the children, teachers were mostly unable to report children's IQ scores. That is the business of psychologists, but psychologists have low visibility and low standing in early intervention programs. Occasionally a psychologist comes into the classroom to establish a behavior modification program, but mostly she is seen as a gatekeeper, someone the family must pass through in order to receive services, but of no use to the family in understanding or improving their child's condition. When parents and teachers talk of "therapists," they are referring usually to language, occupational, and physical therapists. These services are in great demand, and parents want more, but no parent ever told me she wanted more from a psychologist. Teachers are sceptical of evaluations that result in large-scale judgments based on small behavioral samples, especially when those judgments are discouraging.

As we have seen, teachers use developmental inventories rather than psychological tests to evaluate children and write IEPs. But, without reliable information on probable rate of progress, they have no reasonable way of judging how long it will take to accomplish a particular objective. That is, if an average child between the ages of 21 and 27 months learns 150 new words (Gard et al., 1980), how many should a mentally retarded child learn between the ages of 3 and 3½? Only if one knows the rate of development (i.e., the IQ) can one make a reasonable projection. Lacking it, teachers can only guess and, given the psychology of early intervention, usually expect too much too soon. When children do not meet expectations, teachers keep at the task rather than confront the inability. Persistent failures are attributed to disinterest, inattention, or uncooperativeness; small achievements are taken as benchmarks of general improvement.

To recapitulate, the alliance between parents and teachers adds subtly to acceleration pressure. Given the absence of any respected basis for predicting the child's rate of progress, and the tacit agreement among parents and teachers not to discuss such matters, there is little to curb turning wishes for rapid progress into objectives, and then explaining away failures. The system nourishes the hunger of parents for improvement and satisfies that hunger by having children memorize "advanced" preacademic facts (colors and numbers) through repetitive drills. Of course optimism is a good thing, but spiraling optimism can be as oppressive as spiraling pessimism (Gruber, 1973, p. 103). The pressure to accelerate is further strengthened by the professional traditions of teachers.

THE SPECIAL EDUCATION TRADITION

Didactic Instruction

Early intervention classes are usually headed by teachers with special education certification. Only 2 of the 10 states, both without early intervention mandates, did not require such training. Some states demand add-ons—early childhood or master's degrees—but special education is the fundamental certification.[3] The tradition of special education in this country is "clinical" and "behavioral": the teacher locates the deficit in the child and tries to remedy it by actively inculcating skills. Remediation is carried out by focused adult direction on specifics, using drill and rote learning rather than "discovery" methods. The vision of teacher as "facilitator," responding to children's self-initiated actions rather than demanding skill improvement, is not part of this tradition (Carta et al., 1991; Mowder & Widerstrom, 1986). Teachers teach, children learn; teachers provide, children receive; teachers have knowledge to impart, children have ignorance to eradicate. Teachers look to children for correct responses, not for personal discoveries. That learning is "constructed" though action (Kamii & DeVries, 1977; Kohlberg et al., 1987), that children must "make meaning" themselves (Kegan, 1982), that children learn only by actively transforming the material and by staking a claim on it, not through recitation, and that receiving information is not equivalent to learning—these are notions alien to the special education tradition.

Teresa has an instructional agenda for each child. She knows what they know and can do, and she knows what she wants them to learn. She cannot leave accomplishing the goals to chance encounters between a child and instructor. She cannot wait until Molly *asks* to be taught circle, square, triangle, and diamond. Molly might never ask. As another teacher put it: "I'm impatient. I don't want to wait for their discoveries. That's why I'm in education and not psychology." To meet her objectives Teresa must plan formal didactic sessions balanced with breaks, for she recognizes that young children have short attention spans and find long periods of sitting intolerable. But even during the free play and movement periods Teresa, as a conscientious instructor, tries to advance her teaching agenda. During obstacle course, for example, children learn to follow directions, sequence movements, attend, recall, wait, take turns, and inhibit impulsiveness. To balance all the program requirements, Teresa has developed a daily schedule similar to those of other programs: six activities over 2½ hours— free play, circle time for group instruction, art for fine-motor improvement, snack, small group for IEP work, gross-motor play, all interspersed with dressing and toileting instruction.

Group Instruction

In addition to organizing the day's activities into several brief time periods, special education teachers like, and are accustomed to, group instruction. It is a comfortable conventional operating procedure, and they believe in it. Even though the wide disparity of children and the obligation to teach IEPs make group teaching difficult (and despite the fact that high teacher–student ratios make individual instruction theoretically feasible), teachers cling to large- and small-group instruction. As we saw at Midwood, except for free play, teachers try to keep children doing the same things at the same time. The use of group instruction and minimal individualization with a wide diversity of children once again requires teachers to gear work to the more advanced children, to put pressure on the slower ones, and to vigilantly monitor progress. In Teresa's Midwood class, Molly, Heather, Doreen, and, of course, Carl, are constantly failing to answer questions that are much more appropriate for Larry and Stephen.

Group instruction with teacher direction is supported by the staffing arrangements. In every program I visited, the staff consisted of a teacher, one or two aides, occasionally therapists (for parts of the day), and from time to time, volunteers. Aides rarely have any professional training or certification beyond high-school degrees. The role relationships are symbolized by circle time. Typically, the teacher sits in front directing activities while the aides control the children from behind their chairs. During small-group time, the teachers orchestrate the IEP work and enlist the aides' help in specific tasks. Aides do most of the cleaning up and toileting, teachers most of the planning and parent contact. It never takes more than a moment of observation to spot the teacher of the class. With eight children and three staff (plus therapists in and out), Teresa could, in principle, have a looser classroom structure that gives children both more freedom for their self-chosen pursuits and frequent adult contact. This, however, would mean bringing aides into co-equal roles, along with a lot of other changes. The hierarchical structure of the staffing, with aides relating to children through teacher requests, and the perceived inequality of competence, due to differences in education, pay (aides usually are paid by the hour with no benefits), and job descriptions, work against truly collaborative efforts.

A modest amount of individualization occurs, even within the framework of fairly permanent schedules and groupings, by modifying group tasks to fit better an individual's level. During circle time Teresa permits the slower children to peek before labelling an object from the grab bag. Heather is asked merely if it is sunny or cloudy (she has a 50% chance of being correct), whereas Larry is asked for the month of the year. A profoundly retarded nonambulatory child like Carl is carried to circle, and his name tag is placed low enough for him to reach it. However, he is expected to "participate" in the calendar and weather sequences, just like all the other children, even though he does not understand the first thing about the subject matter. There are two groups for art and two groups for IEP work. For art, Teresa gives her low group an easier task than her high group, but everyone is doing art, and it is not OK for Molly to slip away and play in the cubbies. Teresa has somewhat different IEP objectives for each child. Even within groups and during IEP time she and her helpers will do some one-on-one work. In the low group, Doreen is learning off, on, under, etc., Heather is concentrating on colors, and Molly on shapes. But everyone is doing IEPs. One rarely sees greater diversity than this. Group instruction in short time blocks is a given.

Naturally, within this basic convention of group instruction through scheduled periods, there is variation in the detail of teachers' lesson plans, in the extent to which they stay "on schedule," in the amount of one-to-one instruction, and in the degree of individualization. Some teachers who say they individualize "all the time" do so exclusively in group contexts, as do many who say they "never" individualize. A common pattern is for teachers like Teresa to work individually, but briefly, with children on IEP goals either daily, or almost daily. Sometimes a child may be excused from a group requirement because he cannot be managed adequately, because he is inciting other children, or because the attention he receives just makes matters worse. Almost never, however, are schedules altered for specific children so that a few are left to play while others clean up, and very rarely are children *supported* in their withdrawal from a group activity such as circle.

Because teachers must squeeze their individualization into group lessons and preset routines, the between-child variation is inevitably limited. An autistic child like Austin, who has no grasp of elemental social intercourse, who would pass his mother on the street without acknowledging her, who "sees" hallways as textured surfaces for tactile contact rather than passageways for groups of children and teachers, is learning "preacademics" along with the rest of the class. Teresa, confined by school, classroom, teacher's roles, schedules, group teaching, and staff patterns, is hardly in a position to spend the day making personal contact with him or playing peek-a-boo with Carl.

The viewpoints teachers hold about individualization are illustrated in the following collection of remarks:

"We individualize in the context of the group." . . . "I modify circle time for each child and scale down the demands for the lower children." . . . "I divide my class into small groups by ability, and then work with individuals on their objectives. Each child has his own folder with a sheet for each skill (colors, matching, identification, sequencing, categorization) and his own basket of materials for teaching the skill." . . . "I have different expectations for different children, even within the same task. One child needs special scissors, a larger crayon; one child will cut, another just tear paper; one child has to match colors, another label them; one sings the song, one does the gesture, one child says the word, the other signs it." . . . "Mostly the children have the same sort of goals: learning their colors, shapes, increasing their vocabulary. We don't need to do one-on-one because we have two groups for instruction and give the slower children more prompting and simpler materials such as larger pop beads and puzzles with fewer pieces." . . . "It's not necessary to do individual instruction, but I praise children differently and have different expectations; one child is rewarded for making a sound, another for using a sentence; for Ethan, just looking at me is progress." . . . "I don't like pulling children out individually. They need to handle routines and participate in groups, so I try to pick an activity with enough range to include everyone." . . . "It all depends on the kids. Some need constant individualization because they don't learn like the others; for instance, one may need auditory input, another tactile." . . . "I have to prioritize with each child. Some children have so many problems I need to ignore a few of them. For example, if we're working with Roger on keeping hands to yourself, I might ignore his leg swinging, but everyone has to follow the routine, like come to circle. A child would only be left out of circle if his negative behavior gets reinforced by my attention and I wanted to extinguish it by keeping him away."

Group instruction would be easier, and pressure on the slower children lessened, if Teresa did not have such a wide range of children. Partly by design and partly through circumstances, all the classes I visited were highly diversified. Handicapping conditions are at once rare and varied. The classes I visited included children with sensory handicaps (primarily deaf and blind); children with motor handicaps (primarily cerebral palsy); children with mild, moderate, severe, and profound retardation (IQs from 0 to 70); children with speech and language delays; children with behavioral disturbance (primarily autistic, hyperactive–distractible, and aggressive); children with known, and more with unknown, medical disorders; children with abnormal, and more with

normal, appearances; children with damage resulting from diseases or accidents; children who have been neglected, abused, or
impoverished. The low incidence of each condition, coupled with
the wide variety among them, would result in extremely heterogeneous classes even if teachers and parents did not regard this as a
virtue, which, of course, they do.

The instructional problems arising from the disparity in levels
is partially hidden because all the children are "preschoolers"—
little children, none of whom do very much—and rarely exceed a
3-year chronological age span. At Midwood, for example, Teresa's
children range from 3- to 5-year-olds. Thinking only in terms of
chronological age, however, misrepresents the true disparity. The
mental age range for Teresa runs from 6 months (Carl) to 4 years
(Larry, at the 4-year level in speech, otherwise at the 5-year level).
But even thinking in terms of this enlarged span does not portray
the true picture. Because development is so rapid in the first years
of life, 3 or 4 years at these early ages is a much bigger "real"
developmental gap than 3 or 4 years during later childhood.

To clarify the point, consider two 5-year-olds in Teresa's class:
Heather with an IQ of 40, and Larry with an IQ of 80. The current
difference in functional level or mental age is only 2 years (Heather's mental age is 2, Larry's is 4). This absolute gap between them,
however, will continue to increase even if the relative (i.e., IQ) gap
remains constant. Assuming no spurts or slowdowns, when Heather is 10, she will be functioning at the 4-year level; when 15, she
will be functioning at the 6-year level; Larry at 10 will be functioning at the 8-year level, and at 15 will be at the 12-year level. Would
we expect any teacher to bridge that range? Yet in terms of relative
competence, the difference between Heather, with a mental age of
6, and Larry, with a mental age of 12, is, proportionally, *just the
same* as the current mental age difference of 2 years. And for a
child like Carl, of course, the increased separation will be even
more dramatic. At age 15 Carl will be at the 30-month level.[4]

Carl is not remotely like Larry, or even like Heather, Molly, or
Doreen (who themselves are very far from Larry and Stephen).
Think back to the classroom. Carl basically watches and gives no
indication that he is taking in anything. Larry follows and participates in everything. Although Teresa tries to reduce the demands
on the lower children, she cannot keep interest alive, in part because only two can keep up.

It would be easier for teachers to accommodate the range of
individual differences, even in a group format, if they did not feel
obliged to keep pushing the curriculum forward. Occasionally a

teacher does use circle for noninstructional purposes. In one program, for example, a teacher spread out a cloth "parachute." Each child grabbed hold of a fringe and waved it more or less rhythmically as a record was played. When one child let go and crawled under the parachute, the teacher had the others alternately bring the parachute down to cover her and then lift it up. When another placed his stuffed animal onto the parachute's surface, the group's play shifted to throwing the bear up and catching it in the parachute. It was informal togetherness with no performance requirement. But mostly circles are a time for turn-taking and question-answering—what's the name, what's the color, what's the shape, what's the size (big or little), how many, etc.

Behind what teachers do and the constraints imposed by habits, traditions, relationships, and laws, lies a belief system about the nature of learning and teaching as applied to this special population. Beliefs are inevitably used to rationalize the givens, but beliefs also generate change.

EDUCATIONAL THEORY AND THE NATURE OF MENTALLY RETARDED PRESCHOOLERS

Teachers were asked about their educational philosophy in the context of instructing handicapped children. They are, after all, special teachers trained to deal with special children in special ways. To what extent do their teaching practices derive from the peculiarities of this particular population? More narrowly, do they view mentally retarded preschoolers as just like younger learners (the developmental position) or, alternatively, as defective learners, unlike normal children of any age (the defect, or difference, position)? Presumably, teachers subscribing to the developmental position teach the retarded as they would teach a normal child of the same *mental* age; adherents of the defect position adopt special methods for the retarded. Let us look at teachers' opinions about the retarded, and how they fit their philosophy of instruction to actual practice.

Teachers and the Nature of Mental Retardation

Teachers agree that to be retarded is to be slow. But what does "slow" mean? It could mean permitting a child to linger twice as long in a particular activity and exposing him to a skill only when his mental age catches up to the chronological age at which most children learn it. This would be a delay position. Or "slow" could mean a child is dull, inert, inattentive, and requires more teacher effort, a more intense bombardment of instruction, if he is to learn. This would be the "defect" view. The teachers were largely in agreement with each other, but their shared position was ambivalent. At first blush they seemed to take a delay position; when asked if the retarded learn differently from nonretarded children they typically replied, "No, only slower." To my follow-up question, however—"Then you treat them like a younger, normal child?"—their response was "No." Over and over they stated that compared to normal children, the retarded require a much larger amount of teacher direction, control, and structure to treat their inattentiveness and distractibility; simplification, repetition, multisensory approaches to treat the dullness. Unlike younger, normal children, the retarded do not make wise purposeful choices, seek out knowledge, recall or generalize what they have learned. In short, while teachers initially favor the "no different, only delay" characterization in the abstract, and perhaps as a matter of ideology, their concrete pedagogical judgments seem more in keeping with the "defect" or "difference " view of retardation. They reach this pedagogical conclusion reluctantly, realizing, apparently, that it goes against their abstract ideology. Their unease and ambivalence is apparent in the following quotes, where often "no difference" is reversed when elaborated:

> "The mentally retarded are more similar than dissimilar to normals, but they need more practice, drill, and repetition. I make them do things like dress, put hands in shaving cream. I tell Peter, 'Say "Peter".' You need to make him; otherwise, he just perseverates." . . . "They just learn at a slower rate, need more prompts, and more adaptation of material. They're not that different and don't require radically different techniques—more modelling and repetition, much more repetition, and direct experiences. They don't pick things up on their own like typical children, don't transfer, don't generalize to home, but can learn the same skills and don't need a separate curriculum. You have to go step by step, use flash cards a lot, model." . . . "They're slower. It could take years for them to write their name so you have to present it 500 ways." . . . "There's no difference except they take more time, need more practice, so most of their time is instructional. I only give them 15 minutes' free time, and I control the agenda." . . . "They don't have the language base to understand what we're saying. They don't generalize, and they

resist change. We have to give them the same goals over and over.
They forget what they learn, so you repeat the same thing day
after day. Patricia has been on 'sorting colors' and Anthony on
'single-word utterances' for 3 years." . . . "They can't figure things
out. They'd never learn colors, shapes and numbers without direct instruction." . . . "They need more diversity, not just more
repetition, so you introduce the same skill in many ways, give
them experience in more modalities. When I read a story about
alligators, birds, and water I use props. When I teach 'red' I put
plastic on the window so light comes in red, we wear red clothes,
paint red, make red trees." . . . "They need structure, repetition,
and focusing, fewer distractors. They would be all over the place
unless directed to specific chairs and activities. They don't have
impulse control. They must be trained concretely. For example,
you don't just send them to the bathroom, but tell them to pull
down their pants, wipe, wash hands, walk them through activities. Regular children don't need so much direction. You have to
feed this stuff because they don't pick it up from the environment." . . . "You need to be structured more. They're very distractible. They won't adapt to the freedom of the nonhandicapped.
Routine and structure will lead to independence. They don't need
more structure than for a 2-year-old but more than for a 5-year-
old. No, they *do* need absolutely more structure. Normals pick up
more from the environment, regardless of level." . . . "They need
more training in play. They don't come up with combinations.
They're not spontaneous or curious. They have to be taught to be
purposeful. Peter would bang on the door for 30 minutes if I let
him." . . . "You model something, then have them repeat, then
back out. Often you have to do hand-over-hand to get them to
change." . . . "You need to train them in play sequences, but you
have to be careful not to overtrain. Don't want to turn them into
robots." . . . "Left to their own devices, Mark and Susie would stay
with simpler things and wouldn't get anything out of exploring
on their own."

A few teachers took the position that special practices are
needed only for particular children:

"Years ago I would have said they're the same, just slower. Now I
think that maybe there are qualitative differences, certainly for
the autistic and some of the Down syndrome children." . . .
"Basically they learn the same, but at a different pace. You teach
them by touching and showing. That's how I treat my toddler.
Really, only the disturbed need behavior modification."

The message of the interviews is that teachers believe these
children fundamentally cannot generate the normal mental pro-

cesses that allow for learning—maintaining attention, controlling impulses, recollecting the past, producing ideas. Because their own spontaneous processes are unproductive, others must do the generating for them. Teachers have come to this position not from books but from experience.

It is clear that when confronted with retardation, teachers prefer to revise their teaching techniques rather than to reduce their demands. Better to teach colors 12 different ways than not to teach colors at all. Everything the teachers say about the children—need for direction, structure, task clarification and simplification—goes against a child-centered open classroom. The children are likely to be unproductive when left on their own. Teachers have to give them everything, from facts like "red" to ideas for play. Behaviorism is justified for these children, even when not appropriate for children in general who "pick things up on their own." Yet when asked about their educational models, behaviorism was not the most common selection. Let us turn to their educational principles to see how they rationalize their pedagogical model and their understanding of retardation.

Teachers' Educational Philosophy

Of all the questions posed, the one about educational philosophy was most irksome to teachers and administrators. On the whole, they had not given the topic much thought; it is not a priority in their work. Administrators explained that fealty to a particular orientation has nothing to do with hiring.

> "I don't care about educational philosophy. Highly structured and teacher-directed works with some teachers, others are looser. Both styles are OK. When hiring I don't ask about educational philosophy." . . . "I don't look for ideology in hiring. I look for an energetic, enthusiastic, flexible person who loves children and has had good training and experience. I use whatever works."

When pressed, teachers' responses were more varied and less clear than to other questions. Many claimed to be "developmental," but the term turns out to be sufficiently plastic to fit any model. Developmental is an "in" buzzword, so it is widely adopted, but depending on the interviewee, it can mean freedom from intervention, as in the romantic model; supported learning, as in the Kohlberg meaning of developmental; or sequenced learning, as in the behavioral model. And sometimes it refers to nonacademic curriculum objectives rather than to how children learn and teachers instruct. For the most part teachers subscribe to additive or blended views and refuse to be pigeonholed into a single orientation; then there are some who find the question to be meaningless. The result is a range of thinking that is wider than the range of practice and more pragmatic than systematic.

As always there are the outliers with clear allegiances. The reader will note the variety of meanings given to "developmental":

> "I believe in short-term behavioral goals like 'sit in a chair,' 'come to the table'; also specific cognitive tasks. The way to help these children is through behavioral management, especially positive reinforcement." . . . "A special education teacher should not be paid to let children play. If they can learn from proximity, they don't belong in special education." . . . "I believe in consistency, structure, and schedules, rules, firmness, not a lot of free play. School is not the place for emoting. I stay away from the touchy-feely. We have specific responsibilities and objectives to accomplish." . . . "Following a child as he goes from thing to thing doesn't work with the IEP. If we're doing 'springtime' and they want water play, tough. We have a busy schedule: opening, snack, gross-motor, large and small groups for IEPs, story, song. We use lots of behavior modification (attending charts, verbal prompts, rewards like happy faces and stickers)."

> "I'm a developmentalist. I look at the concepts and skills a child has and see what comes at the next age." . . . "I'm a strong developmentalist. A program can be loose or structured as long as you start with a child where he is and follow developmental guidelines." . . . "I believe in following developmental sequences. You break things down into developmental steps (not like Piaget). First you have children match, then identify, then name. In matching you start with one-to-one correspondence with no choice, then two choices, then add distractors." . . . "I'm a developmentalist, not big into academics, but that's what you'll see." . . . "I believe in active learning, experience, Piaget." . . . "I follow Gesell and Piaget. I stress exploration, movement and no prepared curriculum." . . . "Young children grow through play. You set up environments, that's how they learn. We need to adapt to them. I like to set up environments that elicit what I'm after."

Many teachers want to put two models (behavioral and developmental) together additively. It is often unclear whether they are joining two sets of objectives—preacademic and non-academic—or two models of instruction—teacher versus child-directed. Thus advocates of an additive model say:

"You need both, freedom and structure, developmental and behavioral." . . . "I believe in preacademics and free choice." . . .
"Home is the place for free play and creativity; at school you
learn from a teacher. Sometimes we need to back off and be
child-centered. We facilitate at water play, for example, by pouring water with a child." . . . "You need a balance of behavioral and
developmental. To manage behavior I use timeout, praise, ignoring the negative; learning comes mostly from play." . . . "I like to
plan, but I like child-directed activities too." . . . "I strive for a
balance between teacher and child-directed. Like a typical preschool we have circle time and station time that are teacher-
directed, outdoor and option time are child-directed. I believe in
active, not passive, learning and play as a vehicle for learning."

Some teachers opt for a fusion:

"I use a special education model in a normal preschool
framework. I like behavioral modification but press language and
concepts through experiences not through drill. I don't just go
with the flow. There is a teacher-directed activity for 45 minutes
each day. We set out a task, such as identification of animal
pictures, and give food for the correct response. I also give a lot of
choices within an activity. That's the High Scope piece. It's important for their self-esteem and concept development to make
decisions." . . . "I teach concepts through play. Keep it structured,
but kids don't realize it's not free." . . . "Our district stresses High
Scope, centers and play. I do classification, seriation, numbers,
but integrate it into play, like bowling." . . . "I'm not rigid, but not
as loose as child-oriented programs. We need to prepare the
children for the next environment. That means sitting. Can't just
allow free play. Next week we'll bring in desks so the children get
used to them. But you have to be flexible, too. When a loaf of our
bread got moldy, we shifted our plan and began growing molds."
. . . "I'm a developmentalist. Learning comes through doing,
exploration, interest centers, but Piaget doesn't work with these
children; they need to be directed to make choices, ask questions,
find what they want appropriately, learn preacademics."

Teachers of combined loyalties do not consistently associate a
developmental or behavioral model with particular objectives,
such as behavioral with self-help, and developmental with self-
esteem. Many believe that behaviorism is compatible with all goal
areas. Independence, for instance, is translated into teacher-
determined self-help objectives such as picking up toys and following directions, rather than developing initiative. Socialization
means following the rules or, as one interviewee put it, "teacher-

pleasing." Self-esteem is boosted by a teacher's praise for a correct performance.

A number of interviewees were uncertain and restive; they sensed change is in the air, a shift away from the traditional behavioral model, paralleling the theoretical shift away from pre-academic goals:

> "Twelve years ago everything was behavioral. We believed in a teacher-proof curriculum. Now we're modifying this, see peer relationships as more important than counting." . . . "High Scope is influencing me. Things are still too teacher-directed." . . . "Ten years ago everything was behavioral. I realize that's wrong. We just drilled and drilled. I like learning through play." . . . "The district is moving away from academics. There's not so much of a need to run prep school for kindergarten." . . . "I like child-led, playful environments, but there is pressure to do the curriculum (numbers, colors, shapes, letters). Our program is assimilated into the elementary-school curriculum." . . . "Summerhill, that's where I'm at: child as active learner, child-directed, child-centered. I'd like to give up circle, but no one else agrees. The problem is the job description that states 'prepare child for the public school system.' " . . . "School should be more like day-care. We impose ourselves too much, but are bound by the IEP. I like child-directed but there is not much time for it once you have IEP time, gross- and fine-motor, lunch, therapy pull-outs, and story."

My reading of these responses, in the context of teacher practice and reflections, is that "developmental" usually means either age-graded, sequenced objectives (hence behavioral) or opportunities for child freedom (hence romantic). Teachers believe children need time to play, a recess from training. Most do not, however, advocate a curriculum centered on children's choices, with teacher intervention built around those choices. They would not see their primary role as sharing in the child's interests or enlarging spontaneous interests through suggestions. Most, therefore, do not mean "developmental" in Kohlberg's sense.

SUMMING UP

As with all educational endeavors, what goes on between child and teacher is a mix of what society wants, what families want, what educational professionals want, and what children can deliver. In the previous chapter we looked at those determinants of early intervention that express broad social sentiments (national legislation, the IEP, mainstreaming, and conventions of public schools). The current chapter focused on four determinants that express the sentiments of parents and teachers. What unites all these forces is the expectation for developmental acceleration; this expectation makes almost inevitable the creation of programs that work on a narrow band of agreed-upon skills pulled from nationally used inventories through a teacher-directed behavioral model. The uniformity in the classes visited—in Massachusetts, Georgia, Nebraska, and California—finds its original source in this pressure to accelerate, to which all teachers are captive (though some resist). Let us review briefly the sentiments of parents and teachers that drive programs.

Above all, parents want their children to be more skilled at socialization and independent living, with increased speech a closely linked subsidiary. Teachers agree, but add self-esteem as an important goal. On inspection, it turns out that independence does not mean assertiveness and initiative but conformity and compliance, so that, somewhat curiously, this goal supports a teacher-directed curriculum.

Parents and teachers collude with each other to stress what a child can, not what he can't, do; to avoid labels and down-play prognosticating tests that deal with growth rates (i.e., IQ); to inflate accomplishments and camouflage delay. Teaching to test items supports the inflated estimates of development, reinforces the belief that children are more capable than meets the eye, and, in turn, produces higher expectations.

Teachers of special education inherit a tradition that emphasizes didactic instruction and limited individualization in the context of small-group instruction. This pedagogy, particularly when combined with the wide ability gap of the children, forces teachers into strong executive roles. Their only other choice—to give up on the daily schedules and establish radically different expectations for the slower children (for instance, freedom not to attend circle or snack or art)—does not fit their teaching traditions.

Most teachers, though very reluctant to say so, subscribe to the "defect" or "difference" position of mental retardation. The children they teach are not like normal younger children: they are impulsive, inattentive, don't generate activities, don't learn incidentally, and forget easily. Although teachers tend to describe their pedagogy as "developmental" and believe children need time to play and make choices, the urgency to advance children's development forces them to break down tasks into small, successive

components, hold children to task, and control interfering behaviors (inattention, forgetfulness, intellectual passivity, dis-
ruptiveness) through structure, clear demands, repetition, reinforcement, and discipline.

From the outset teachers are set up for the "defect" position.
Children come to early intervention programs because of identified problems that teachers are supposed to fix. The children's
thick folders describe in great detail what they are missing: they
can't make a particular sound, they don't use the negative, they
only follow a one- not two-part command, they are having difficulty with prepositions, and so on, page after page. The portraits,
drawn largely from failed items on inventories, are the descriptions of defective, not younger, children. More importantly,
all the pressures already reviewed make it impossible for a teacher
to treat 4-year-olds like 2-year-olds. To do so would sabotage the
object of intervention—normalization. So, teachers work with
them as 4-year-olds, not 2-year-olds, and in doing so *may* unwittingly *produce* just those negative behaviors that teachers have
come to believe are indigenous in the retarded.

Consider a normal toddler age 18 months to 2 years at an early
intervention program. Would he not, like the children in Midwood,
finger the clothes and hair of another child, take a hat on and off
his head, pull objects out of backpacks, dump blocks into a sandbox, and wander? Would he not leave circle, resist clean-up, not
learn to count, not label the months, not identify the weather, and
require endless repetition to learn shapes and letters? Few adults
would have the interest or patience to pursue these objectives with
a toddler. They would intuitively know time was on the child's
side. But a retarded child does not have the luxury of time, not if he
is to be mainstreamed, not if he is to be accelerated. So when he is
inattentive to number instruction, it is proof of congenital rather
than acquired "distractibility"; when he can't learn his numbers it
is proof of "bad memory" and "need for repetition"; when he can't
do anything with numbers, even after they're memorized, it is
proof of "failure to generalize"; when he doesn't do more with
blocks than dump and fill, it is proof he has "no play ideas," "can't
sequence," isn't "purposeful."

There is an irony here. Teachers, the supreme advocates of the
retarded preschooler, would be the last people on earth to hold a
wrongful, deprecatory belief about them. But it is possible, it
happens all the time, that circumstances elicit behaviors that
observers attribute to the actor not the setting.[5] The external
climate stresses acceleration through achievement. Teachers try to

meet unrealistic expectations. Children resist and fail. Teachers locate the problem in the child and try to banish it by reforming the child. He must be made (usually through praise) to pay more attention, not wander off mentally or physically, recall what he is taught, etc. The teacher has to be ever more vigilant, has to double—not withdraw or reduce—her efforts to promote learning.

The above scenario is possible, but it also may be true that retarded children are defective, not just mentally young. This critical question, the nature of the retarded, is pursued further in the next chapter.

CHAPTER NINE

Developmental Principles and the Retarded

Constructiveness is another great instinctive tendency with which the schoolroom has to contract an alliance. Up to the eighth or ninth year of childhood one may say that the child does hardly anything else than handle objects, explore things with his hands, doing and undoing, setting up and knocking down, putting together and pulling apart . . . The result of all this is that intimate familiarity with the physical environment, that acquaintance with the properties of material things, which is really the foundation of human *consciousness*. To the very last, in most of us, the conceptions of objects and their properties are limited to the notion of what we can *do with them* . . . The more different kinds of things a child thus gets to know by treating and handling them, the more confident grows his sense of kinship with the world in which he lives. An unsympathetic adult will wonder at the fascinated hours which a child will spend in putting his blocks together and rearranging them. But the wise education takes the tide at the flood, and from the kindergarten upward devotes the first years of education to training in construction . . . Living things, then, moving things, or things that savor of danger or of blood, that have a dramatic quality—these are the objects natively interesting to childhood, to the exclusion of almost everything else; and the teacher of young children, until more artificial interests have grown up, will keep in touch with her pupils by constant appeal to such matters as these.

—JAMES (1892/1958, pp. 53–54, 73, italics in original)

NATURE OF THE RETARDED

Opinions and Observations

Opinions about the retarded have been remarkably steadfast. The ideas of professionals a century ago are very reminiscent of teachers today. Then, as now, the "defect" view prevailed. For example, using a two-type defect typology, A. F. Tredgold, an early expert whose text on the "feebleminded" went through nine editions, described "aments" as: passive, inert, sluggish, *or* restless, mobile, impulsive, instinctive (animal like), inattentive (Tredgold, 1908, 1st ed.); and, in a later edition, simply stable–apathetic or unstable–excitable (Tredgold, Tredgold, & Soddy, 1952, 9th ed.; see also Note 5, Chapter Three). The defects justified cultural transmission instruction—as today's teachers (cited previously) put it: "practice, drill, repetition," "prompts," "adaptation of material," "modeling," "go step by step," "practice," "structure," "fewer distractors," "direction" because the children are "distractible," "resist change," "perseverate," "don't generalize," "don't pick things up," "not spontaneous or curious." These opinions are buttressed by authoritative writings in special education that *still* tend to describe the retarded as inert and unresponsive on the one hand, and as inattentive and restless on the other. Specifically, they are described as having diminished intrinsic motivation (Bailey & Wolery, 1984; Harter & Zigler, 1974; Haywood, Meyers, & Switzky, 1982; Zigler & Balla, 1982); as being relatively unresponsive and low in initiative (Brinker & Lewis, 1982; Hanzlik & Stevenson, 1986; Jones, 1978, 1980; Mundy, Sigman, Kasari, & Yirmira, 1988; Odom, 1983; Rosenberg & Robinson, 1988), rigid (Linder, 1983), poor at exploration (Garwood, 1983), play (Anastasiow, 1978), and spontaneous learning (Fewell & Kelly, 1983). They also show limited self-regulation and planning abilities (Naglieri, 1989; Whitman, 1990). The picture of an empty, drifting, unresponsive, impulsive organism, when combined with the acceleration pressures, makes it clear why "few programs for exceptional preschoolers employ this [the developmental] approach" (Neisworth & Bagnato, 1987, p. 26). Are they right?

At one cut, the retarded are defective by definition. If they were not slow to learn, they would not be retarded. Even if we match Doreen at age 4 with a younger, normal child, say age 2, Doreen, because she is retarded (learning in 1 year what another child learns in 6 months) will respond more slowly. At the point of initial comparison, the two children may have achieved the same amount—that's what it means to have equivalent mental ages—but they will be unequal in processing new material. After all, if Doreen learned like a normal child, she would not stay retarded for long! That means in any instructional situation with the 2-year-old, Doreen is unlikely to catch on as quickly, be as responsive, see as many alternatives. It will take her twice the time to learn something new, she will be less alert, more will pass her by. The slowness with which she observes, processes, reacts, and recalls gives the impression, certainly at times, of a dull, passive, rigid, child. Teresa, quite naturally, sees her endless preening at the mirror as "nonproductive," not considering that she needs twice as long to complete her play. Research studies have actually measured how long it takes a retarded child to absorb fully a novel stimulus. Children with Down syndrome, it has been shown, take much more time than normal infants to become familiar with a stimulus and organize a response. At a biological level it has been documented that they have a less reactive central nervous system (Ganiban, Wagner, & Cicchetti, 1990). Contrariwise, there is some evidence that fast reactions are associated with higher intelligence.[1]

Problems of attention manifested by distractibility and impulsivity are less obviously intrinsic to retardation, but plausible. Cognitive psychologists consider attentional control to be the highest aspect of intelligence; no wonder, then, that it should be weak in those with low intelligence.[2] Here again, in any given situation, the child with a 50 IQ should not be expected to have the attention, impulse control, and interests even of the normal younger child who is at the same developmental level. David, at Midwood, exemplifies the child who cannot set a goal, order his activities sequentially, or keep his mind on the task at hand. Playing with Play-Doh during gross-motor time, he is everywhere and nowhere, running back and forth between the "oven" and the table, using trays, dolls, spatulas, and timers at random. Happenstance, not planning, calls the tune; whatever his eye or hand falls upon, that is what captures his attention. But while distractibility is blatantly apparent in early intervention programs, its causes are less so. It may be a consequence of the children's slow processing, a reaction to excessive school demands, or neither of the above.

As discussed in the last chapter, we cannot disregard the "environmentalist" argument that children acquire such qualities as passivity, rigidity, and inattentiveness as a protective defense against environments poorly calibrated to their developmental level.[3] Molly and Heather, for example, are distractible at circle time when they cannot follow all the calendar talk, but Molly is not distractible when emptying out the backpacks, nor Heather when she is "shopping." When a teacher "redirects" the children from these "off-task" activities to difficult tasks, they, overwhelmed, may narrow their foci and block out adult entreaties (appearing rigid or slow); or, without a good match for their interests, "float" (distractible). If we keep in mind that these children are functioning at half their age, the possibility of overload seems plausible. By analogy, consider a 4-year-old alone at Grand Central Station in New York City. Is it not likely that he would either roam distractedly or hunker down and become absorbed with a toy or with his body? Indeed, do we not all either space out or pull in when the demands of a situation get too great? Of course, we would not subject a 4-year-old to the challenge of Grand Central Station (but we might an 8-year-old). Are the usual preschool demands not equally overwhelming to a 4-year-old functioning at the 2-year level? In short, is it not possible that these children's failures—to absorb instruction, to learn spontaneously, to initiate activities; their unresponsiveness, rigidity, and perseveration—signal distress from excessive demands, not, as teachers would have it, defects requiring extra repetition and control of attention?

Finally, it is possible that we simply misread the children; the distractibility and rigidity may be in the eye of the beholder. "Inattentive" behaviors may be "off-task"—for example, Molly attending to her socks, dumping toys, rummaging through backpacks—only according to *our* definitions of "on-task." And "rigid" may simply be *our* characterization of plodding, repetitive behavior that, for the child who works slowly on a small palette with fewer colors, may be rich in discoveries.

> For example, Danny, a 4-year-old child with Down syndrome, takes a mallet and begins to bang under a "sink" (a wooden preschool representation). The teacher is pleased and comments on how he is fixing the pipes. Danny leaves the sink and starts to bang on each toy lined up on a shelf (truck, busy box, shape-sorter, etc.), twisting them about in his free hand to find new surfaces for banging. The shape-sorter spills. He then picks up a plastic square and bangs it against the mallet. The teacher interrupts the banging, perceiving it as rigid and repetitive, but for Danny it is appropriate exploration.

Research on Development in the Retarded

Researchers, by studying a broad spectrum of characteristics in the retarded starting from infancy, and looking at their expression in a wide variety of situations, have made a stab at answering

the tough question: Are the retarded innately different from children of like mental age, and if so, how?

Once again, the variability found in children defies our conceptual dichotomies. The broad conclusion, largely but not entirely drawn from studies of children with Down syndrome, is that the
retarded go through the *same stages* in the *same sequence* as normal children and, from this molar perspective, are accurately
described as developmentally delayed rather than deviant. But
when it comes to their moment by moment *processing* of information, they are indeed deviant (as would be expected). More specifically:

> Delayed young children achieve major milestones in a similar
> order and with a similar organization as their normally develop-
> ing peers, the main reliable differences being that the rate of
> development is slower and the appearance of achievements is
> later. This general finding applies to socioaffective development,
> selective attention, sensorimotor development, language and
> symbol formation, pretend play, and attachment behaviors . . .
> [On the other hand,] differences appear in situations where (a) a
> primary   task   involves   acquisition,   encoding,   retention,
> transformation, or transmission of selected information, and (b)
> the information is either not immediately obvious or there are
> competing stimuli from which the child must select . . . [The
> differences may produce] a slow rate of development or increas-
> ing constriction of the repertoire of responses that are available,
> [that is, rigidity]. (Krakow & Kopp, 1983, pp. 1143–1144)

The growth of language and play well illustrate the delay-only
position. Children with Down syndrome, for example, like the
nonretarded, do not use language referents until they have a clear
grasp of the conceptual category to which the word applies; that,
in turn, requires understanding that objects are permanent even
when not immediately visible (object permanency); early referents
are to action and function words (Bruner, 1983; Mervis, 1988,
1990; Nelson, 1973; Warren & Rogers-Warren, 1982); symbolic
play does not emerge until the child is "preoperational" (can mentally represent experiences in which he has participated) (Cicchetti
& Beeghly, 1990; also Rondal, 1988, with severely retarded children). Further, there are strong play–language correspondences:
Retarded children without language have no symbolic play; at the
one-word stage they manage single symbolic schemes; complex
play combinations await word combinations (Spiker, 1990). The

content of play and language in children with Down syndrome also parallels that of their mental-age peers. They use as many toys, play out as many roles with just as much imagination (Fewell & Kaminsky, 1988; Krakow & Kopp, 1983; Loveland, 1987; Motti et al., 1983; Seibert, Hogen, & Mundy, 1984, in a diagnostically mixed population). Their first words come from the same categories—toys, food, clothing, animals, vehicles (though language acquisition is slower than one would predict; Mervis, 1990); and, when "mean length of utterance" (MLU) is held constant, they produce very similar vocabularies (Leifer & Lewis, 1984). The same parallelism characterizes their emotional development. They become attached to caretakers, fearful of strangers, and negativistic in the same sequence and at the same mental ages as nonretarded children. They laugh or smile at the same circumstances and in the same order—first to being touched, then to seeing incongruous situations, such as mother sucking on baby's bottle (Cicchetti & Beeghly, 1990).

But there is a hitch; a close look reveals differences. In the humor study, children with Down syndrome smiled more and laughed less than the controls, presumably because they "simply could not process the incongruity with sufficient speed to produce the tension . . . required for laughter" (Cicchetti & Sroufe, 1976, p. 927). Their emotional expression was muted: both initial arousal and recovery from arousal were slower (Cicchetti & Beeghly, 1990; Emde, Katz, & Thorpe, 1978). Studies have shown that attention in the young retarded child (at least in those with Down syndrome) is more poorly deployed, sustained, or controlled than in children of the same mental age. The deficiency shows up in both restricted and impulsive behavior. Compared to children of the same mental age, their play patterns are more stereotypic, repetitive and rigid, and they are less likely to monitor their environment (Krakow & Kopp, 1983; Mundy & Kasari, 1990). In a frequently cited study, Claire Kopp asked a group of preschool children with Down syndrome and a matched nonretarded group of equivalent mental age *not* to go after a raisin the experimenter hid under a cup and *not* to touch an appealing red plastic telephone while she went out of the room. On both tasks the retarded were less restrained (Kopp, Krakow, & Johnson, 1983; Kopp, Krakow, & Vaughn, 1983; Kopp, 1990).

Because these findings—normal stage progression with some differences in information processing—are largely derived from studies of children with Down syndrome, a group relatively easy to study because they are diagnosed at birth and etiologically homogeneous, we cannot be certain how far to generalize the findings. Certainly they do not apply to autism, classified in the *Diagnostic and Statistical Manual of Mental Disorders* of the American Psychiatric Association (1987) as a pervasive *developmental disorder.* All the systems reviewed above—play, language, attachment, affect—are distorted in children with autism, as are perception (of objects, self, and others) and cognition (for a review see Cohen et al., 1987). The deficits of a child like Austin at Midwood go well beyond those recognized in children with Down syndrome. And the same may be true of the extreme hyperactivity of a child like Heather. The developmental pathology of such children contrasts sharply with the relative developmental normality of other slow children and, as discussed in the next chapter, requires different treatment.

Despite these caveats, the research evidence is that most retarded children appear to develop in the same manner as the nonretarded.[4] That being the case, we need to consider, at least briefly, those widely accepted developmental principles that are relevant to programming for this population. I shall note six which, if taken seriously, would cause a major shift in our early intervention efforts. First, psychological growth is integrated, holistic, organic; subsystems (e.g., motor, cognitive, emotional, social) do not develop independently of one another. Second, intelligence develops through repetitive acts instigated by children upon their world; repetition in variation breeds mastery. Third, it is the child's active engagement with the environment (exploration and play) that propels early development; knowledge is constructed by the child, not handed over by the adult. Fourth, growth is sequenced and ordinal; each stage depends on the passage through a prior stage. Fifth, the drive to mastery is intrinsic. Sixth, the process of instruction is a mutual, flexible, tightly interlocked and intimate collaboration; a successful educator kindles interest and fills in blanks opened by a child's quest and questions.

DEVELOPMENTAL PRINCIPLES AND THEIR PROGRAMMATIC IMPLICATIONS

Holistic and Syncretic

No one has more vividly described the holistic patterned nature of development than Heinz Werner (1948), whose theory in broad outline is comparable to Piaget's. According to Werner, mental development proceeds from the nondifferentiated and global to the differentiated and integrated. Nondifferentiation means both poor separation of the subsystems within a child and poor separation between the child and the outside world. At the outset of life the child acts globally; when stimulated, arms, hands, and body all move simultaneously. Gradually, he learns to move just legs, just arms, then one arm at a time; the movements of the several parts become coordinated (the eye spots the object, the hand reaches for it, the other hand acts as a supporter), and the totality is organized around an end or purpose (Werner calls this process "hierarchization"). Perceptions are similarly global. Objects are recognized only in their context (a duck in the water, a cup on a plate).[5] The first drawing done by a child will be a circular glob out of which, over time, will emerge arms, legs, body parts. The first words of a child may be overinclusive (e.g., duck and water both called "qua-qua"; "ball" employed for "give me," "look at," "take away," or "find").

The child as a global actor blurs visual, auditory, tactile, somatosensory, and affective experiences. Werner (1948) uses the term "syncretic" to describe this fusion of internal subsystems.[6] The following anecdote illustrates the phenomenon: Asked if his mother was good, a child retorts, " 'No! She's sour!' " (p. 84)—syncretism of affect and taste. A child remarks, " 'The leaf smells green!' " (p. 89)—syncretism of visual and olfactory. Another demands, " 'Open up your eyes or you won't hear' " (p. 89)—syncretism of visual and auditory. On seeing a broken zwieback, the child proclaims, " 'poor zwieback' " and a tipped cup, " 'poor, tired cup!' " (p. 73)—syncretism of vision and emotion, what Werner calls "physiognomic perception."

The child, unable to separate himself from the world, is egocentric and subjective in his judgments. Others exist only as extensions of himself; objects cease to exist when the child cannot see them, even space and time are personalized through action. For example, a child, asked to describe the location of his room, responds: " 'You first go through the play-room, and then the steps go down, and then you're there' " (Werner, 1948, pp. 173–174). Behind, in front of, next to are understood, if at all, in relationship to the child's own body rather than any independent referent. Time, too, is equated with experienced events and may be controlled by one's actions. Summer, for example, occurs whenever it is hot, and time can be made to pass by tearing sheets off a calendar (Werner, 1948).

Acknowledging the oneness of development would require

several changes to typical early intervention programs: eliminating separate domains for instruction, increasing intersensory connections, and enlivening the affective dimension, among others.

As pointed out in earlier chapters, teachers develop instructional objectives in a number of separate domains such as language, cognition, gross-motor, fine-motor, social–emotional. Except perhaps for purposes of assessment, these domains would be abandoned in a holistic program. With an understanding that domains, from the child's position, are syncretically fused, our newly sensitized teacher would introduce novel experiences in the context of ongoing child-meaningful activities. And, to the extent possible, she would make these experiences vivid, intense, charged, "multimodal"; she would relax the affective and motor restraints; and she would allow children to vent and explore their feelings, both sensory and emotional. She, too, would have to "let go," permit children to experience—not just talk about—happy, sad, and even mad. This would be a radical departure from current practice and hard to pull off given the bureaucratic and pedagogical reasons for keeping children calm, orderly, restrained, their physicality and emotionality under wraps. Early interventionists are not yet convinced that learning is greased by full-bodied involvement, and that the highly visual–verbal atmosphere of our programs do not speak to the sensorimotor character of our charges.

It would not, however, be a radical departure from past practice. Jean Itard, the French physician who won fame in the first decade of the 19th century for trying to tame Victor, the wild child of Aveyron, had as one of his five objectives: "To awaken his nervous sensibility by the most energetic stimulation, and sometimes by *intense emotion*" (1801/1962, p. 14, italics added). Itard, noting that "in the force of his [Victor's] passion his intelligence seemed to acquire a sort of extension" (p. 17), was not beyond promoting anger as a stimulant to learning: To instill in Victor a sense of remorse after he was returned from a runaway attempt, Itard turned "a cold and displeased expression" to Victor's outreached arms. When the boy began to cry

> I [Itard] increased his [Victor's] emotion by my reproaches, spoken in a loud and threatening tone. The tears redoubled and were accompanied by long, deep sobs. When I had carried the excitement of his emotions as far as possible, I went and sat on the bed of my poor penitent. This was always the signal of forgiveness. Victor understood me, made the first advances towards reconciliation, and all was forgotten. (p. 90)

His equally famous disciple, Edward Seguin (1866/1907), was no more sheepish. Confronted by an "idiot" who could not or would not use his hands, Seguin advocated suspending the child on a ladder and letting him fall again and again until "the child, understanding better, and feeling where more comfort may be found, holds on with his hands" which are "slightly bruised, and heated by the process they have been through." The "frightened grasp" alone, however, is inadequate. It must be made functional so into the hot hands Seguin puts a "bright apple." The child "partly to feel the coolness on all the burning surfaces, partly not to let the apples fall, will contract his fingers and get a circular, equable, prehension of them" (pp. 78, 80).

One need not endorse the tough love techniques of Itard and Seguin to see room for affective expansion in early intervention. More tolerance for noise, touching, moving, anger, and sadness would provide an environment better adapted to the child's syncretic means of learning. As pointed out in Chapter Six, teachers I observed often tried to elicit engagement by dramatizing and clowning. Children responded by becoming good spectators but not actors, because the activity, unlike the teacher, did not invite participation. Teachers also introduce emotions by asking children if they are happy or sad, often as a language lesson. And they introduce sensory stimulation by having children identify objects by touch or smell. But these exercises, abstract and isolated, are not fused into meaningful happenings. Activities dictated by a holistic approach would be sensually and emotionally rich, use real rather than symbolic materials (e.g., real animals, real babies, real weather, real stoves and sinks, real experienced feelings), invitations to syncretic responses. Schools, to their credit, do often have water–sand tables, cooking opportunities, adult clothing for dress-up, and sponsor trips for greater reality. Still the atmosphere is more "schoolish" than life-like, particularly in those settings where even three dimensional representations are pushed out by two dimensional paper-and-pencil tasks.

Repetition

Repetition, says Piaget, is the most elementary fact of psychic life, the indispensable means by which a child moves from the twilight zone of infancy where the boundaries and properties of self and non-self are obscure and into an objective world. It is through repetitive encounters with the environment that the child sorts out what he can do, what he can make other people and things do, how the animate is different from the inanimate. Piaget uses the term "circular reactions" to describe the repetitive moves through which children make the "discovery and conservation of the new" (1952, p. 138). Repetition is not always an instrument of intelligence: Sometimes children engage in repetitive acts just for fun; sometimes it secures for them a sense of self and place. And not all repetition is constructive: Beyond a certain point, environmental repetition deters growth (e.g., teachers hammering away at the same lesson); so, too, does child repetition, or "perseveration" (e.g., when it becomes an analogue to obsessive–compulsive behavior). Early interventionists, therefore, need to dissect repetition—its good uses and abuses.

Circular reactions, according to Piaget, are a combination of assimilation—incorporating new objects and experiences into existing child schemas (e.g., sucking on everything)—and accommodation—modifying schemas to the demands of the environment (e.g., raising the hand to support the bottle). The first brings the new into the known, the second modifies the known to fit the new. Danny (above), banging his mallet on everything in sight, is exhibiting what Piaget (1952) calls "reproductive assimilation" (trying out a known schema on new objects).[7] When he later shifts and bangs two cars together, he is accommodating the banging schema to the properties of cars. He will go back and forth between the two kinds of banging, changing his movements—perhaps push and pull, as well as hit—and changing objects—perhaps blocks and dolls—before he has fully mastered a small set of simple actions and before he coordinates movements, such as pushing the car and the doll into each other. And then it will be longer still, and after more repetition, before he "pretends" to be using a mallet to fix a pipe! These repetitions or circular reactions are adaptive ("an active synthesis of assimilation and accommodation"; Piaget, 1952, p. 61). The child is affecting his environment by absorbing it into himself and adjusting himself to it; in the process he stretches existing schemas and invents fresh combinations.

Repetition does not always serve adaptation; familiarity seems to appeal in its own right as seen in this description by Piaget (1951/1962) of his daughter Jacqueline.

[At 10 months:] J. put her nose close to her mother's cheek and then pressed it against it, which forced her to breathe much more loudly. This phenomenon at once interested her . . . She quickly complicated it for the fun of it: she drew back an inch or two, screwed up her nose, sniffed and breathed out alternately very hard (as if she were blowing her nose), then again thrust her nose against her mother's cheek, laughing heartily. *These actions were repeated at least once a day for more than a month, as a ritual.* (p. 94, italics added)

[At 16 months:] She had her leg through the handle of a basket. She pulled it out, put it back at once and examined the position. But once the geometrical interest was exhausted, the schema became one of play and gave rise to a series of combinations during which J. took the liveliest pleasure in using her new power. (p. 94)

[At 14 months:] She amused herself by making an orange skin on a table sway from side to side . . . She did it again *as a ritual, at least twenty times;* she took the peel, turned it over, put it down again, made it sway and then began all over again. (p. 95, italics added)

Then there is repetition in the environment that children, dominated by "qualities-of-the-whole" (Werner, 1948), seek and need. Children insist on routines in eating, dressing, going to bed, and woe to the parent who tries to interrupt or provide a substitute routine. "Preschool" is not a series of independent activities, but an indivisible experience; take out the greeting and departure songs and the child may be disoriented, just as she is if the bed in her room is moved or mother comes home with a different hairstyle. For the young child each element is a part of the whole; any small change fractures the unit and is disorienting; it is a matter of "all-or-nothing" (Werner, 1948).

When exaggerated, the child's requirement for environmental regularity becomes "insistence on sameness" and his personal repetitious acts, "stereotypies"—both hallmarks of autism. There is a difference between the repetitions of a child like Austin (running back and forth from the window to the beanbag chair), clearly not a mechanism for improving his information about the world, and the adaptive repetition of Danny's play (above). Austin's rote recitations and ritualistic movements do not accommodate to the properties of objects or demands of the setting; Danny's do.

Teacher repetition, like child repetition, can evoke adaptive schemas in a child or produce only rote responses. For example, in Chapter Five I described a teacher who engaged in a repetitive game consisting of rounds in which a child placed a cow on the teacher's head, the teacher then tilted her head to let it fall off, and the child picked it up and returned it to the teacher's head. In this reciprocal game the teacher became part of the child's circular reaction. As suggested, to enlarge upon the child's schema, she might have stretched the up–down routine by subtle shifts— placing the cow on other surfaces, or dropping other objects from her head. This sort of repetition, premised on mutual engagement and the child's existing behavioral repertoire, is worlds apart from repetitive reviews of object and color names, even if the teacher varies the stimuli. The imposition of the same exercise day after day is a teacher version of child perseveration: it neither enlarges nor stabilizes the child's grasp of the world (as some routines do); nor does it provide any fun. At best, the memorized facts float in mental space, recalled when the teacher requests them but not used in an ongoing elaboration of adaptive schemas. There is, then, child, adult, and environmental repetition; much of it essential but some of it bad.

When teachers talk about repetition, and it is much on their minds, they refer to all three kinds—the repetitive daily routines (what they usually call "structure"), their own repetition of in- struction, and the repetitive behaviors of children. The first is clearly acceptable to them and provides a rationale for their sched- ules. The second concerns them. They do not like endlessly repeat- ing lessons but see no alternative given the children's slow uptake. The third they regard as an obstruction to the learning process and, as we have seen, they try to interrupt repetitive play be- haviors not considered "productive." A new look at repetition would recognize that some of the child repetition is adaptive (Do- reen in the mirror, Molly removing and returning blocks from a shelf), others not (Austin's TV commercials); and that some of the environmental and teacher repetition supports adaptation, while some curtails it. A teacher needs the flexibility and sensitivity to alter her input, rather than relying on repetition, when her instruc- tion is not picked up by the child.

Knowledge through Action

Fundamental to the theories of both Piaget and Werner is that the young child's world is made up of "things-of-action" (Werner, 1948), the natural movement of objects, and the movement of the child upon the object. As Piaget succinctly explains: "To know an object, to know an event, is not simply to look at it and make a mental copy or image of it. To know an object is to act on it. To know is to modify, to transform the object, and to understand the way the object is constructed" (1964, p. 76).[8] The growth of language, logico-mathematical concepts, causality, space, and time all emerge from early sensorimotor schemata. Language acquisition, well documented in the research literature and a major activity in early intervention, serves as a good example of this progression.

Jerome Bruner, in his wonderful book *Child's Talk* (1983), describes the mapping of early language onto early action patterns. Little children do just a few things (he mentions reaching, taking, banging, looking); they then apply a single act (schema in Piaget's terminology) to a wide range of objects (recall the banging example above), or use their entire action repertoire on one object. Mimicking this pattern, early word combinations consist of a large assortment of words linked to a class of just a few words (open-pivot). More complex language, constrained by rules requiring the proper placement of an agent–action–object sequence, does not emerge until a child is goal-directed in his play and understands that he acts upon objects to make things happen. Roger Brown's classic, *A First Language* (1973), makes the same point. The first two- and three-word sentences produced by a child describe a limited number of relations among an agent, action, and object. To use them a child must have distinguished an object as separate from the action upon it and distinguish different causal sources. He must know, for example, that a dog can hit a leg, a leg can hit a dog, and a person can hit a dog. Or, as Bruner puts it: "The aspiring language learner already knows the so-called argument of action: who performed the action, on what object, toward whom, where, by what instrument, and so on" (1983, p. 34).

The content of language also is function- or action-oriented. Katherine Nelson (1973) found that the first 50 words acquired by children ages 18 months to 2 years are names of things that move independently—dog, cat, baby, car, truck, mama, dada—or things that can be manipulated—shoe, sock, hat, ball; not static and abstract qualities such as form, color, and number. Letters and numbers make up only 1%, and attributes such as red, big, and pretty another 1%, of the initial 50 words. A further indication of the action-oriented life of small children is that imperatives rather than declaratives dominate early language (Newport, Gleitman, & Gleitman, 1977).

Early categories also are organized by functional or event relationships, not taxonomic ones. For example, jeans, shorts, and skirts are joined together into a category labeled "clothes," and peanut butter, milk, and juice into one labeled "food," because the child recognizes that they share the same function or fill the same slots (hence it is that linguists use the term "slot-fillers" for the early development of categories; Nelson, 1983, 1988; also Fivush, 1987; Lucariello & Nelson, 1985).[9] Without the experiential base, the meaning of new words and concepts cannot be absorbed. The child takes in only that small portion of the linguistic environment that matches schemas he already possesses (Mervis, 1988; Newport et al., 1977; Nelson, 1973).

Even after a word is learned, it changes its meaning as a consequence of experience. A bike is one thing when it is known by observing stationary bikes in store windows or bicyclists passing by, something else when one has mastered the skill of riding, and something still more when one purchases, maintains, and repairs it.

The theory that language normally maps onto prior sensori-motor knowledge is supported by a major exception that helps prove the rule: autism. Austin, at Midwood, like other autistic children, has echolalic language—words and phrases picked up by echoing others. His vocabulary may be larger than that of a child like Molly, but her speech expresses intentions, requests, reactions, and interrogations, whereas his is largely noncommunicative, usually triggered by associations to other words (e.g., Teresa invites Austin to play with an airplane, to which he responds, "Fly the friendly skies of United," and does not follow her play suggestion). David, a Down syndrome child at Midwood, learns words normally but also enjoys (and is rewarded for) learning word strings that are detached from experience (numbers and letters, in particular). As this "splinter" skill becomes more and more central to his life, he looks more and more autistic-like, and that is worrisome because symbol training independent of experience, as Dewey has noted, is "dead and barren," like learning a "hieroglyph" (1902/1959, p. 106). Would he not be better off mastering things-in-action?

Children at early intervention programs are active. In addition to their work periods, they have regularly scheduled periods for play, art, gross-motor, music with gestures and movement, songs, snacks, etc. These activities, however, are not valued, primarily at least, as good in and of themselves, but as either a break from "work" ("They can't work all the time," said a teacher) or as another means for infusing the core curriculum (recall how the teachers at Midwood point out color and size distinctions at free play, snack, art, etc.). And the core curriculum is not the stuff of action. Consider how many times letters, numbers, and shapes are removed from a child's experience: Letters, for example, are abstracted from printed words, printed words from spoken language, spoken language from the representation of experience, finally the representation from the experience itself. There is no life to a letter, number, or shape, no context, no personalization, no action potential, no meaning until a child can move through the several derivations. Early interventionists are committed to "teaching" language and logico-mathematical knowledge to the child; they do not see this knowledge as emerging from the child acting on objects, making discoveries, setting objectives, resolving problems.

Much of the "preacademic" curriculum at early intervention reverses normal sequences.[10] It takes static objects (e.g., vocabulary words) and attributes of objects (colors, shapes, numbers, size) and tries to build up a context for them. With red on her mind, Teresa introduces it into as many of the "doing" activities as she can. Another teacher selects the word ball for a child to learn, presents a card illustrating a ball, labels a real ball, tells the child to get the ball. Letters are featured as parts of words ("A is for apple"), words are found in books, books are sometimes dramatized, and the dramatization is a representation of experience. Were teachers committed to a "developmental" sequence for letter teaching, they would do the opposite: start with the child's activity and expand on (or abstract from) it as the child's mastery and curiosity permitted. From the experience comes the pretend enactment, from the enactment an elaboration through stories, from the story the words, and finally, and not for a long time, the letters. As Bruner (1972) puts it, the natural course of learning is from "knowing how" to "knowing that." Reversing the direction is likely to produce alienation and confusion.[11]

Stage Progression

The child's movement toward a more differentiated and objective world occurs gradually and in an orderly fashion through the stages made familiar by Piaget. Children cannot be rushed through the stages (Kohlberg, 1968; Whitehead, 1929/1959), and attempts to skip or accelerate understanding in preschoolers have been unsuccessful.[12] Educators, eager for their diligent instruction to "take," particularly in the language area, are deceived by children's mimicking and memorizing feats into believing that the rote recollection of answers to specific questions amounts to major progress. Yet research has shown time and again that an unready child will reject adult instruction (e.g., a label) until she has a prelinguistic sensorimotor understanding (Brown, 1973; Bruner, 1983; Mervis, 1987; Nelson, 1973); the influence of adults in this growth is very modest (Newport et al., 1977). The teacher's stimulus prods a child "only to the extent that it is significant, and it becomes significant only to the extent that there is a structure which permits its assimilation" (Piaget, 1964, p. 182). David, at Midwood, may know his letters and letter sounds and count as well as a 5-year-old, but he does not understand that words are constructed of letters, the content of stories, or the relationship of quantity and numbers.

The moderately retarded children described in these pages are functioning at the end of the sensorimotor stage (roughly mental age 0 to 2) and the beginning of the preoperational stage (roughly mental age 2 to 7). Although children at these levels are beginning to represent experience (hence language and symbolic play), they do not understand abstract concepts (e.g., more, small, even animal). To do so requires the formation of a stable objective reality, impossible for these children who are still *perceptually dominated, egocentric, preconceptual, and preoperational* (Piaget, 1951/1962).

Because young children's thinking is perceptually bounded, they have difficulty understanding concepts. They do not grasp that a "concept is general and communicable" as distinct from an "image [which] is singular and egocentric" (Piaget, 1951/1962, p. 223). The child does not see the unity underlying multiple appearances, or the multiplicity in things that look the same. At ages 2 and 3 the image is all-consuming; concepts lacking constant perceptual referents—and that includes all words that are generalizations of specific instances—are not understood. At the age of 31 months, Piaget's daughter Jacqueline believed the same individual was several distinct persons according to the clothes she had on:

> Seeing L. [Lucienne] in a new bathing suit, with a cap, J. asked: *"What's the baby's name ?"* Her mother explained that it was a bathing costume, but J. pointed to L. herself and said: *"But what's the name of that?"* (indicating L.'s face) and repeated the question several times. But as soon as L. had her dress on again, J. exclaimed very seriously: *"It's Lucienne again,"* as if her sister had changed her identity in changing her clothes. (1951/1962, p. 224, italics in original)

At the same age, she also believed several identical slugs were a single one:

She cried: *"There it is!"* on seeing one [a slug], and when we saw another ten yards further on she said: *"There's the slug again."* I answered: "But isn't it another one?" J. then went back to see the first one. "Is it the same one?"—*"Yes"*—"Another slug?"—*"Yes."*—"Another or the same?" . . . The question obviously had no meaning for J. (1951/1962, p. 225, italics in original)

Concepts that are defined culturally rather than visually—such as animal, food, toy—are particularly difficult. As Katherine Nelson notes: "There is no animal that includes dogs and cats and tigers" (1988, p. 4). But even harder are concepts that refer to attributes of things or relations between things. Such terms—including colors, antonyms, and prepositions, all early intervention favorites—modulate meaning rather than making reference (Brown, 1973). Children do not consistently name colors accurately until ages 3 to 4 (Bornstein, 1985). At these ages children still cannot distinguish more from less and same from different, but assimilate the negative to the positive word, treating them as synonyms (Clark, 1979). Similarly, Clark found the word in was overextended to include on and under until age 3. The easiest of the antonyms, big versus little, is only distinguished at age 3½.

Conceptual thought also requires disentangling a personal from an objective viewpoint, impossible for the egocentric child who confuses his own activity with the independent activity of people and things. This confusion produces animism—the attribution of living personal qualities to the inanimate (e.g., the wind sings, the boat sleeps, the moon hides in the clouds when it is cold). As Piaget and Werner explain, natural processes are assimilated to, and not independent of, the activities of the subject or of another person. As long as the child does not separate his doings from those in the external world, his perceptions of the two will be fused, and he will not be able to structure an objective and constant reality.

During the period when children infuse the personal and perceptual into their worldly constructions, they remain preconceptual and preoperational. Organizing objects with different appearances into a greater unit that incorporates the differences (e.g., animals) requires mental "reversibility" (e.g., a bee and a slug are both animals, animals include bees and slugs) not available to the child who is so image-dominated and egocentric. Reversibility is also the key to manipulating reality through "operations" (e.g., in arithmetic: if A plus B equals C, then C minus B equals A).

The preoperational child presented with two rods of equal

length will identify as longer the one that "sticks out" more. Presented equal numbers of beads in two clusters, she will identify the one that is spread out on the table as containing more. The dominance of the perceptual and the absence of internal mental operations means that the child in the preoperational stage cannot seriate objects because she does not understand transitivity (if A is larger than B, and B larger than C, then A is larger than C) and cannot add or subtract because her thought is irreversible. Confronted with a series of increasingly long sticks, she will identify the little one, the big one, and the middle one, but will not recognize that the middle one is both big (compared to the smallest) and small (compared to the biggest) (Piaget, 1967, 1970, 1971). During the preschool years, therefore, even a normal child will have difficulty fully understanding relational words such as big versus little and number meaning.

For small children something is absolutely either big or little depending on how it compares to a typical example of such an object. In one experiment, for example, 2- to 3-year-olds called a shot glass "little" even when it was compared to smaller eating implements in a doll tea set (de Villiers & de Villiers, 1978; Reich, 1986). They do not see that the same thing can be small in one context and big in another. That awaits a mental age of approximately 7 years, when they move into the stage of concrete operations.

Once again, rote skills such as counting should not be confused with the understanding of basic mathematical principles. Rachel Gelman and Melissa Cohen (1988), studying the math skills of young children with Down syndrome ages 10 to 13 (matched with 4- to 5-year-old normal children), found that, though excellent rote counters, they did not grasp basic counting principles well understood by the nonretarded—for example, that each item in a series can be tagged only once (one-to-one correspondence); the last item tagged represents the total count (cardinal value); counting is the same regardless of the item (item indifference); and the order of counting is immaterial (order indifference). Unlike the preschoolers, the children with Down syndrome failed to generalize solutions, succeed with novel tasks, self-correct, or vary solutions flexibly as conditions were changed.

Play also cannot be advanced beyond the child's stage. At the end of the sensorimotor stage, as they approach 2 years of age, children begin to pretend, but only to a limited extent. They will go through sleeping, eating, drinking routines with themselves or with a doll. They may even develop a few sequences (e.g., feed the doll and put her to bed), but they cannot take on roles of other people until they are more cognitively decentered and better able to grasp the lives of others (ages 3 to 5) (Fein, 1981; Fisher, Hand, Watson, Van Parys, & Tucker, 1984; Rubin, Fein, & Vandenberg, 1983).

Molly, Doreen, and Heather fit the levels described above. They are beginning to put a couple of words together though their vocabularies are small. Play is at an early symbolic stage, mostly related to their own bodies and limited in the number of sequenced acts. Much of their time is still spent in typical sensorimotor activities—delighting in their agency powers (Doreen pulling apart a diaper, Molly pulling apart the backpacks, Heather throwing sand); repeating a simple schema with small variations such as building up and knocking down; gathering, depositing, arranging, moving, and recovering objects; experimenting with disappearance and reappearance. They operate on what they see by doing, but they cannot operate abstractly.

A teacher, acknowledging the limits set by developmental stage, will realize that much of the core curriculum should be modified. Notwithstanding the impressive rote memory responses of a child like David, there is no possibility that these children understand seriation and large time dimensions (both reviewed daily with the calendar), the relativism of size, and objective spatial concepts. It is therefore educationally unproductive to do daily calendar drills, counting and sequencing exercises, teach antonyms (like more and less, big and little), colors, and prepositions. Aside from the fact that this material is not embedded in any meaningful natural context, learning it requires a degree of decentration that is a long way off for the child.

Also beyond the grasp of these children are the frequent exercises in abstract categorization, so foreign to their "irrational" sorting systems. Rather than following the common request to put together "all the vehicles," "all the foods," and "all the people," the preoperational child is likely to put together "child," "bus," and "hot dog," with the explanation that the doll wants to eat the hot dog on the bus. The criteria she uses are personal identification (with the doll figure), normal juxtaposition (person and bus rather than airplane and motor scooter), linked actions (riding and eating), or common appearance. Suspending these principles would be tough even for the nonretarded preschooler who is also preconceptual and preoperational.

Intrinsic Motivation

"Virtually all of learning comes down to incentives" says Ted Sizer (1984). The trick is to get the right mix between extrinsic and intrinsic for children who by nature are responsive to both (as recognized a long time ago by both Rousseau and Locke; see Chapter Three). Because early intervention programs tilt strongly toward extrinsic motivation, we need to reconsider the nature and value of intrinsic drives.

The Piagetian infant who bats his mobile and shakes his rattle, who later gets "into everything" as he pulls, pushes, dumps and fills, is propelled by his own curiosity and drive for mastery (notably described by Bruner, 1966; Hunt, 1961, 1965; Kohlberg et al., 1987; White, 1959). He does not wait for approval from the environment, indeed is not easily deterred by disapproval. Play, in the early years, is the ideal expression of intrinsic motivation. In its reliance on flexibility, divergent thinking, freedom from a specific objective, it is antithetical to external reinforcement, which constrains behavior (Bruner, 1972). In fact, there is research to suggest that external reinforcement of play actually degrades invention.[13] Play satisfies because it calls upon personal direction, invention and control. These together produce a sense of competence, and competence for young children (who do not have a generalized sense of self) is essential to self-esteem (Erikson, 1977).

Intrinsic motivation powers cognition. In the first months of life, as Piaget points out, children will repeat a simple action over and over (e.g., swinging a mobile) just for the "pleasure of being the cause" (1951/1962, pp. 91–92, quoting Groos). In the process they will experiment with new movements that bring about different ends and thus is established a broadened repertoire of behaviors. Driving the growth of intelligence is the simple pleasure of following one's interests. As Alfred North Whitehead put it: "There can be no mental development without interest. Interest is the *sine qua non* for attention and apprehension . . . Without interest there will be no progress . . . We eat because we like a good dinner" (1929/1959, p. 48, italics in original).

Dewey, taking a similar position, instructs his readers that there is no learning without "craving," "need," "demand." It is "need" that

> supplies motive for the learning. An end which is the child's own carries him on to possess the means of its accomplishment. But when material is directly supplied in the form of a lesson to be

learned as a lesson, the connecting links of need and aim are
conspicuous for their absence. What we mean by the mechanical
and dead in instruction is a result of this lack of motivation. The
organic and vital mean interaction—they mean play of mental
demand and material supply. (1902/1959, p. 107)

But intrinsic motivation cannot operate alone.

Children also need and respond to external reinforcement.
Without the drive to please teachers and parents, children would
not submit to the unpleasant tedious labors that skill development
and social conformity often require. Divergent creative thinking
will not get a child to set the table or use "please" and "thank-you."
The more one wants to instill specific skills, information, and
conventions, the more one will tilt towards using external motivation.

Early intervention programs, more concerned with knowledge
transmitted than interest released, are heavily invested in cultivat-
ing extrinsic motivation. If one did a count of the most frequently
repeated words, "good" would likely top the list. The lavish use of
positive reinforcement results naturally from programmatic
attachment to core skills, and from conceptions of the retarded as
passive. Positive reinforcement (when it works) constrains and
focuses behavior onto what the teacher wants. The problem is that
praise (for satisfying a teacher rather than for personal initiative)
reinforces extrinsic motivation in a group who, by nature, are
supposed to lack intrinsic drive. As we have seen, teachers not only
praise children for accomplishing tasks but for attending and submitting (e.g., "nice listening," "nice sitting," "nice waiting," "nice
being quiet"), and for repressing their own imperatives. "Nice
sitting" is a thin disguise for telling a child she is good for not
doing what she wants to do. A child may like the approval, but it
does not stimulate exploration, independent learning, spontaneity—traits perceived as diminished in the retarded—and it does
nothing for any "I'm-OK-as-I-am" sentiments. Even when we con-
gratulate a child for doing something on his own, the act of praising undermines ownership of the act. As Herbert Kohl notes, in
reflecting on his son's love of music, singing and dancing, "the
music is his—we corrupt it with our praise" (1978, p. 65).

Excessive praise is just one ploy that undermines child initiative in early intervention. Teachers fill the vacuum left by passive
inactive children with talk, directives, and a heavily structured
ritualized day that has only narrow opportunities for child initiatives. Each day at Midwood Teresa goes through the same greet-

ings, calendar routine, and songs; she plans out the IEP instruction and art project in great detail. The role of the children in Teresa's day is to fill the narrow slots that she opens (name a color, count a sequence, paste a turkey). Reinforcement, dispensed before and after responses, primes attention and binds answers, but it leaves the child no room for self-expression. The teachers' belief that their energy and organization will ignite the children may be an activist fallacy; quite possibly the more active the teacher, the more passive the child.

Intrinsic motivation must be encouraged, released, tapped—not demanded or coerced. Enticing the child to be more expressive suggests a teacher role that is more suitor than sergeant. To win affection, the suitor invites and solicits participation, lures his beloved by understanding what she likes and what she can be persuaded to like. He must be flexible, explorative and creative, open and free from traditional constraints. Most of all, courtship involves mutuality: one partner learns from, and builds on, the strength and needs of the other; in the process new interests and discoveries are released, there is an expansion of heart and mind. This romantic approach toward learning, as Alfred Whitehead has beautifully described, is particularly important for the novice learner who requires considerable freedom if he is to discover the effects of his own initiative, formulate questions, seek answers. The help and discipline administered must be subtle so as not to undermine the child's zest and confidence that he can trust himself to make order out of confusion. Ideally, a teacher's guidance

> answers to the call of life within the child. In the teacher's consciousness the child has been sent to his telescope to look at the stars, in the child's consciousness he has been given free access to the glory of the heavens. Unless, working somewhere, however obscurely, *even in the dullest child*, there is this transfiguration of imposed routine, the child's nature will refuse to assimilate the alien material . . . My point is that a block in the assimilation of ideas inevitably arises when a discipline of precision is imposed before a stage of romance has run its course in the growing mind . . . Without the adventure of romance, at the best you get inert knowledge without initiative, and at the worst you get contempt of ideas—without knowledge. (1929/1959, pp. 51–52, italics added)

To release initiative in passive, inattentive children, without the use of authority, a teacher must be very resourceful. Like a suitor, she can entice by providing fetching materials, making suggestions, offering demonstrations, setting up challenges that invite (but do not demand) participation, attracting the child by the force of her personality, but she has to stop short of dominating the child's will. To be successful she, like the successful suitor, must be an expert on the child's condition and nature; she must be flexible and creative, ready to "read" the child from his reactions and shift accordingly, or, absent those reactions, ready to search for the spark that will ignite an indigenous interest. She will have to make plans and revise them when they fail; she must know his developmental destination and gently lead but still await his timetable and follow his proclivities.

Giving up substantial amounts of authority, having teachers become slot-fillers to children rather than the reverse, would inevitably introduce disorder into a program and make IEP instruction, as currently carried out, virtually impossible. Would it be a productive trade-off, at least in those areas where strict cultural compliance is not the goal, at least for some of the children more of the time?

Collaborative Teaching: The Example of Language

The five principles elaborated earlier require a realignment in the relationship between teacher and student. The leadership and guidance of the teacher has to be filtered through the availability and reactions of the child. The child's intent can no longer be dismissed as irrelevant; it has to become foreground, while the teacher's intent becomes background. Parents, teaching their nonhandicapped preschoolers to talk, intuitively assume a more collaborative and less dominant role, although parents of the retarded, like early intervention teachers, respond to slowness with production demands.

Language growth is a high priority to teachers as well as parents, one which occupies a great deal of program time and IEP space. At home, however, it is carried out much more informally and collaboratively than at school. In the home setting, children attain language through a complex child-centered approach that includes continuous adult–child reciprocity, thick redundant contexts, sensitive fine-tuning of the child's productions, and negotiation. Language, at least at the outset, is not "taught " by a parent selecting the words and speech parts that she wants the child to learn and then training acquisition; language, like an ingredient in a thick stew, is absorbed into a mix that is already substantially complete. It is an add-on, dropped into a communicative context.

Language has its origins in the nonverbal mutual mother–child interchanges, what Werner and Kaplan have called the "primordial sharing situation" (1963, p. 42). It begins, writes Jerome Bruner (1983), in the first reciprocal parent–child eye-to-eye contact. Mutual gaze is succeeded by "joint attention," the child following the mother's visual regard as she points out and names an object of interest to the child. In the next incremental advance, the child searches for an object when alerted by mother's vocal intonation alone, and finally he is able to discriminate by word meaning. Parents intuitively recognize that language is not a matter of seeking or giving information but of communication between two people locked closely together in preverbal reciprocal routines.

First words come to be absorbed by children, says Bruner, because they are embedded in familiar repetitive contexts such as games. A game format constrains content, meaning, and intention because it is ritualized, predictable, and script-like. In peek-a-boo, for example, there is a script (appearance, disappearance, reappearance) that is restricted to just a few moves and patterned interactions, or "turn-taking," between an adult and an infant with demarcated, mutually contingent roles for each (i.e., the response of each partner depends on the response of the other). The shared and familiar game structure provides a "scaffold" that supports the meaning of language (Wood, Bruner, & Ross, 1976). In language scaffolding, the adult assists the child by controlling "those elements of the task that are initially beyond the learner's capacity, thus permitting him [the learner] to concentrate upon and complete only those elements that are within his range of competence" (p. 90). It involves recruiting the child's attention; keeping the task simple, repetitive and familiar; reducing alternatives and maintaining direction; filling in gaps for the child when needed and, as the child advances, reducing the scaffold. In peek-a-boo, for example, the meaning of "Where's Mommy, find me, here I am" is already built into the game by the parent, the language layered onto existing nonverbal understandings. Another example of parental scaffolding is the practice of leaving out words from oft-repeated stories for children to fill in.[14]

Parents further contribute to language growth by gradual and modest adjustments, or fine-tuning, of the child's productions (Bruner, 1983; Snow, 1989). Baby talk ("motherese")—characterized by shorter sentences, limited vocabulary, slow and careful enunciation, good grammar, repetition, here-and-now content, amplification by pointing, more questions, different intonation

(Chapman, 1981; Gleitman, Newport, & Gleitman, 1984; Newport et al., 1977)—is a prime example of fine-tuning. This universal language pattern is literally "child-centered," for it originates in parents imitating the talk of babies (Brown, 1977). Using the baby's talk as a starter, parents go on to "recast," "expand," "correct," and carefully check, through questioning, what the child takes in.

Rather than lose the child in a conversational interchange, parents are willing actually to negotiate and compromise on word meaning. Bruner (1983) points out that if a child rejects a recasting by parents—insisting the picture is a squirrel not a mouse—the parent accedes. Or the parent will indulge the child's special vocabulary (e.g., night-night for sleep) or the child's own errors (kitty for leopard) to keep her engaged. This is done through negotiation; the parent does not didactically select words or phrases she wants the child to acquire, or insist on the child's acceptance of an expansion; rather, a mother will check to see if her child accepts the suggestion and shifts if she does not.

Increased language development, researchers have shown, is associated with "contingently responsive" verbal interactions between parents (also teachers) and children, rather than adult direction and control (Girolametto, 1988; Hanzlik & Stevenson, 1986; Mahoney, 1988a; Mahoney, Finger, & Powell, 1985; Mahoney, Fors, & Wood, 1990; Nelson, 1973; Snow, 1989). Although this is true for all children, parents of the handicapped (once again studies focus on those with Down syndrome), like their teachers, respond to deficiency by taking on a more directive and less collaborative role. Specifically, compared to parents of normal children at the same language level, they make more requests (900% more; Mahoney, 1988b) and demands, control conversational topics, talk faster and longer, and interrupt their children. Parents, in poor synchrony with their retarded children, ask questions unrelated to the child's current focus, talk at levels that are too difficult, do not promote conversational turn-taking, and may respond less to child overtures. The children, in turn, participate less in mutual exchanges. Even at the preverbal level there is less referential looking (glancing at an object and then back to mother), less back and forth vocalization, and less verbal initiative. The finding is strong, the explanation problematic.[15]

Once again we have a chicken-and-egg difficulty. Parents (like teachers) may dominate language exchanges in response to their children's *pre-existing* low initiative, passivity and limited interests; they fill in for their children's impoverished contributions and keep making suggestions to keep an interaction alive (Cunningham et al., 1981; Maurer & Sherrod, 1987; Tannock, 1988). On the other hand parental interference, growing out of pessimism over their child's abilities (Cardoso-Martins & Mervis, 1985), difficulty in reading their child's levels (Mundy et al., 1988), inappropriate expectations (Brooks-Gunn & Lewis, 1982; Mervis, 1990), or general anxiety and eagerness, may inadvertently increase the passivity (Mahoney, 1988a). In an effort to tease out which of these alternatives might be correct, Mahoney et al. (1990) found that, even when all children had the same amount of initiative, mothers of children with Down syndrome were more directive than mothers of similarly functioning normal children. Regardless of whether parental intrusiveness creates, responds to, or supports low child initiative, it seems fair to conclude that young retarded children, both at home and school, are receiving less of the nourishing reciprocal relationships accorded to the nonhandicapped.

SUMMING UP

Imagine an infant alone at sea in a row boat. You, concerned that he will drift into danger, sidle up next to his boat and tell him to start paddling; just follow you and he will reach the shore. Your instructions and modelling fall on deaf ears. In his original state of global nondifferentiation, he cannot distinguish the water from the boat, the boat from the oars, the oars from his arms, to say nothing of movement through space to an invisible destination; all is fused. But because he is "directed towards knowing" (Werner & Kaplan, 1963, p. 12), the child keeps moving his arm–oar and looking about. After months of repetitious fumbling, he begins to distinguish the topography of self and nonself. It dawns on him that his arms cause the displacement of the oars and that the movement of the oars drives the boat. More months, more repetitious fumbling and he can represent an event. "I row the boat" — agent–action–object. Now he is ready for an instruction to row; now the words will overlay an understood plan of action (though understanding the destination still awaits the experience of getting there); now he can imitate.

So we have some basic developmental principles: growth is holistic, domains within the individual and attributes outside the individual are gradually distinguished; growth is a long slow process and takes a lot of repetition; growth is accomplished through the child's own actions, it cannot be transmitted without his involvement; growth is stage-based and stage-limited, symbols are not understood before the referents are known; growth requires intrinsic motivation and is driven by a child's desire for mastery; growth is accomplished by representatives of the culture staying close to the child's position, offerings she cannot put to use will be rejected.

As far as we know, the above principles apply generally to the majority of moderately retarded children—although we have noted repeatedly the exceptions exemplified most clearly by those with autism—and therefore should serve as our guide in early intervention programs.

If heeded, the principles enumerated above would take early intervention down a reconstructed road. Methods of instruction would become more informal, more affectively colored and intense, more flexible, with teachers soliciting the involvement of children and shifting when that involvement waned. The content of instruction would become truer to life, concrete and real rather than conceptual and abstract, derived from what the child does spontaneously, not a watered down version of the first-grade curriculum. Much of the core curriculum and IEP objectives—numbers, shapes, colors, letters, big and little, antonyms, prepositions, vocabulary lists—would be abandoned. A truly "developmental" program would honor the natural way in which retarded children grow and respect their pace, not force them through a set of attainments from developmental check lists that may or may not represent a normal sequence and have little to do with children's interests, actions, motives, and manner of sorting out their world.

One possible objection to the proposed shift is that it ignores the finding of deviance. The retarded are not good boat operators; they play with the water, lose their oars, forget the objective, sit and do nothing. As much as possible teachers want to be proactive, give lots of rowing lessons, and head off the drifting. I have suggested that the twin problems of retarded children—passivity–rigidity and distractibility–impulsivity—may be, in part, a reaction to incomprehensible demands. Insofar as they are intrinsic characteristics, it is still preferable to offer better support—shorter broader paddles, sharper distinctions between child and oars, oars and boat, boat and water, a calmer sea, more obvious landmarks—than to take away from the child her captainship. She will learn, albeit slowly, by doing and self-correcting. And only her active engagement can correct (as opposed to temporarily cover up) the passivity and distractibility.

"All very well and good," another critic complains, "but what of the child who uses freedom to bang his head, stare into space?" This is a legitimate and realistic concern. Some children cannot use freedom adaptively; that is, in a state of freedom they do not advance their own growth. Although adults will disagree on what constitutes a productive use of freedom, no one, I should think, would accept persistent head-banging. But pot-banging is different. When it is explorative, shows some variation (as in the example of Danny above), is appropriate to the child's mental age, game-like, and not an exclusive behavior, it serves development. Granted, where there is no adaptive use of freedom, the teacher must intercede and become controlling. In these instances we are forced to settle for training rather than educating, without abandoning the ultimate goal of bringing the child into a state of productive self-determination. Even though training does not create changes in the child's understanding of the world, it is the right choice for some children all of the time and for others some of the time. For those few children cut off by the nature of their disorders from adaptive interchanges with the environment, the most we can do in the short run—and it is no mean accomplishment—is to establish rote conformance to reasonable social demands, eliminate behaviors that are destructive, and inculcate those that make children more acceptable and adaptive. Everyone needs to learn the rules and regulations of our society. However, we must be careful and recognize "that training is apt to kill initiative" (Whitehead, 1929/1959, p. 56).[16]

In her redesigned classroom, Midwood II, Teresa will have to do it all—establish a program based on developmental principles that also makes use of the cultural transmission model for her "deviant" children and for those skills of adaptation she wants grafted onto all children.

CHAPTER TEN

Midwood II: The Family as Model

> To imposition from above is opposed expression and
> cultivation of individuality; to external discipline is opposed
> free activity; to learning from texts and teachers, learning
> through experience; to acquisition of isolated skills and
> techniques by drill, is opposed acquisition of them as means
> of attaining ends which make direct vital appeal; to
> preparation for a more or less remote future is opposed
> making the most of the opportunities of present life; to static
> aims and materials is opposed acquaintance with a changing
> world.
>
> —DEWEY (1938, pp. 19–20)

SETTING THE STAGE FOR A SLOWDOWN

Teresa's head is spinning. She just informed her principal of a tempting job offer in a nearby school devoted exclusively to the preschool handicapped. He, upset by the prospect, promised her a free hand to develop an ideal program at Midwood (assuming approval of the special education director). She will be given permission to have any classroom in the building, any schedule, any type of IEPs that meets code requirements, any method of instruction. Teresa, having just read this book, is interested in rethinking her work, perhaps moving toward a more child-responsive, less accelerated program, but she remains wary. She is unsure that the proposed reforms will work, that she wants to relax demands, and she has a gnawing sense that it is somehow unprofessional to intrude less.

Doubts about a more child-centered, nondirective strategy

working are important to raise, but premature; first, we need to clarify the characteristics of a "good" outcome. I have argued for substituting broader developmental goals—such as sustaining interest, exercising initiative, exploring options, recognizing problems—in lieu of the conventional narrow preacademic ones. Since it has not been customary in early intervention to evaluate comparative goals, and since we have no information on the long-term outcome of the handicapped regardless of goals, we will need to do some controlled experimenting before the evidence is in hand.[1]

The concern about professionalism is widespread. Conscientious teachers have been taught to exert continuous leadership in the classroom, to construct lessons carefully and leave little to chance; informality, tentativeness, child input, observer status, a plan-as-you-go approach do not sit well. For Teresa, teaching is not courtship. Acting the suitor by watching children for leads, insinuating stimuli, or opening up explorative opportunities feels too passive to a prepared and determined professional. My reply is that it takes more expertise, not less, to understand a child's world construction than to force-feed into resistant minds objectives drawn from a preestablished list. A teacher's expertise is enlarged when she assembles the same detailed knowledge of her subjects as she has of her subject matter, and when she responds to each in a thoroughly individual manner, rather than merely adjusting difficulty level. In so doing, she adds the role of therapist to that of educator.

It will take all the professionalism the staff can muster to resist pressures for acceleration; to require not more, not the same, but less of these children than is expected by their parents and "the system"; to help parents adjust their manner and expectations to the child; to turn classrooms into slowed-down havens specially designed to move at half-speed. To stay in synchrony with the children's pace, teachers must vigilantly monitor their own speech, movements, reactions, and demands, making sure no more is asked than the child grasps. It means using child feedback, not external criteria, to regulate moment-by-moment behaviors. It means distinguishing child repetition that is rigid and stereotyped from repetition that is adaptive. It means overcoming one's own restlessness and boredom as the children slowly and ineptly use materials, seeing with professionally sensitized sympathetic eyes that in the child's fumbling lies his struggle for mastery. In thus bending toward the nature of the child rather than the demands of society, Teresa defends and protects her clients' interests—the first commandment of a professional—against less knowledgeable nonprofessionals.

Teresa is fearful that if she gives up an instructional model that is not teacher-directed and behavioral, the children will fall further behind. The belief that nurture should provide what nature has withheld is part of her professional identity, and she knows that parents will complain if she abandons her way of teaching the current set of core objectives and adopts looser objectives taught less directly. Admittedly, Teresa is intrigued by the possibility that her children may accomplish more over time if she lets up in the short run, but it is a risky wager.

By way of encouragement, what follows are suggestions on how Teresa might diversify rather than divest. Her many tasks and variety of children require a sophisticated match of technique to objective and child. I am not advocating *merely* lowering demands or installing a program approved by the National Association for the Education of Young Children. As previously indicated, there are retarded children who do not use freedom well because deficient mental structures prevent them from perceiving, manipulating, organizing, and controlling their environment. At Midwood, Austin is our best example, Heather another possibility. Furthermore, while we can slow up our special environments, we cannot control the wider world. Parents want to take their children (retarded or not) to the homes of friends, stores, restaurants, zoos, and playgrounds; they have enough to handle without the added embarrassment of a child who does not conform to public rules. Training must be done, and done through a teacher-directed cultural transmission model. The question comes down to how much, with which children, and when.

As mentioned in the introduction, the extent to which educators, parents, therapists, and the general public impose a cultural agenda on children is always a matter of taste, tolerance, and values. A moderately open society has room for some variety, and marginal groups keep pushing at the boundaries of acceptable social behavior, but generally not much room is made for the retarded. How comfortable are we when, at a restaurant, a small retarded child comes over and touches us in unfamiliar places (fingers our clothes, pulls our leg, or rubs our cheek), grabs our food, makes funny noises, messes up our place (pulls food and silverware off the table)? Do we stop to think, "Oh, this is a retarded child. That means she has a big body relative to her babyish mind, so I should expect her to act infantile?" No, unless there are telltale signs (and usually there are not), we do not even realize the child is retarded but inwardly condemn the mother for the unmanageable behavior. Even if we know the child is handicapped, we are embarrassed, irritated, and disapproving, not because we are mean-spirited but because we are thrown off guard, frightened by these unexpected and unpredictable actions; and fright turns us against the perpetrator.

Teresa is beginning to appreciate the complexity of her task. She wants to respect the developmental pace of her children—though she still cannot completely give up on pressing for those signs of progress that make them seem normal. At the same time she wants her children to be socially presentable. Maybe a slow child in a big body gets away with immaturity in a protected environment, but the demands of the outside world (even the demands of kindergarten) needle her conscience. How does she balance the social necessity for table manners and the inhibition of impulses as against the value of a prolonged, sometimes funny-looking explorative odyssey? And how does she adapt her balancing act to the differences in diagnoses and developmental rates? Teresa needs some benchmarks, although in the end she will (and should) adapt any formula to her particular set of families and her own value system.

A FAMILY MODEL

An adequate model must be supple and rich enough to make a number of distinctions and fit comfortably the variety of handicapped preschoolers. It must separate those who can and cannot profitably use freedom, the areas in which self-directed behavior is appropriate, and the levels that are right for each child. An adequate model should include all three of the Kohlberg schools differentiated by instructional objectives. Cultural transmission methods (behavioral training and teacher-selected objectives) are appropriate for what Kamii has called social-conventional learning, progressive methods for cognitive development, and romantic methods for hedonistic satisfactions. An adequate model must further allow for changing the balance struck among the "schools," depending on the child's disability and level—Austin, Carl, and possibly Heather are candidates for more cultural transmission instruction than Doreen, David, and Molly, and Carl's training has to be pegged way below Austin's. And an adequate model must envelop children in an ambience of honesty and acceptance.

We do not have far to look for an institution that provides a model for all the above: freedom and rules, expectations and interventions tailored to the child's interest and aptitude, latitude for discovery, and lots of affection and fun. We find it in the ordinary, well-functioning family. I hear Teresa resisting: "No, parents and teachers have complementary, not parallel, roles; in no way do I want, or have permission, to be like a mother." Such an objection might validly be made by a high-school biology teacher (though even she is now supposed to teach about matters formerly in the parental domain, such as safe and unsafe sex), but in early intervention the similarity of home and school tasks makes similarity of approaches a logical choice. Like parents, teachers are responsible for keeping children safe, clean, and fed; for training them to be independent in eating, toileting, and dressing; for helping them to control their impulses, cooperate with others, give and receive affection; for supporting them emotionally and building their self-esteem; for increasing their development in everything from sitting, walking, and talking, to knowledge of the cultural fundamentals. I am not suggesting that teachers become parents; teachers inevitably will be more objective, realistic, controlled, deliberate, purposeful, and self-conscious, but parents are quite amazing teachers in the early years and provide a brand of child-centeredness—melding with, yet molding, the child; bending to, yet shaping, him—that serves as a useful intervention model, *not* as a blueprint. And, more than teachers, they abide by the developmental principles elaborated in the last chapter.

Parents, at least initially, court their children, entice them to respond in a way that is foreign to early intervention. They become highly attuned to their child's communications, indulge and foster her interests, do extravagant, crazy things to attract and attach her to them (what linguists call "attention recruitment"), are truly "nutty" over their kid. They stick out their tongues, make nonsense noises, poke and tickle, gurgle and coo, fling themselves and baby about, return objects to be hurled again, any antic to get and maintain a response. The motive and objective seem clear. They will do whatever it takes, and it takes much more than praise, to elicit from the child an active interest in themselves (and in their surroundings). By intuition, by trial and error, they discover what movements and shifts in movements, what expressions and changes in expressions, what objects and object happenings most delight their child and maximize prolonged attention. They learn she prefers noisy to colorful mobiles, rough to gentle handling, sleeping with background music to silence. The experimentation with methods to arouse and comfort the child creates a deep knowledge of her—what positions are comforting; what tastes, movements, smells, and sounds delight; what inputs will tempt, excite, overwhelm, frustrate, or bore her—hence a great intimacy.

Parents do not just pamper and evoke responses, they subtly shape them as well. In this early "bonding" there is a mutuality of adaptation, each party shifting in the interest of the other. Soft rhythmic sounds, more to parental liking, may be substituted for the loud noises; nuzzling the child's tummy substitutes for rough tickling; a partially open door substitutes for the nighttime record. If the child cannot adapt to the changes, other procedures are tried, the parents watching the child's reactions as indicators of how they might shift tactics without full submission to the child's demands. The mutuality is, of course, lopsided (and here the romance analogy falls apart) because the enterprise is so child-centered.

Acting as custodian of the culture and protector of her child's safety, the parent also sets an agenda, dominates instruction, and suppresses alternatives (again, the extent varies depending on parental values). In many instances the mother offers her child few options: "You must stay in bed all night and cannot come into mine . . . You must drink from a cup, not a bottle . . . You must use the toilet, not the diaper . . . You must wear clothes that match and no dresses because you are a boy . . . You cannot go outdoors looking for Daddy . . . You cannot sit on the stove . . . You cannot climb on the car . . . You cannot eat the kitty litter." She does not much care if the child agrees, is engaged in the enterprise, or has interesting alternative notions. She wants skill acquisition and habitual unquestioning conformity. If the child resists she may delay the demand, or she may break the task down: "Just pull off your sock . . . Just pull down your pants." And she is quite prepared to use plenty of positive and negative contingent reinforcement: "One more bite and I'll give you dessert . . . No, you can't leave the table until you've had your eggs . . . You peed in the toilet, won't Daddy be proud."

Above all, the family individualizes; developmental level is always kept in mind. The 2-year-old and 4-year-old have different toys, different schedules, different adaptive requirements, and different amounts of parental attention. The 2-year-old, for example, is given more latitude, but also more supervision, than the 4-year-old. The former is allowed to pull toys off the shelf, eat sloppily with a bib for protection, cannot go out of the house alone; the latter must put her toys away, use napkins not bibs, can go to the neighbor down the street.

Parents as indulgent suitors winning their child's affection partake in the romantic model. They also do so by permitting great freedom. For much of the day the child is playing as he wishes, doing whatever comes naturally (though restricted, more or less, by family standards of appropriateness), the parent merely assuring he is safe. When parents establish and enforce behavioral requirements, they are partaking in the cultural transmission model. As collaborative partners supporting and embellishing their child's responses, negotiating novelty, watching for openings where they may insert a suggestion, they partake of the progressive model. In my travels, I noticed how natural it is for parents to teach in this "progressive" way, perhaps because they do not see themselves as teachers! Here are a few ordinary everyday parent–child exchanges to remind us.

> *(Father and son at an airport.)*
> CHILD: See the man, is he walking to the plane?
> FATHER *(expands):* Yes, he's walking. He's the pilot.
> *(Child looks confused.)*
> FATHER: *(reverting to a word already in the child's vocabulary):* He's the driver. He drives the airplane.
> CHILD: He goes up?
> FATHER: He makes the airplane go up. He sits in the cockpit.
> *(Child looks confused and starts to move away.)*
> FATHER *(realizes "cockpit" was too much so, trying to hold him):* The cockpit is where he drives the plane. Want to see the man [no longer called "pilot"] in the cockpit, where he pushes lots of buttons?"
> *(The child's face lights up at the word "buttons," and the conversation continues about how they will try to see the pilot and the buttons he pushes.)*

> *(Mother and daughter in a restroom. Mother assists child in washing her hands and pulls down a paper towel for her.)*
> CHILD: More wash.
> *(Mother goes through an abbreviated rewash.)*
> CHILD *(moves to extract towel from waste bin):* More towel.
> MOTHER: Those towels are dirty. *(She pulls down a clean one.)*
> CHILD: More wash.
> MOTHER: Time to see Daddy.
> CHILD: No, I'm cleaning. *(Rubs towel around sink.)*
> MOTHER: Time to leave.
> CHILD: No, have to clean.
> MOTHER *(negotiating their mutual demands):* Come clean Daddy's chair.
> *(Child, towel in hand, goes off with mother.)*

(Mother and son at a natural history museum, standing by a diorama.)
 CHILD: Is that a lion?
 MOTHER: No, it's a cheetah, the fastest running animal in the world.
 CHILD: Faster than me?
 MOTHER: Yes.
 CHILD: Faster than Bobby [older brother]?
 MOTHER: Yes.
 CHILD: But not faster than Dad.
 MOTHER: Yes, much much faster, fast like a car.
 CHILD: No way, an animal can't go as fast as a car. I bet I could go faster if I really tried.
 (Mother smiles and does not push the point. She sees that the child's egocentricity prevents his understanding relative speed.)

In these examples, parents differ from teachers in their structure, objectives and methods. They teach opportunistically, as the setting and child's availability allow, not within preselected time periods. They elaborate upon the child's topic rather than initiate their own. They tailor their teaching to the child's activity, not to predetermined IEP objectives. Instruction is collaborative rather than directive; parents back down when a child resists information and, when a tussle erupts, negotiate the impasse rather than securing compliance through praise or punishment.[2]

Early intervention programs, because they are formal places with specified instructional objectives, are not well positioned for a child-centered progressive model. The daily schedule, preplanned objectives, core curriculum, and group teaching limit opportunities to follow and expand upon the child's initiatives. Using the family as an organizing principle, what changes might Teresa make to bring more flexibility and child-responsiveness into her program?

MIDWOOD II

Changing Structure, Individualization, Content, and Methods

Teresa cannot accommodate the tempo of her various students unless she relaxes her schedule. This will not be easy. As previously noted, the daily schedule, an important component in early intervention programs, is multipurpose: It provides a framework for exposing children to a series of activities, each designed to stimulate a separate developmental area; it establishes a routine, seen as

so essential for children with self-control deficits; and, not acknowledged by programs, it is a device for adult authority over
unruly behavior. School would not be school without the regularity of punctuated periods. And that is just the problem. Early
intervention is too "schoolish" for young, slow children. Forced to
shift every few minutes, they cannot develop and explore interests,
feel in control and effective, or receive sufficiently individualized
attention from teachers.

There are several ways to reduce structure. Teresa can limit
the time children spend in prescribed activities, while expanding
their time in elected ones. She can increase her flexibility during
scheduled activities beyond the provisions already made (e.g., providing two Thanksgiving projects at art time, different questions
at circle time, and different demands at work time). She can have
fewer periods, with each one lasting longer. She can excuse children from scheduled activities, or they can choose among several
activities. Loosening requirements on children reduces teacher
time spent in policing and reinforcing behavior, leaving more time
for individualization.

"Individualization," like "structure" and "developmental," is
one of those words everyone subscribes to without agreement on
meaning. In early intervention, individualization is interpreted as
slotting children into appropriate objectives as determined by the
inventories against which abilities are measured; children are
placed on different rungs of the same ladder. Everyone is exposed
to the core curriculum taught according to ability in small groups
or individually (e.g., Stephen, Larry, and David identify and/or
match letters, forms, and prepositions; Heather, Molly, and Doreen fit forms into puzzles, sort colored monkeys, act out prepositions); everyone's day is similarly segmented; everyone receives
the same amount and kind of teacher attention.

This manner of individualization does not adequately respond
to the range of children. The delay-only group (Molly and Doreen)
require much less of Teresa than those with serious additional
problems (Austin and Heather). They will prosper under a strong
progressive approach because they can exploit appropriate opportunities. Not so for Austin, who when left alone, rubs spittle onto
beanbag chairs and windowpanes, recites TV ads, and grazes his
hands along the wall. He requires intensive attention and perhaps
a behavioral approach. The last thing autistic children need is the
core curriculum.[3] Ordered repetitive sequences like numbers,
shapes, colors, and letters are easily memorized by them, but the
exercises do nothing to offset, and perhaps support, their social
remoteness and poor coping. As emphasized in the previous chap-

ter, the dominance of the core curriculum is inappropriate for all the moderately retarded children. How then should it be replaced?

Perhaps because of the IEP, the importance of curriculum content has been vastly exaggerated in early intervention. Fidelity to transmitting a limited set of concepts and skills forces teachers to restrict free choice severely. A more child-oriented program, therefore, requires de-emphasis on specific predetermined content. Eliminating detailed cognitive objectives may be more palatable to Teresa if she bears in mind that until recently children successfully handled first grade (or kindergarten) without benefit of a formal curriculum. Parents, engaged with active children, apparently transmitted the necessary knowledge incidentally—8,000 to 14,000 words by age 6 (de Villiers & de Villiers, 1978). Once again, an exception should be made for children whose problems go beyond slow-only; for them *broad* corrective goals are important (e.g., increase in sustained attention, initiative and interests, communication, self-control). But for the merely delayed, specific child objectives must be extremely limited if spontaneous interests are to dominate programming. Instead of the long lists of learning objectives, Teresa might consider enumerating just how teachers will construct an environment and secure the involvement of each child. This would shift accountability from child achievement to teacher performance, with an emphasis on method greater than, or at least equal to, content.

Teachers at early intervention centers are excellent managers of children; it is rare to see any significant "discipline" problems. If Teresa follows the implications of the previous chapter—encourages children to be themselves, while she becomes less directive—one can bet there will be more "acting out" (reinterpreted as normal), higher noise levels (more child, less teacher, noise), unpredictability, and greater demands placed on teachers. They will have to become expert observers, for "only through the continual and sympathetic observation of childhood's interests can the adult enter into the child's life and see what it is ready for, and upon what material it could work most readily and fruitfully" (Dewey, 1897/1959, p. 29). They will have to expand upon children's activities with such small increments that the child can absorb the novel without labored drill. They will have to make subtle distinctions between activities that do, and do not, need to be interrupted, for not all conflict or repetitive behavior is anti-developmental: children squabbling over toys may reach their own resolutions; the slow child who, over and over, pours water from cup to cup, and transports blocks from shelf to shelf, may bore the teacher, but she is learning. Staying in tune will require self-discipline, patience, improvisation, openness, and conviction. Bearing all this in mind, let us rerun a segment of Teresa's morning and see how she experimentally modifies her practices.

Teresa's Modifications at Midwood II

The classroom is now located close to the school entrance with a connecting bathroom and big storage room. No more long corridors on arrival or lineups to go to the toilet. After watching the children, Teresa decided that what most attracted them were large objects, the opportunities to nest inside or climb on top of furniture, and messy play. To satisfy these interests, she purchased several large wooden boxes (44″ × 44″ × 22″) that can be organized in various formations. Of the six sides to each box, one is entirely open, two opposing sides have circular holes, and three sides are closed.[4] This morning she has put two boxes together (open sides touching to double the height, closed sides making a floor) and filled the bottom with small plastic balls. Another box is freestanding (open side to the floor covered with a mat and pillows, solid side as the top). A smaller cube (22″ × 22″ × 22″) holds a fiberglass tray that is filled with water. To excite the children's curiosity and participation, Teresa has added a live white rabbit and hutch.

As the children arrive (all the same ones, with the exception of Carl, who has been moved to a class for those with severe motor and mental incapacities), Alice works on unzipping, removing, and hanging up their jackets in the assigned cubby. She knows just what each requires and teaches this cultural task behaviorally. When Heather disrobes, flings her jacket to the floor, and takes off, Alice brings her back with the reminder that she cannot play until she hangs it up. When Doreen sits on the floor and refuses to unzip, Alice sits down next to her, pulls the zipper down part way, and remarks, "Now you must do the rest." Alice also assumes responsibility for taking (or sending) Heather and Molly to the toilet on a 30-minute interval schedule.

Anita now spends virtually all her time with Austin and Heather. Today she interrupts Austin's back-and-forth circuit from window to beanbag chair by clasping him under the arms and swinging him around. Catching a flicker of a smile, she continues until, tired, she lowers him to the floor, straddles his body, and begins nuzzling and tickling him. Austin looks her right in the eyes

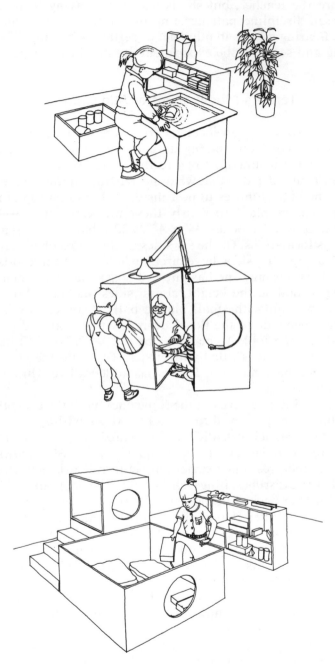

Midwood II.   Drawings by Felix Drury.

and giggles. She then picks up a stuffed animal and presses it against his stomach while he, smiling, watches her every move. Suddenly she stops and raises the animal into the air above his arm; he takes the bait, pulls at her hand indicating "more." At this point Teresa tells the children it is time for circle, but Anita stays on the floor with Austin.

> *Comment:* In Midwood I, a major objective for Austin was to establish age-appropriate behaviors through the normal use of objects. Teresa tried to accomplish this by giving him a helicopter. The intervention failed because it did not mesh with his psychological state. He used it abnormally, as a prop for his twirling interest, and then abandoned it and went back to roaming. In Midwood II, the objective is not to have Austin act more like a 5-year-old, but to participate in those infantile social interactions that are a prerequisite for normal development.

While Anita is occupied with Austin, Heather takes the can of Playskool blocks and starts gleefully slamming them into the water tray. Teresa reflects for a moment on what the behavior means. Is Heather, attracted to water like any small child, innocently indulging in the joy of splashing? (This "delay" interpretation might suggest substituting sponges for blocks.) Has she, jealous of Anita's attention to Austin, or frustrated and angry at a deeper level, deliberately chosen a "naughty" activity? (Such a "disturbed" interpretation might warrant discipline or demonstration of child-acceptance by, for example, asking Heather to be her helper.) Has the brain damage from meningitis resulted in excessively high sensory and motor arousal levels satisfied only by intense violent actions? (Such a "defect" interpretation might suggest finding a more acceptable but equally absorbing activity.) Teresa is uncertain, although she doubts the first interpretation. It will take many months of observing what Heather does at what times and how she responds to various interventions before Teresa understands this enigmatic child.

Before scolding her, Teresa decides to try an alternative activity. Going quickly to the water tray she takes Heather by the hand and says brusquely: "Heather, stop. You cannot throw blocks into the water; you see the water is getting all over the floor and wetting other children. Come with me and see if you like what is in the big boxes."

The suggestion works. Heather climbs through a hole into the boxes with the balls and is joined by Doreen. The girls prance, fall, roll around. Teresa, kneeling at the outside, comments on the activities. "Whoops, Doreen fell down. Heather, I can't see your legs. They are covered with balls." Heather, quite clearly due to excitement, kicks a ball, sending it through a box hole onto the floor. Delighted, she gathers up several more balls and throws them helter-skelter; another one gets out. This time—drawing a distinction between water and balls—Teresa decides not to stop her; instead, she brings over a large pail and invites Heather to throw balls into it. Meanwhile, David is attracted by the action. He recovers a ball from the floor and lobs it to Heather who is hanging out of the hole; so starts an interaction among Heather, Doreen, David, and the pail.

> *Comment:* In Midwood I Teresa handled Heather's "misbehavior" with prohibitions, timeout, statements that distorted her intentions (e.g., "Heather wants help to use the blocks appropriately," "wants to follow the rules"), and regular administration of positive and negative reinforcement. Now she is verbally much more straightforward ("Heather, stop. You cannot throw blocks."), and tries harder to individualize by "reading" the child's behavior and responding flexibly. As a result, at least in this instance, Heather exchanges time*out* for time spent *in* an enjoyable activity that Teresa then exploits to expand language, social, and motor education.

At circle time, now shortened considerably, Molly, as at Midwood I, starts to stroke David's arm during the greeting song, and he returns the touching. Since it is developmentally appropriate, Teresa lets it go on. Even so, Molly slips away and crawls into the solitary box, where she nestles against the pillows, removes her socks, and plays with her feet. After a bit she climbs out, goes to the shelf that houses the cardboard blocks, picks one up, returns to the solitary box, deposits the block in the box, climbs in, climbs out, goes to the shelf for another block, deposits it in the same box, climbs in, climbs out, and continues this routine until five blocks have been deposited into the box. Then, finding the box crowded, she reverses the routine, returning blocks to the shelf one at a time. On one trip from box to shelf she forgets to replace the block and is startled to see it still in her hands when arriving back at the box ready, but unable, to pick up another one. She deliberates (looks at the block in her arms, the blocks in the box and on the shelf), picks up a second block while holding onto the first, drops it on the floor as she returns to the shelf, goes back for it, puts it away, and then back to the box for a remaining block.

Teresa allows all this to continue. However, when Molly removes Larry's candy from his backpack, she intervenes quickly: "Molly, you must put the candy back. It is Larry's. If you want, you may play with your own backpack." Teresa also makes a mental note to bring in some hanging shoe bags with assorted objects for Molly to sort and rearrange.

> *Comment:* In Midwood I "paying attention" meant conforming to group routine. In Midwood II it is reinterpreted as involvement with activities appropriate to a child's developmental level. Molly is learning more, Teresa realizes, through her block trips (about space, size, weight, sequences) than by nonparticipatory passive sitting. But even developmentally appropriate acts are stopped when they are not culturally acceptable (seizing another child's treasure). Taking her cue from Molly's behavior, Teresa decides to encourage the packing and unpacking "schemas" by bringing in shoe bags. Again, in this incident, Teresa does not distort Molly's feelings as she did at Midwood I ("I know you didn't mean to take Larry's candy." "She is sorry, aren't you, Molly?"), but matter-of-factly lays down the rules.

At music time, when the children choose "The Wheels on the Bus" for their song, Teresa asks for volunteers to get on the floor and be a "bus," or "climb" on the "bus" and be the "man" who goes "honk, honk, honk." Following some initial confusion—Doreen wants to be "man-bus"—each child takes a position, either crouching on the floor as a "bus" or sitting astride a "bus" as the "man." To allow for plenty of repetition, Teresa abandons the audiotape in favor of singing without accompaniment. After half a dozen honking verses, the "buses" and the "men" shift positions. Larry, as "bus," starts crawling on the floor and several others (including Austin) follow. Doreen, as "man," is left behind her "bus" (David) and shouts "Stop" to the moving caravan. This prompts Teresa to sing, "The man on the bus says, 'Stop stop stop,' " and the "buses," except for Austin, do so. Seeing the children controlled by this refrain, Teresa continues: "The men on the bus say"—and she pauses for the children's "Stop, stop, stop." The group does a series of stop-and-go verses, appropriately halting and starting at the right signals—except for Austin, who does not stop on cue, and Doreen, who grabs David's hair. Teresa embroiders the action further by pulling on a pretend bus chain at the "stop" command.

Comment: In Midwood I, though there was some choice in song selection, music was a pretty passive experience. The children, unable to keep up with the pace and rapid verse changes on the tape, watched Teresa for gesture clues and often dropped out when they were unable to or uninterested in imitating the teacher. In Midwood II, because Teresa gets her clues from the children, fewer are left behind. Further, rather than singing *about* events that may or may not be meaningful to them, the children now *become* the event—man and bus—stopping and starting one another. By making the song a collaborative event, Teresa allows the children to experience invention and control (in this instance, over one another's movements), while she still exploits opportunities for increasing their behavioral repertoire. The song is a wonderful vehicle for future enactments of traffic life that might include pedestrians and policemen as well as "buses" and "men."

At art time Teresa provides a much broader array of options—one table is completely covered with a large sheet of paper for brushing on glue and collage scraps—and Molly is allowed to continue with her block maneuvers. However, when considerable time passes and the children stay stuck on paste (brushing it on the paper, sticking their fingers in the paste bottles, smacking sticky hands together), Teresa suggests (and demonstrates) that they apply the paste to the collage materials. Everyone must come to snack, and Heather is timed-out when she grabs for extra juice before all are served; table manners, Teresa decides, are another cultural imperative.

Following snack, both play and work time are merged to provide the children a large uninterrupted period. Teresa puts out a few puzzles, stacking toys, peg and form boards, matching and sorting games for the interested. Alice sets up an obstacle course with input from Stephen and Larry. Doreen scampers to the dress-up corner followed by David, Molly, and Heather. As at Midwood I, this group busies itself putting the doll into the baby carriage, along with fistsful of plastic utensils. Heather empties a large plastic tub and stuffs the contents—imitation food and flatware—into a toy oven. Next, she seizes the baby carriage and announces, "Me go shopping." With David and Molly in pursuit, the expedition takes off but stops at the water tray, where Heather dumps the baby.

Doreen, meanwhile, puts the plastic tub over her head, sits down next to the rabbit hutch and, sticking her nose and tongue through the slats, tries to make contact with the bunny. Getting no reaction, she removes her plastic cage and joins the children at water play. Teresa, noticing the children's interests, comes over with several additional dolls, a cake of soap, washcloths, and towels.

David grabs a towel and, wrapping it over his shoulders, struts about the room flapping his arms. Arriving at the big box, he does not notice that Austin and Anita are sitting inside. Anita has been trying to engage Austin in reciprocal exchanges by giving him one end of a rope while she holds onto the other. Earlier, in repeated attempts, he dropped it each time she pulled, so now she has tied the rope onto his wrist and is jerking it hard to get his attention, but with no success. As David arrives, she is wondering if elastic material such as Silly Putty would be conducive to reciprocal pulling. Outside the box, David drapes the towel over one side (thereby covering a hole) and, much to his surprise, it vanishes as Austin pulls from within. Seizing the moment, Anita gets another towel and, with Austin in hand, drapes it over the opposite hole. A peek-a-boo game commences: the two boys pull down the towels, sight each other through the portholes, raise the towels again, and continue. David laughs and says, "Hi, Austin," each time the two heads meet at the openings. The exchange lasts only briefly. When Austin sits on his towel, gets absorbed in twisting a loose thread, and begins to rock, David takes off.

As the girls busy themselves with washing, Teresa watches with interest and *occasionally* comments on their actions with questions, suggestions, amplifications, demonstrations—"How does the hair get shampooed? . . . What parts of the baby need to be washed? . . . What will you do when she is clean? . . . Heather, don't forget to wash inside her ears . . . Do you need more soap? . . . Doreen, how about turning your baby over and doing her back? . . . I think I'll dry my big baby with the big towel. Please hand it to me, Doreen? . . . When the babies are washed and dried, what should be done next?" Teresa is mindful always to wait for responses and adjust her subsequent remarks accordingly:

> DOREEN *(replying to the last question):* Sleep now.
> TERESA: Where will the babies sleep?
> *(Doreen looks around and marches over to the big box, only to find Austin and Anita inside.)*
> TERESA: I wonder if you can find another place?
> DOREEN *(reaching for the top of box):* Up dere.
> TERESA: Good idea. Let's put the babies up on top of the box *(but she does not assist).*

Doreen stretches to reach the top of the box, realizes she is too short, and runs off to find something she can stand on. She first tries to move a table—too heavy. She then brings over a couple of Playskool blocks—too small. Finally she finds the steps by the sink and, with the help of Heather, drags them to the big box—just right.

Teresa asks: "Will the babies sleep just like that? Do they need to be wrapped in a something?" The question sets off more activity.

> *Comment:* Although teachers cite children's short attention span as a primary problem, well-occupied children are often interrupted to meet the schedule. At Midwood I the children were frequently told, before they were ready, to clean up and prepare for the next activity. Beyond the frustration and disappointment the interruptions must cause, they discourage sustained concentration and the enlargement of play repertoires. A bigger time frame permits teachers to pace transitions according to the children's own rhythms—a short time in the doll corner, a longer time with the bathing; or a number of short bursts for Molly, more sustained play for David—and to take advantage of serendipitous events. Even had Anita thought of the peek-a-boo game with the towels—a perfect intervention for an autistic child—it is unlikely David would have cooperated in the game on demand. The enthusiastic vibrations David sent to Austin could only come from spontaneous invention.
>
> The unanticipated towel game turns out to be more effective in establishing reciprocal play than Anita's pulling efforts; but it should be noted that, because he is autistic, Anita is also teaching Austin "reciprocal play" in a self-conscious, determined manner, just as she teaches table manners and dressing to everyone.
>
> To criticism that Teresa has substituted "play" for "work," I would respond that the two are now naturally joined without teachers straining to keep children on task. For example, during the washing scene Teresa naturally alludes to many of the items traditionally found on IEPs—body parts, prepositions (turn the baby over, wash inside her ear), sequencing (first wet, then shampoo, then dry), even big–little and more–less (Teresa requests the little towel to dry the baby, asks Heather if she needs more soap for washing?). Better still, at the big box, Doreen hears the words "up" and "in" while she lives them. And best of all, problems and solutions (where to put the baby, how to get her to the designated spot) are not artificially manufactured but arise in the context of Doreen's interests, stimulated by Teresa's questioning.

The morning ends with a review of the song and dance routine planned for the Christmas assembly. Since Teresa knows it is hopeless for all the children to perform in unison, she is orchestrating appropriate roles. Heather will conduct with a baton, Molly will be in charge of the cymbals, the boys will sing the lyrics, and Doreen will have a simple dance.

Evaluating Midwood II

When the children are gone, Teresa and her aides sit down to review the new program. They all agree it was an exhilarating morning; more fun, less tiring than Midwood I. Anita is jubilant. Did everyone see the David–Austin interaction? Did they agree that it was a tremendous breakthrough for Austin, the first time he had ever participated in social play? What should they do to make sure it happens again? She cannot wait to phone his mother.

Alice is more sober and dubious.

> "I didn't like the free-for-all atmosphere. It was really hard for me to let Molly leave the circle, and when I saw what she did— playing with her toes—I was sure it was a mistake. What if she does that sort of thing in kindergarten? I also didn't like David flying around like Batman. Remember how well he has been doing in phonics? Instead of flapping his arms, he could have have been practicing his sounds. The 'ball bath' might be OK for a child like Carl, or even Austin, but it plays right into Heather's wild behavior. Especially letting her hurl balls out of the box. It will only encourage her to do more throwing. I don't see what she learns from all that. And while I'm at it, the water play seems to me a waste of time. That's the kind of activity parents may do with their children, not teachers. It's no big accomplishment to keep them attentive in water, but that's not our job. We need to keep them attentively listening when someone is speaking."

Anita, boldly:

> "I don't agree. We should go further. The less interference, the better. Teresa, I believe you should have stayed out of the flare-up between Molly and Larry altogether. He could have rescued the candy without help and let Molly know in no uncertain terms that she has to leave his possessions alone. That's a lot better than a teacher lecturing to her. I also thought you should have let the children play with the paste and not suggested a collage. We talk about the importance of sensory experiences and then, when the children indulge themselves, we say no. What's so important about a collage that you pushed them to do it? They'll be making those for years. I thought it was wonderful when Doreen tried to

make contact with the rabbit through her own 'cage.' We could make it easier for her by taking the rabbit out of the hutch tomorrow."

Alice groans:

"And will you clean up after the rabbit, Anita? Look, I understand the idea that perhaps we should act more like parents because we deal with the same developmental issues, but today we went *further* than parents—children inside boxes, throwing balls around, glue, water, rabbits—and now, Anita, you are suggesting we go further still. Maybe we were too restrictive at Midwood I, but now you want the opposite extreme, and that's just as bad. These children are retarded. They depend on us to get them organized, ready for schooling, and I think it's unfair just to let them go wild."

Anita, in spirited defense:

"That's just the point, Alice, they are retarded. They deserve more time to be infantile. We can't organize them; they have to organize themselves. Yes, we are 'going further' than their parents because we have a better, more professional, understanding of their problems. Parents of the retarded overregulate their children and expect too much of them, just as we did in Midwood I; that's what I think is unfair. Besides, look what it produced— passive distractible kids whom we were always controlling. That is not the road to 'organization.' "

Teresa has listened hard. This is an important discussion, not just for her children, but for the education of all children. While less exuberant than Anita, she, too, liked the changes at Midwood II. It felt good to watch more, talk, praise, and direct less; better (i.e., less coercive) to lead children by controlling the environment than by controlling their bodies. She does not mind giving up force-fed accomplishments—recognizing them as paste-ons that drop off when the teacher turns her back—for more active participation by children. Releasing the children from the schedule may have created more havoc, but it opened up space for self-determination and inventiveness. She is convinced that an authoritarian classroom, in addition to sending a you're-no-good message, works against remediating those very deficiencies (e.g., initiative and sustained activity) tagged to the retarded. She was heartened by the constructive chance encounters between children—Heather and David with the balls, Austin and David with the towels—and the way teachers elaborated on them. Reallocating teacher time so that the neediest (Austin) get the most also appeals to her. It was a relief not to be tethered to a lot of specific objectives, to make "educational" materials available but not required, and to exploit naturally occurring events for the expansion of knowledge. What such contingency teaching lacks in systematic presentation, it more than makes up for in meaningfulness, and that should result in a better "take."

The division of models—behavioral for skill instruction in cultural necessities and specific intransigent behaviors, progressive for the construction of knowledge—now makes sense to her. Still, she is uncertain of the details. Heather may need more behavioral controls by teachers. Perhaps the ball throwing is not a good idea. And no, she does not want a free-for-all between Molly and Larry, but maybe the rabbit out of the hutch, with Doreen and Molly on clean-up detail.

Teresa leaves for home knowing she has some fine-tuning of her own to do but converted to a more "parental" role for teachers. The repercussions of authoritarian teaching are graver than she had previously understood; the line between demanding productions of children and exploiting them a narrow one. She sees an analogy to the dispute over farming methods, as discussed by writer–poet–farmer Wendell Berry:

> The exploiter is a specialist, an expert; the nurturer is not. The standard of the exploiter is efficiency; the standard of the nurturer is care . . . Whereas the exploiter asks of a piece of land only how much and how quickly it can be made to produce, the nurturer asks a question that is much more complex and difficult: What is its carrying capacity? (That is: How much can be taken from it without diminishing it?) . . . The exploiter typically serves an institution or organization; the nurturer serves land, household, community, place. The exploiter thinks in terms of numbers, quantities, "hard facts"; the nurturer in terms of character, condition, quality, kind. (1977, pp. 7–8)

Teresa wants to be a nurturer.

CHAPTER ELEVEN

Conclusion—Slow Is Sometimes Fast Enough

In God's eyes the differences of social position, of intellect, of culture, of cleanliness, of dress, which different men exhibit, and all the other rarities and exceptions on which they so fantastically pin their pride, must be so small as practically quite to vanish; and all that should remain is the common fact that here we are, a countless multitude of vessels of life, each of us pent in to peculiar difficulties, with which we must severally struggle by using whatever of fortitude and goodness we can summon up. The exercise of the courage, patience, and kindness, must be the significant portion of the whole business; and the distinctions of position can only be a manner of diversifying the phenomenal surface upon which these underground virtues may manifest their effects. At this rate, the deepest human life is everywhere, is eternal. And, if any human attributes exist only in particular individuals, they must belong to the mere trapping and decoration of the surface-show.

—JAMES (1892/1958, p. 177)

Those responsible for the lives of young children draw from three child-care traditions—cultural transmission (children are empty organisms who learn through behavioral conditioning), romantic (children are preformed and learn through maturation), and progressive–developmental (children's learning is a combination of preset structures and stages and appropriate environmental interaction). The "schools," according to Kohlberg, encompass complete world views—each with its own morality, epistemology, psychology, and set of educational objectives—and are irreconcilable . For example, a commitment to learning through child *construction* (progressive–developmental) is incompatible with teacher *instruction* (cultural transmission). One cannot, therefore, combine a child discovery methodology with preset objectives, or conversely, behavioral methods with developmental objectives. The model selected depends as well upon nature-of-the-child beliefs. Progressivism, for example, with its assumption of the child as an "inquiring knower" (DeVries & Kohlberg, 1987) sits poorly with those who hold a "defect" view of the retarded.

I have argued, as an amendment to Kohlberg's irreconcilability claim, that although some within-model links seem virtually indissoluble—for example, educational objectives and methods—both the knower and the known are of such complexity that mixing the schools is possible, indeed necessary. As was obvious to the "schools" founders (Locke, Rousseau, Dewey–Piaget), children make meaning autonomously *and* are conditioned by social experiences. The capacity for independent learning, however, varies as a function of individual differences and informational content. Within the category *retarded*, the "delayed" children learn better on their own than the "deviant" group; progressive methods, therefore, are apt to be more effective with children who have Down syndrome than with children who are autistic. Within the various knowledge domains, physical and logico-mathematical knowledge require more active child participation than social-conventional knowledge. Progressive methods, therefore, are better for understanding one's relationship to a world of moving and movable parts; behavioral methods, for self-help and social compliance.

This broad theoretical framework does not get us very far into early intervention practice. It leaves unspecified the extent to which children are perceived as "defective," how a knowledge realm is partitioned, and which realms are selected for instruction. Under pressures to accelerate learning, early intervention centers tend to recast physical and logical knowledge into the social-conventional domain. To increase his acceptability in a less restrictive environment, the child learns counting, prepositions, and the days of the week, without grasping number, space, and time concepts; learns labels for objects and events that are not within his world of operative knowledge. A behavioral model, required for this instruction, gains further credibility from the belief that all retarded children are more or less "defective" and will not learn under their own impetus.

The hegemony of the cultural transmission model and the "defect" interpretation of retarded children owe more to political and social than to psychological considerations. The public has been captured by an optimistic spirit of reform. Enthusiastic teachers join parents in the hopeful expectation that if they just try hard enough, early enough, they will reverse or minimize developmental delay. Trying hard means instilling, through an ordered, intense, self-conscious regime, a "core curriculum" (e.g., shapes, colors, numbers, puzzles, big and little) normally acquired informally by nonretarded children. Teachers are encouraged in their mission by a set of powerful beliefs and circumstances that make it difficult to hold a different vision. These include: the high expectations for restoration of function established by law; the obligation to project in advance on an IEP the specifics of what a child will accomplish; the anticipation of family and professionals that children will be mainstreamed; the demands for orderly, controlled behavior natural to a school environment; the shared parent–teacher expectations for behavioral improvement; the collusion between parents and teachers to inflate progress in order to preserve their intimate alliance; the didactic pedagogy traditional to the field of special education; and the intellectual understanding that bifurcates the nature of retarded and nonretarded children.

For the most part, the curriculum seems too hard and remote for children functioning at only half their age. They respond to the difficulty with failure and resistance, thereby forcing teachers to take on excessively restrictive and repressive roles. The burden of this book is that from every standpoint—psychological, empirical, and moral—a corrective shift toward a freer, more child-centered (i.e., progressive) model is needed.

Piaget and his interpreters have taught us that adults have a somewhat limited educational impact on children. Particularly in the early years, children's learning is constrained by developmental mechanisms that restrict their "take" to what they can actively process and make sense of; nourishment in excess of the child's appetite will not be digested. An instructor can fill some open slots, support evolving structures, refine developing skills, offer opportunities—and all this is not insignificant—but the child is essentially her own teacher: She learns that which slakes her curiosity, answers her acknowledged problem; the rest is ignored or repeated by rote. The vast amounts children learn in the preschool years—as much as eight words a day—is acquired informally, on an as-needed basis.

So far as we know (and admittedly research has been restricted largely to Down syndrome populations), the constraints operating on normal children operate on the retarded as well. The principal distinction between them is rate rather than manner of learning, and attempts to speed up stages, or short-circuit self-generated learning will be no more successful with one group than the other. In the eyes of a teacher, however, a slow child may look uninterested, repetitive, passive, inattentive, and distractible—that is, "defective" in addition to "delayed." It is easy to forget that a retarded child, even in comparison to a younger normal child, will absorb stimuli slowly, repeat actions, display fewer and weaker interests; otherwise, he would not be retarded for long. The withdrawal of attention, expressed either by distractibility or passivity, will be accentuated when retarded children are placed in demanding environments poorly calibrated to their slowness. And the requirement to learn discrete bits of information with no intrinsic appeal month after month, sometimes year after year, only increases the passivity and distractibility.

Admittedly, some retarded children fit a "defect" model. Autistic children, for example, are cut off from their environment and substitute ritualistic repetitive behaviors for productive exploration. They do not go through the normal stage progression; an interest in print often precedes verbal communication. Even scaled down nondemanding surroundings will not stimulate adaptive activities in this group. The intervention research literature suggests that their "defects" require much more rigorous teacher-mediated instruction. To "individualize" adequately teachers need to give more time and directive intervention to the Austins than to the Doreens. But even with Austin, the goal is to establish sufficient social and perceptual connections with the world so that he will learn autonomously.

Professionals in the field, as devoted and conscientious a group as one is likely ever to encounter, believe accelerated learning through behavioral instruction is "for their own good" because it enhances self-esteem. If retarded children improve sufficiently to be accepted in the mainstream, and thereby avoid labeling and rejection, they will feel good about themselves. This view of self-esteem—as a derivative of the approval society gives for one's success in meeting its general standards and expectations—is valid but incomplete. Self-esteem flows also from being one's natural self without regard to social comparisons. For this to occur among the retarded, society has to withhold its normal standards and judgments. And therein lies a tension.[1] To promote both sources of self-esteem simultaneously is often very difficult, as every teacher has discovered. Acceptance of the slow child as-is (romantic model) often means not holding him to the same standards that are applied to other, higher functioning, children. When a conscientious but weak student does poorly and, according to the grading criteria, merits an F, the teacher can uphold social standards and give the low grade, or uphold the child, lower the demand and thereby raise the grade. A low grade may injure self-esteem. Reducing the demands dissolves the distance between child and social (teacher) expectation and may increase self-esteem but at the cost of separation from other, higher achieving, children. This is what occurs when retarded children are not entered in the races most children run, but, instead, have a Special Olympics of their own.

In an ideal situation, socially acceptable expectations are attractive to children's natural interests and not too far a reach. In meeting them, children can then receive *both* social approval and personal fulfillment. The larger the gap between child and criteria, the harder it is for a child to achieve social and personal acceptance. At early intervention—because of the alien, difficult and uncompromised work requirements—children are largely deprived of both. Teachers, to keep the child motivated and on task, rely on effusive praise (lowering demands is not an option). The problem is that with children who mostly fail and resist, it is hard to find acts worthy of praise. So the teacher handles failure by "cheating"—for example, she puts the right answer under the child's nose and then praises her response—or ignores it and praises the effort. She handles resistance by replacing a child's impulse with her own demands—for example, "You want help sitting" when the child wants to leave. (In the same way a "regular" teacher may "cheat" by coaching a child on an upcoming exam, attribute failure to lack of application, or grade on effort rather than accomplishment.) The problem with this dissimulation is that it deprives the child of an objective standard against which to measure herself. When guesswork and pretense are encouraged, failures ignored, and feelings distorted, the child can only be confused about who she is and what she must do. Teacher-pleasing becomes an end in itself rather than a means to an end. The child is working for praise, not for accomplishments, and so loses out on self-esteem from attainments. The shift in the child's goals—from socially acceptable standards to praise—may seem slight until one witnesses children blindly guessing, searching the teacher's face for clues, and clapping for themselves as if to bring on, or mimic, her approbation. It is hard to imagine the possibilities for self-respect in such truly rudderless children.

   The other means of supporting self-esteem—a genuine tolerance and respect for the child as-is—is even more neglected. Children in early intervention programs are rarely far from a teacher's
reach, either physical or verbal. Their moves are carefully monitored when not prescribed, their initiatives regularly "redirected,"
their opportunities for free choice narrowly curtailed. The sadness
of so much repression is heightened when one considers what
happens to this population with age.

   Situated in a society too complex for their adaptive skills,
most moderately retarded adults will have very circumscribed
choices: where they live and are employed (if they can do anything
gainful at all), with whom they live, and how they spend leisure
time will largely be determined for them. Their big choices may be
a coke or milkshake at McDonald's, a brown or blue sweater at
Sears. Given these unenviable social prospects—in part the necessary consequences of a limited mentality but also the circumstan-
tial consequences of our elaborate society—must we also deny
them freedom in the preschool years? Must they do penance because they are handicapped? Are not the retarded entitled to *at
least* as much freedom as the nonretarded child? One could argue
they are entitled to more. Those of us without mental limitations
have ongoing opportunities throughout our lives for self-definition
and self-renewal. But for the retarded, who will be marginalized
by a society that is too hard and too fast, the early years—when
they are unaware of their pariah status, when social demands are
less, and indulgence for immaturity greater—may be their one
chance to acquire self-esteem through approval of who they are,
not what they should achieve.

   Genuine noncontingent acceptance requires an earnest commitment to the popular adage: "They are children first who happen to be retarded." It will be easier for the child to overshadow
her retardation if we relax our reformist agenda. Like all children
the retarded are naive, innocent, affectionate; willful, whiny, demanding, and disagreeable. Like all children they experience the
elemental pleasures of the senses, the good feelings of intimate
attachments, and the revelations of discovery. Like all children
they bring joy to caretakers through their dependency, "bonding,"
and small steps towards independence—made more precious
when so belated. To appreciate these qualities we must join in
their natural pace. We can no more expect a 4-year-old, functioning at the 2-year level, to master "story listening skills," shape and
number knowledge, sitting and attending, than we would expect a

9-year-old to master the social–sexual skills of a high-school senior. The more teachers accommodate to the children's special needs, the less they will have to censor and distort their behavior.

The go-slow message should not be misinterpreted as support for benign neglect. To emphasize the point once more, retarded children and their families need and deserve professional intervention in the preschool years. It takes savvy, sensitive, and well-trained personnel to circumvent passivity and distractibility in the children and excessive intrusiveness and demands by the parents; to provide an environment that invites prolonged productive participation; to spot and enlarge upon nascent interests and skills. Not any old environment or caretaker will do. We need a different, not a lesser, vision. Rather than getting children prepared for the next environment, we need to prepare present environments that intrigue and appeal. Rather than dictate behavior to children, we must find dictates in their behavior. Slowing up will give these children, like other children, the opportunity for mastery and discovery, for fulfillment of their own drives while they meet expectations set by adults. Paddling with the tide, guiding rather than coercing, should result eventually in greater conventional achievements. The burden of change, however, does not rest on teachers alone.

No child can say with dignity, "I am mentally retarded," without a "so be it" from the rest of us.

Notes

CHAPTER ONE

1. Although all moderately retarded children were by no means institutionalized at this time, it was a common choice. The number of retarded children in institutions rose steadily from 1940 until the 1970s when the deinstitutionalization movement started to reverse the trend. Of the residential institutions for the retarded in the United States, 75% were built after 1950 (Scheerenberger, 1983; see also Robinson & Robinson, 1964, for a discussion of the institutionalization movement).

2. "Early intervention" refers to educational and quasi-educational services for handicapped children ages 0 through 5. In many states the administrative structures and methods of service delivery are divided at age 3, with the older children often educated in public schools, the younger children in other facilities or at home. Programs for 3 and older have existed for some time, in some states as long as 10–15 years, and so are more "jelled" than programs for the younger population. As of 1991, under Public Law 99-457 all children ages 0 to 6 are entitled to a free, appropriate education if their state agrees to the conditions for accepting federal funds.

3. Diana Baumrind (1967, 1968, 1971, 1975), in a mammoth longitudinal study, observed three major types of parenting (with subtypes within each style)—authoritative, authoritarian, and permissive (she later added a fourth, nonconforming). They differ markedly from one another on the freedom–restraint dimension.

Baumrind characterizes the authoritarian parent as one who attempts:

> to shape, control, and evaluate the behavior and attitudes of the child in accordance with a set standard of conduct, usually an absolute standard,

theologically motivated and formulated by a higher authority. She values obedience as a virtue and favors punitive, forceful measures to curb
self-will at points where the child's actions or beliefs conflict with what
she thinks is right conduct. She believes in inculcating such in-
strumental values as respect for authority, respect for work and respect
for the preservation of order and traditional structure. She does not
encourage verbal give and take, believing that the child should accept
her word for what is right. (1971, p. 22)

The authoritative parent, by contrast, attempts

to direct the child's activities but in a rational issue-oriented manner.
She encourages verbal give and take, and shares with the child the
reasoning behind her policy. She values both expressive and in-
strumental attributes, both autonomous self-will and disciplined conformity. Therefore, she exerts firm control at points of parent–child
divergence, but does not hem the child in with restrictions. She recognizes her own special rights as an adult, but also the child's individual
interests and special ways. The authoritative parent affirms the child's
present qualities, but also sets standards for future conduct. She uses
reason as well as power to achieve her objectives. She does not base her
decisions on group consensus or the individual child's desires; but also,
does not regard herself as infallible or divinely inspired. (pp. 22–23)

Finally, the permissive parent attempts

to behave in a nonpunitive, acceptant, and affirmative manner toward
the child's impulses, desires, and actions. She consults with him about
policy decisions and gives explanations for family rules. She makes few
demands for household responsibility and orderly behavior. She presents herself to the child as a resource for him to use as he wishes, not as
an active agent responsible for shaping or altering his ongoing or future
behavior. She allows the child to regulate his own activities as much as
possible, avoids the exercise of control, and does not encourage him to
obey externally-defined standards. She attempts to use reason but not
overt power to accomplish her ends. (p. 23)

The effects on children of these three styles are too complex and qualified
to be adequately summarized but, without doubt, Baumrind finds the
children of authoritative parents to be the most competent—self-reliant
and assertive, but controlled and respectful of group standards.

4. The priority given to the early years, both for correcting and
damaging children, has an intuitive resonance to our post-Freudian ears
that is not well supported by research. Head Start, according to Ramey
and Suarez (1985), was built on the early experience and critical-period
paradigm. It seemed reasonable: give an educational boost to the dis-

advantaged during the early years when the mind is most pliant and learning most rapid (Bloom, 1964) and they will be prepared for school, "inoculated" against the possibilities of future school failure (Sarason, 1990, and Zigler, quoted in Holden, 1990—both describe the inoculation theory of Head Start). Today researchers criticize this thinking as over-simplified: Early positive experiences do not necessarily have the lasting beneficial effects, nor early negative experiences the lasting deleterious effects, formerly attributed to them. The issue of human malleability is, of course, highly contested, enormously complex, and hard to study because the number of intertwining variables cannot readily and ethically be isolated and controlled. Consequently, there is a tendency for the pendulum of opinion to swing. (For a good recent review of various viewpoints, see Gallagher & Ramey, 1987.)

To a large extent, contemporary work suggests, the development of early cognitive and sensorimotor processes await physiological maturation (Brownell & Strauss, 1985). Development is strongly canalized, resilient and buffered against permanent alteration either for good or ill (Kopp & McCall, 1982; Wilson, 1983). According to Sandra Scarr (1982), a highly respected investigator in the field, specifically designed remedial environments have little impact on the broad array of generally acquired infant and child behavior. Narrow skills, of the kind often taught in early intervention, may be more susceptible to tutoring and less likely to be "picked up" through the general environment, but there is no evidence that such skills are the basis for, or related to, later skills; even assuming a relationship between early "preacademics" and later reading or math, there is no reason to believe that accelerating one will lead to acceleration of the other. As Scarr plainly puts it, "I do not know of any evidence for an early critical period for the development of component reading skills" (p. 475). Specific instruction may be required by some children to learn some skills, but the results will not be as facile or generalizable as that which is learned naturally. In other words, it is probable that the more narrow and explicit the instruction, the less its general adaptive utility.

If early development is less reversible than the environmentalists have held, later development may show greater plasticity. The story of Genie illustrates the remarkable recuperation of an adolescent youngster after a desperate childhood. According to Susan Curtiss (1977, 1981), who worked extensively with this child,

> From the age of 20 months on, Genie was confined to a small bedroom in the back of the family home. There she was tied to an infant potty seat by means of a harness which allowed her mobility only of her lower arms and hands, and lower legs and toes. She was frequently removed from this harness at night and "dressed" in a sleeping bag with sewn-in arm restraints, and therein placed in a wire mesh crib with a wire mesh

cover. She was fed only infant food . . . Light mainly came from a bare
ceiling light bulb . . . There was no TV or radio . . . and Genie was beaten
for making noise. Genie's mother developed bilateral cataracts shortly
after Genie's birth; thus, Genie's care fell on her brother who, together
with the father, never spoke to her. When Genie was 13½ years of age,
her mother arranged to escape from the home with Genie, after which
she applied for welfare . . . She [Genie] could neither chew nor bite; could
barely walk; had flexion contractures at her hips, knees, and elbows; was
incontinent; and could neither speak nor understand language. (p. 151)

With intervention Genie learned to eat, walk, use the toilet, relate warmly
to others, and, most remarkably, speak, although her language was not
normal and lagged behind other functions.

Clarke and Clarke (1976), in an influential book, cite other cases of at
least partial recovery from extreme deprivation. In a chapter of that book,
Jerome Kagan argues against a strong critical-period position that, he
believes, has improperly overgeneralized from animal to human experiences. He summarizes his reading of the literature in the following balanced remarks:

> For most of this century developmental psychology has been friendly
> toward the pole of the irreversibility–reversibility theme that posited
> irreversible effects of early experience. The extreme form of that position
> is as unlikely as the opposite pole that assumes complete capacity for
> resilience of all dispositions at any age . . . The first messages written on
> the *tabula rasa* may not necessarily be the most difficult to erase. (Kagan,
> 1976, p. 121, italics in original)

We can surmise from the above that little children are both more and
less easily influenced than older children and their susceptibility to
change depends upon the targeted area. It is easier for them to learn a
foreign language during the preschool years but easier to learn to read in
the elementary ones. Offsetting the findings of early plasticity are those of
stage and physiological readiness.

5. David Elkind's (1988) position is that efforts to accelerate development are not merely harmless, but detrimental, to development. Beyond
failing to meet their stated aims, such efforts actually inhibit children's
desire to learn.

6. For discussions of deaf education see Furth (1973), Lane (1989),
Liben (1978), Meadow (1980), Medoff (1980), Sacks (1989), and Schlesinger
and Meadow (1972).

The effort to "normalize" extends beyond the mentally retarded and
deaf. R. D. Freeman (1976) describes instances of other disabled populations pushed, against their preferences, to obscure their handicap.
Thalidomide children, for example, have rejected the introduction of

upper-limb prostheses, preferring to use their feet or abnormal arms. Cerebral palsy children have resisted professional efforts to give them a normal-looking gait, preferring their own abnormal, but more comfortable, one. As an individual quoted by Freeman put it:

> They [the public] seem to impose upon the disabled person, or upon his or her parents, the obligation to do everything possible to "improve" the disabling condition and bring about "progress." To my doctors and parents, for instance, my ungainly walk appears abnormal, in need of correction, and "wrong." For myself, it's the way I most naturally get about . . . I simply . . . do not share the overwhelming interest . . . in doing everything possible to ameliorate my disability at the expense of other things important to me. (Freeman, 1976, pp. 112–113, quoting Blumberg)

And for a hundred years there were efforts to withhold braille from the blind because it isolated them. Freeman questions the prevailing assumption that the handicapped are, or should be, grateful for efforts to make them more normative.

7. The reader may object to the analogy between the education of deaf and retarded children. The argument might go as follows: For the deaf, who have a circumscribed limitation, signing is a good substitute for "normal" education; for the retarded, with their overall limitations, no such substitute is available. Accordingly, the best way to advance the deaf is through sign language; the best way to advance the retarded is through acceleration. In response—although, admittedly, the analogy between deaf and retarded children is not perfect—there are two striking similarities. First, for the deaf formerly, as for the retarded now, educators have stressed conformity to the mainstream over acceptance of differences. Second, for both groups, the resolve to restore normality has proceeded without documentation of likely success; it may be as difficult to accelerate the retarded as to teach oral language to the deaf.

Harlan Lane, by contrasting the positions of Laurent Clerc, a 19th-century advocate of signing, to that of Alexander Graham Bell, a 19th-century advocate of oralism, sets up useful, if exaggerated, alternatives that are relevant to the essential question of this book—to what extent do we try to remake the child according to our specifications, and to what extent do we remodel the surroundings for the child's comfort?

> Where Clerc saw difference, Bell saw deviance; the one had a social model of atypical people, the other a medical model. For Clerc, deafness was, above all, a social disability; the great problem of the deaf was the hearing world in which they were a minority; he hoped for a day when hearing people of goodwill would remove the handicap by accepting deaf culture and language. For Bell, deafness was a physical handicap; if it

could not be cured, it could be alleviated by covering its stigmata; hearing people of goodwill would aid the deaf in a denial of their particular language and culture, in "passing" as hearing people in a hearing world. Addressing a conference of speech teachers, Bell said of deaf children, "We should try ourselves to forget that they are deaf. We should teach them to forget that they are deaf" . . . While for Clerc the overriding purpose of education was personal fulfillment, for Bell it was integration with the hearing majority. (Lane, 1989, pp. 340–341)

8. Estimates on the number of children eligible for early intervention services vary from 1 to 12% if states elect a narrow definition of developmental disabilities, but that jumps to 20–30% if the "at-risk" population is included (Harbin, Terry, & Daguio, 1989). Even a conservative 3% rate yields an estimated 571,350 handicapped children ages birth through 5 (based on 1987 live births; Bureau of the Census, 1990). No figures are currently available on the projected costs of educating this preschool population. However, using the 1991–1992 projection of $10,064.00 per special education pupil (Sylvia Feldman, Planning and Budget Office, Department of Special Education, personal communication, October 1991), and multiplying that by 3% of the 0 to 5 population, early intervention would cost *$5,750,066,400*. This may be too low, if the states consider more than 3% as "developmentally disabled," and it may be too high, if services are limited and costs kept below special education generally. Estimates done for the National Early Childhood Technical Assistance System (Bowden, Black, & Daulton, 1990) are based on case studies of particular states and tend to be somewhat lower. (One should, however, be wary of lower figures that may not include transportation.) From all estimates, it is clear that if the initiative is carried out seriously, it will be very costly.

Head Start, by contrast, projected a 1991 budget of *$1,951,800,000* to serve approximately 596,295 children (Project Head Start Statistical Fact Sheet, 1991). Thus, unless Head Start grows, we can expect early intervention to serve approximately the same number of children (because it extends from ages 0 to 5, whereas Head Start is a 1- to 2-year program), but at much greater cost. Even if per child costs for early intervention were as little as $5,000.00, it would carry a price tag of *$2,856,750,000*.

CHAPTER TWO

1. The National Association for the Education of Young Children (NAEYC; Bredekamp, 1987) endorses "appropriate developmental practice" as the approach of choice for normal preschool children. Authorities

in preschool education for the handicapped, because of the special nature of their population, tend to favor a more prescriptive approach (e.g., Bagnato & Neisworth, 1981; Bailey & Wolery, 1984; Carta, Schwartz, Atwater, & McConnell, 1991; Fewell & Kelly, 1983; Hanson & Lynch, 1989; Neisworth, Willoughby-Herb, Bagnato, Cartwright, & Laub, 1980). However, this division is by no means uniform. There are emerging voices, albeit still a minority, that support the NAEYC approach for handicapped, as well as for normal, preschoolers (Astman, 1984; Ballard, 1987; Heshusius, 1982; Poplin, 1988a, 1988b).

2. As of 1989, Iowa, Minnesota, and Nebraska offered services from birth; Virginia, from age 2; Connecticut and Massachusetts, from age 3. Arizona, California, Georgia, and Pennsylvania had no educational entitlement until age 5 but offered a variety of programming (for services listed by state, see Thiele & Hamilton, 1991).

3. On my behalf, Jill Greenberg carried out the enormous task of contacting leaders in 10 states, finding appropriate programs for me to visit, and coordinating dates for a cross-country trip.

4. The concept of prototypes and the distinction between prototypes and averages has been thoughtfully analyzed by Eleanor Rosch and her colleagues (Rosch, 1975, 1977; Rosch & Mervis, 1975). The prototype, they point out, is the best exemplar of a category—for example, apple is a prototypical fruit and robin a prototypical bird. It is more a set of correlated features that come together and create saliency or distinctiveness for people, than a list of criterial or average attributes.

CHAPTER THREE

1. The notion that knowledge depends on self-generated action may have been systematized by Piaget, but long before Piaget it influenced the child-study and kindergarten movements in this country through the work of Froebel (Weber, 1984; White & Buka, 1987). Writing in 1826, he advanced the critical importance of "self-activity" (Froebel, 1826/1887). According to Froebel, development moves "from within outward" through the spontaneous activity of the child. By acting on the world, largely through the medium of play ("the highest phase of child-development"), inchoate feelings become differentiated and the world is made real. Froebel cautions against learning that occurs from the outside in: "To have found one-fourth of the answer by his own effort is of more value and importance to the child than it is to half hear and half understand it in the words of another; for this causes mental indolence" (p. 86). A case in point—relevant to the instructional programs in early intervention—the

learning of numbers. At first the child spontaneously groups similar familiar objects, say, apples, pears, nuts, beans.

> Let, now, the mother or some other attendant add the explanatory word; in other words, let them join the visible with the audible, thus bringing it nearer the child's insight and knowledge, nearer his inner perception by naming these objects . . . e.g.: apple, apple, apple, apple etc. . . . At no time should the numerals be given to the child as empty, unmeaning sounds and be thus repeated by him. (pp. 81–83)

2. Both Dewey and Piaget analogize learning to eating. Dewey wrote, for example: "Subject-matter is but spiritual food, possible nutritive material. It cannot digest itself; it cannot of its own accord turn into bone and muscle and blood" (1902/1959, p. 95). In a similar vein Piaget believed that the mind has to be nourished, not furnished. External reality provides "aliments" (food) to be digested (assimilated), but the child has to do the work of digesting (1952, 1970).

3. For interesting accounts of, and explanations for, the success of Japanese education see the following: Barrett (1990), Garden (1987), Leestma (1987), McKnight et al. (1987), Miyake, Campos, Kagan, and Bradshaw (1986), Simmons (1990), Stevenson and Lee (1990), Tobin, Wu, and Davidson (1989), White (1987), and White and LeVine (1986).

Students of Japanese child-raising and early education agree that Japanese mothers, who spend considerably more time in that role than their American counterparts, encourage dependency and intimacy, rarely threaten, warn, or punish, and consider it a duty never to oppose the child's wishes. It is a true Rousseauean world. Children are perceived as born good, their instincts to be trusted; the task of mothers is to protect the child from influences that may inhibit that goodness. At preschools—attended by 40% of the 3-year-olds and 90% of 4- and 5-year-olds—children receive a nonacademic curriculum: music, games, physical activity, origami, group cooperation, and chores. They are expected to be "lively and boisterous" (Simmons, 1990, p. 60), although short periods of time are set aside for repetitive instruction in songs and rituals. White (1987) reports that in a survey of elite private kindergartens thought by parents to encourage preacademics, only 13% taught even a few written characters and only 8% provided work with numbers; neither activity occurred in public kindergartens. As good Rousseaueans, the Japanese do not raise blithe spirits; they believe that enduring hardship toughens character, but not during the preschool years. Despite all this early indulgence, by first grade the children are academically ahead of their American counterparts (Stevenson & Lee, 1990).

4. The Middle Ages might have been a more fertile time for the

"romantic" school. A leave-alone policy was then compatible with various popular perceptions of the retarded—innocents and children of God, possessed by the devil (some burned as witches in the Inquisition), or buffoons and jesters (Scheerenberger, 1983).

5. The division between under- and overactivity, that today we often see as aspects of a single child, goes back at least 100 years when it was used to categorize types of individuals. Martin Barr, chief physician of the first training school for the retarded, located in Elwyn, Pennyslvania, described, in 1899, two types of low-grade retarded children: "one good, docile, obedient, having little or no will power . . . the other, obstinate, perverse and indolent, needs always a strong hand to keep him at constant occupation . . . He would be the tyrant of a household—the terror of a community" (1899, p. 206). Other authorities classified the retarded as "apathetic" and "excitable" (Wylie, 1901), as "passive" and "restless" (Tredgold, 1908), or as "dull and apathetic" versus "nervous and easily excited" (Nash, 1901/1902).

6. The absence of executive (or metacognitive) skills is another explanation for the reduced mental flexibility found in the retarded. Inattentive to their own performances, they are apt not to recognize when a particular strategy is failing and another one, one that even may be part of their behavioral repertoire, is required. Their failure rates could be reduced if they took more control over learning by organizing, elaborating or reducing their own previously acquired information (Brown, 1974; Campione, Brown, & Ferrara, 1982). Along similar lines, it has been suggested that the retarded are poor planners, they lack foresight; this problematic characteristic is found in samples of the retarded, even when equated with control groups on mental age (Goodman, Fox, & Glutting, 1986; Naglieri, 1989).

7. One well-developed curriculum for preschool retarded children, High Scope (Hohmann et al., 1979), is derived from Piaget's work. It stresses the value of child-initiated activities and defers the presentation of new material until the child has reached the appropriate cognitive stage. However, the curriculum is criticized by leading developmentalists (DeVries & Kohlberg, 1987; Kamii & DeVries, 1977) as violating Piaget's theory because it sets out instructional activities in domains—such as classification, seriation, time, numbers, spatial relations—that are essentially unteachable. The critics claim that these knowledge areas merely illustrate the end points of a reasoning process and it is the reasoning—which cannot be taught—rather than the content, that is important. Children may learn the appropriate words associated with the domain areas, but not the more essential conceptual underpinnings. The result is the appearance, rather than the substance of learning; what Kamii and

DeVries (1977) call "school varnish," a shiny superficial gloss not integrated with the child's cognitive structures.

8. For good general references on autism see Cohen, Donnellan, and Paul, (1987), Rutter and Schopler (1978), and the *Journal of Autism and Developmental Disorders.*

9. Philip Strain has also carried out intensive and impressive behavioral interventions with autistic preschoolers (see Strain, 1990; Strain, Jamieson, & Hoyson, 1986; Simeonsson, Olley, & Rosenthal, 1987). His method is to teach nonhandicapped peers how to interact with autistic children in an integrated program. The children participate several hours a day, five days a week, and parents continue the efforts at home. In one such program, after 2 years of work, the six experimental autistic children were at age level on a learning scale and were equal to their nonhandicapped peers in positive social interactions. Combining a series of studies, Strain found that autistic preschoolers who received peer-mediated instructional treatment in integrated classes, improved at twice the rate of a comparison group not receiving the treatment.

10. The importance of the abstract principles that infuse practice is not meant to preclude the obvious need for decision making based on pragmatic case-by-case considerations. A teacher, for example, committed to the progressive school selects "child explores" as a goal, but if the child lies still or roams without engaging, she shifts to the cultural transmission school and selects as an objective "touch on command." Conversely, if the teacher has a preacademic goal of learning three colors in a year and the child makes no progress, she may shift to a more free-play objective.

CHAPTER FOUR

1. The song "The Wheels on the Bus" has a wide variety of verses accompanied by gestures—for example, "The baby on the bus goes wah-wah-wah," "The mommy on the bus goes shh-shh-shh," "The horn on the bus goes honk-honk-honk," "The wheels on the bus go round and round," "The driver on the bus goes 'move on back' "—each verse ending with "all through the town."

2. The song "Hokey Pokey" asks children to move various parts of their bodies—for example, "You put your left leg in, you put your left leg out, you put your left leg in and you shake it all about; you do the hokey pokey and you turn yourself around; that's what it's all about. You put your right arm in, you put your right arm out . . . ," etc.

CHAPTER FIVE

1. Acknowledging happiness is important in early intervention programs. At circle time children are asked to indicate if they are happy or sad; stickers of "happy" faces are given to, or drawn for, children as an indicator of approval; children are asked to identify from a series of drawings the "happy" child; often there are songs about being happy (e.g., "If you're happy and you know it clap your hands."). Yet because the emotion is reified—children are instructed in happiness regardless of what they are feeling—the obviously sincere effort to generate it falls flat. This is but one example of how early intervention programs, trying to preserve a peaceful pleasant atmosphere, replace spontaneous and authentic experiences with derivatives and abstractions.

2. In my talks with teachers and administrators "preacademic" always referred to elements extracted from early academic skills—principally reading, writing and arithmetic. Teaching them is seen as building a foundation. Thus shape and color naming refine visual discrimination, which is needed for letter discrimination; rote counting is a prerequisite for adding. "Preacademic" does not refer to prior stages a child must pass through to be conceptually ready for meaningful participation in the three R's. Teachers may believe that reading readiness relies on a child's understanding stories, which relies on the ability to represent a prior experience, which relies on representation of present experience, etc., but that is not what they mean by "preacademic" and, therefore, the developmental sequence is not as likely to be stressed.

3. The determination to graft the cognitive curriculum onto preschoolers is not, of course, limited to early intervention with the handicapped. Valerie Polakow Suransky (1982), in a critical account of a nursery school program for children of professionals, points out that even free play is used "to reinstill the cognitive. When a child was coming down a slide or playing with a boat, they [teachers] would ask, 'Good, what color is the slide?' or 'What shape is the boat?' Although this period was labeled 'free play,' the children were not *free to play*, nor were they free *not to play*" (pp. 62–63, italics in original).

4. Increments in language are difficult to gauge and estimates therefore differ, but there is no disagreement on the rapidity of word acquisition in the early years. According to a group of speech and language experts who put together an expectancy chart from the research of linguists, an average child at 19–24 months comprehends approximately 300 words and speaks 50; at 25–30 months he comprehends 500 words and speaks 200; at 31–36 months of age he comprehends 900 and speaks 500. That would translate into an increment each month of 50 new com-

prehended words and 28 new spoken words for the normal child, except
that he picks up speed with age (Gard, Gilman, & Gorman, 1980). The
Columbia University College of Physicians and Surgeons (Stillman, 1990),
in its pediatric encyclopedia, estimates 12 new spoken words a week from
ages 2 to 3, Dunn et al. (1976) suggest 14 new words per week from ages 3
to 4; topping them all, Nelson (1988) puts the figure at 10 to 20 new words
daily.

   5. In the only longitudinal study I located that followed retarded
(Down syndrome) children who had attended educational programs from
preschool to 21 years (Carr, 1988), most of the 41 adults fell below the
6-year level in reading and could not score even on a primary test. Of the
16 who achieved a "reading age," their average accuracy level was 7 years,
8 months and their average comprehension level was 6 years, 9 months.
Only 5 read at all for pleasure. Arithmetic ages were still lower: over half
could only recognize numbers and count; the highest score achieved was 7
years, 11 months. If this is David's fate, think of the repetition he will have
to endure!

   Another British study (Shepperdson, 1988) that looked at teenage
accomplishments of Down syndrome children, two thirds of whom had
received education before age 5½, reports similar academic accomplishments. Of 50 children evaluated in 1981, nine read at the 6- to 7-year level,
and nine at the 7- to 9½-year level. More startling was the extreme
dependency of these children. Only a fourth could dress and bathe themselves; only 20% of the girls could manage their menstruation; only half
were independent in the bathroom; only 38% were left alone at home, and
then for only an average time of 36 minutes; for the group as a whole an
adult had to be in attendance almost all the time.

   Although we do not have longitudinal data for handicapped children
in this country, there is reason to be concerned about the 300,000 students
leaving high school each year. It was estimated, according to testimony
before a Senate Subcommittee on the Handicapped in 1985, that 67% of
those between the ages of 16 and 64 were unemployed (and this, of course,
includes mildly retarded, learning disabled, and emotionally disturbed,
along with the moderately retarded) (Rusch & Phelps, 1987). Most of those
employed had only part-time jobs.

   Studies on the quality of life paint no brighter a picture. According to
Parshall (1991), only 13% of students who had been classified as educable
mentally retarded met an index of success developed by Halpern (1985)
that includes: participation in more than three leisure activities, employed full- or part-time, living independently or with a friend, and paying
more than half the expenses of living. Using similar criteria, Frank, Sitlington, Cooper, and Cool (1990) found only about 8% of 318 former
special education students had a successful outcome.

While the handicapped are not getting jobs, schools are *decreasing* vocational training (Edgar, 1987), this despite suggestive evidence that students with vocational training do better than those without it (Kerachsky & Thornton, 1987; Hasazi, Johnson, Hasazi, Gordon, & Hull, 1989). One cannot but wonder if the academic stress that starts in preschool, and continues thereafter, has been at the cost of valuable vocational training. Researchers studying the postschool adjustment of the handicapped are critical.

[Hardman and McDonnell:] Follow-up studies [since PL 94-142] indicated with increasing regularity that graduates of public school programs were not employed, did not utilize community services and resources effectively, and tended to be isolated from handicapped and nonhandicapped peers. (1987, p. 493)

[Parshall:] Special education programs have not taught their students the adjustment skills they need for successful acclimation in the adult world. (1991, p. 25)

[Haring and Lovett:] The scenario for adults with disabilities described in this community is not optimistic. (1990, p. 472)

CHAPTER SIX

1. While a teacher obviously must take the lead when introducing a novel activity, it is customary to shift authority from the adult to the child as learning proceeds (Dunst, 1986; Tharp & Gallimore, 1988). There is no getting around the fact that at some point in the learning process the child must grab hold of the material.

2. The problem of praise inflation is not limited to early intervention. Suransky (1982) notes that the lavish expenditure of praise distorts children's intentions in regular nursery school. She gives as an example a child, Myron, standing in a corner, sucking his fingers while holding a block. The teacher comments: "Oh, you found a block, very good," and leads him off to build. At another moment, the teacher approaches him standing by a wooden wagon and comments, "That's a nice toy to play with; that's a good idea." In the first instance Myron "had clearly displayed no enterprise in 'finding' a block; nor did he seem particularly interested in building with the block." On the second occasion "Myron was not playing *with* the toy, nor did he after Teacher Sally's remark" (p. 63, italics in original). Suransky also criticizes the tight schedule as a means to deny children freedom and to institute the "bureaucratization of children" (p. 106). The domination of the schedule interferes with child–child

engagements and the natural rhythms of play. The schedule also "facili-
tates a dependence on teacher authority to control their [the children's]
experiences" (p. 65).

Stipek and Sanborn (1985) criticize the help and praise given in
greater abundance to handicapped than to nonhandicapped children: the
excessive help because it undermines the child's development of frustration tolerance, the excessive praise because it undermines the child's
connection of effort and achievement.

CHAPTER SEVEN

1. There is a tendency to lump together the multiple initiatives this
country has taken on behalf of young disadvantaged children. We need to
distinguish the massive number of programs grouped under Head Start
(Haskins, 1989, cites 1300), the small number of programs (11) loosely
organized together into a consortium for standardized longitudinal
evaluation, and early intervention for the handicapped. The best results
have come from the consortium. Although there was substantial variation
among these programs, as a group they offered more services to children
than the Head Start programs — better adult–child ratios, more home
visiting, and longer duration (many years versus a single year).

The most robust finding from the consortium programs is that graduates were less likely to be assigned to special education, to drop out of
school, and were somewhat less likely to be retained in grades (Haskins,
1989; Lazar & Darlington, 1982). IQ, reading, and math scores showed
initial spurts that declined over the years. Within the consortium, the
most optimistic findings have come from the Ypsilanti Perry Preschool
Project (Berreuta-Clement, Schweinhart, Barnett, Epstein, & Weikart,
1984). In comparing, at age 19, an experimental group of 58 children who
attended preschool against a control group of 63 children who did not, the
authors found that the Perry Preschool students were superior on several
indices: they had better scholastic achievement; more graduated from
high school, enrolled in post-secondary programs, and were employed;
fewer had records of delinquency and crime, teenage pregnancy, assignment to special education, or to welfare. These findings, however, have not
been replicated (Haskins, 1989).

Results have been less favorable for the more substantial number of
children enrolled in other programs for the disadvantaged (mostly Head
Start). Although Head Start has lacked the resources to do careful
systematic follow-up, existing findings are: an immediate rise in IQ and
achievement scores that disappears within 3 years, no long-term benefits

in school achievement, and only slight evidence for lower rates of grade retention and assignment to special education. (For recent reviews see Farran, 1990; Haskins, 1989; McKey et al., 1985.) In a summary of 99 studies with disadvantaged preschoolers, White (1986) concludes that there is an immediate gain of half a standard deviation in IQ and achievement (about 8 points), but this washes out after 5 years. The combination of less academic retention or assignment to special education, despite no IQ or achievement gains (Perry Preschool excepted), suggests disadvantaged children with preschool education have achieved more social, than intellectual, accomplishments.

Studies of handicapped preschoolers given early intervention are all short-term. Here, too, in the better done research, there is an immediate rise of something on the order of 6 to 7 IQ points and, for the less methodologically rigorous work, 10 to 11 points (Casto, 1987; Casto & Mastropieri, 1986; Casto & White, 1985; Farran, 1990; Guralnick, 1988; Shonkoff & Hauser-Cram, 1987). One long-term study from Australia (Crombie, Gunn, & Hayes, 1991) has tracked two groups of children with Down syndrome, one of which received early intervention. When tested at the age of 11, there was no difference between the groups on cognitive or adaptive measures.

2. For a review of the IEP history, see Goodman and Bond (1990). For influential articles that set the stage for the IEP, see Abeson, Burgdorf, Casey, Kunz, and McNeil (1975) and Gallagher (1972).

3. Accountability has been a driving force in the special education reform movement and, as Carta et al. say, it "is a bedrock principle in early intervention practice" (1991, p. 7). Although one could imagine a variety of criteria by which teachers and programs might be measured, in the present climate, accountability is demonstrated by improved child competence. If improvement is not documented, the teacher should try something else (Carta et al., 1991). Accountability is thus linked both to acceleration and to didactically taught, narrowly prescribed objectives (Wise, 1979). In practice, the theory that professional accountability rests on child progress gets subverted. The earnest teacher who tries and tries without results, naturally turns the blame on the child, who is perceived as not trying, not attending, not learning.

4. The authors of a recent study of 3- to 6-year-old special needs children from Connecticut report that teachers like to use structured activities for primary instruction. Only 13.8% preferred play. My observations were similar. The investigators find this "startling in light of contemporary and unrefuted theories of child development [that young children learn through play]" (Mahoney et al., 1989, p. 267).

5. Of the seven developmental inventories analyzed in this study, five suggest using the instruments for both evaluation and IEP objectives: Brigance, HELP, HICOMP, LAP, and Portage.

6. Teachers are long-suffering. Research reviews of their attitudes indicate, as I found, a general satisfaction with the IEP (Smith, 1990). Yet according to one study of 75 teachers in a suburban Pennsylvania region, the average special education teacher spends 6.5 hours in developing an IEP per student, and that does not count time spent in evaluating outcome. As these were not preschoolers, teachers had an average of 12 students per class (Price & Goodman, 1980).

7. For an impassioned plea in support of mainstreaming see Strain's keynote address at the Division for Early Childhood Conference (Strain, 1990b). Guralnick, another major leader in the field, is equally enthusiastic. "*Perhaps the single most significant achievement in the field of early childhood mainstreaming in the decade of the 1980s has been the repeated demonstration that mainstreamed programs can be implemented effectively* ... the political question as to whether 'mainstreaming works' at the early childhood level has been answered in the affirmative" (1990, p. 3, italics in original).

8. Programs for the 3- to 5-year-olds are usually school-based and more likely to be half- than full-day (Moore et al., 1988). This arrangement means that the retarded have no chronological-age peers within the school. Even if public schools begin admitting younger children, the preschool retarded child is still unlikely to have any mental-age peers.

CHAPTER EIGHT

1. Teachers frequently use the word "functional" to refer to real life skills. These are the sorts of items that psychologists usually organize under "adaptive" skills: principally self-care (e.g., dressing, feeding, toileting) and self-sufficiency (e.g., shopping, traveling, cooking). In this study, I am equating "functional," "adaptive," and "independence."

2. It has been shown repeatedly that parents overestimate the IQ of their handicapped children, especially when they are little (for a summary, see Miller, 1988). Although this is hardly surprising, given the parents' hopes and their relative isolation from nonhandicapped preschoolers, the overestimation tugs on the teachers to meet parental expectations.

3. Of the 31 teachers who informed me of their professional training, only 2 did not have a special education background. Several had

more than special education—early childhood, guidance and counseling, elementary education. Eight teachers had master's degrees, 19 had a BA or BS, and 4 had special education certification only.

4. Mental growth should be thought of as a rate: amount of progress over a specific time period. The average child makes mental gains of 12 months in one year. Carl grows at one sixth his chronological age, so each year he advances 2 months; Larry grows at four fifths his chronological age, advancing 9 to 10 months in 12; Heather grows at two fifths her chronological age, advancing 4.8 months in 12. We used to determine IQ (before we shifted to developmental indexes based on standard deviations) by using a ratio of mental age to chronological age (and multiplying by 100). Ratio IQs for retarded children still appear to be quite stable and better predictors than a standard deviation IQ in preschoolers (see Goldstein & Sheaffer, 1988; Goodman & Cameron, 1978). Carl, with a mental age of 6 months, at 3 years has a Ratio IQ of 17; Larry, with a mental age of 4, when he is 5 has a Ratio IQ of 80; and Heather, with a mental age of 2, when she is 5 has a Ratio IQ of 40. These large IQ differences mean very different rates of progress and a swelling discrepancy in the chronological years that separate them. Studies have consistently shown that retardation is quite stable in retarded children, at least until adolescence (Goodman, 1990), so that the examples of ever increasing age gaps are realistic.

5. It is common, according to a body of psychological research, that when judging responsibility for an event (e.g., academic failure) observers overestimate the responsibility of the person and underestimate the role of the situation. In the case of early intervention, failure to attain an educational objective is perceived to be the fault of the child (person) rather than the fault of the instructional material and methods (situation). Psychologists call this the "attribution error" (Billig, 1982; Ickes & Kidd, 1976; Jones, 1979; Kelley, 1972, 1973; Ross, 1981; Snyder, 1976). It occurs because it is easier (more salient) for an observer to "see" the person than the setting. Attributing cause to the person is particularly likely when the subject's behavior does not vary from one occasion to the next (high consistency), when there is little behavioral fluctuation as a result of changing stimuli (low distinctiveness), and when other people behave differently in the same or similar situations (low consensus). In the context of early intervention, when a child fails regularly in a lesson on colors (high consistency), and fails also at other learning tasks (low distinctiveness), while other children are succeeding (low consensus), it is altogether natural to blame the child. And since "the perception of cause is intimately linked to the exercise of control" (Kelley, 1972, p. 24), the instructor is likely to insist that the child assume responsibility for learning the material, rather than change the material for the child.

CHAPTER NINE

1. To measure how long it takes infants to "learn," researchers use a habituation model. By this they mean the number of trials required before a child is satiated with a given stimulus and attracted to a novel one (Cohen, 1981; Gunn, Berry, & Andrews, 1982; Lewis & Brooks-Gunn, 1984; MacTurk, Vietze, McCarthy, McQuiston, & Yarrow, 1985; Miranda & Fantz, 1974). In a study comparing mirror play of children with and without Down syndrome matched by mental age, Loveland (1987) suggests that the longer involvement of the Down syndrome group may have resulted from their failure to habituate to the mirror.

The slow processing of retarded preschoolers is supported by a preliminary intervention study in which researchers, after asking a question, waited 1 to 5 seconds before either giving an answer or moving on to another child (Lee, O'Shea, & Dykes, 1987). The investigators found that while the delay was of no aid to the one normally progressing child, it did improve the frequency and accuracy of responses in the two delayed children. This line of research suggests that we must modify our pace, as well as our expectations, when working with delayed children.

For a recent review of the general relationship between speed of processing and intelligence, see Vernon (1990), who states that over 50% of the variance in intelligence scores can be accounted for by reaction time.

2. According to the influential Russian neuropsychologist Aleksandr Luria (1966), the brain is organized hierarchically with regulation and planning of behavior located in the highest level, the third unit of the brain (frontal lobes). He states there is evidence that "*the frontal lobes synthesize the information about the outside world received through the exteroceptors and the information about the internal states of the body*" and that "*they are the means whereby the behavior of the organism is regulated in conformity with the effect produced by its actions*" (p. 233, italics in original). It is this unit that mediates most of the skills found on intelligence tests (Golden & Wilkening, 1986; Naglieri, 1989). Therefore, it is to be expected that those with retardation will have deficits in this function. (For a related comment see Note 6, Chapter Three.)

3. It is not within the power of psychology to determine precisely the extent to which the observed passivity and distractibility in the retarded are due to nature or nurture since, by the time we observe the traits, both have been at work. However, an adult causal role in these problems—called iatrogenic illness when brought on by doctors—cannot be ruled out. At the very least, it is possible that parents and teachers are exaggerating a native deficit by pressuring children beyond their capacity.

A study by the Michigan Department of Education on the status of former handicapped students notes: "Special educators press their students with basic academic skills and submissive classroom behaviors well into secondary education. This promotes a passive response and places value on dependency. Passivity and dependency are often major post-school problems of students who leave special education" (Parshall, 1991, p. 26).

4. The broad implications for the whole range of retarded children of the normal-but-slow findings are well summarized in the following quote from Seibert, Hogan, and Mundy (1984):

> That stage-related patterns, reported originally for normally developing children at specific chronological ages, occurred in parallel for at-risk and handicapped children at roughly comparable MA's, supports the applicability of the developmental model to heterogeneous samples of organically impaired children. Apparently, a predictable coherence of behavioral systems characterizes developmental organization even in severely retarded and multiply handicapped individuals. (p. 26)

5. A somewhat counterintuitive by-product of the child's pattern of global responsiveness, of perceiving "qualities-of-the-whole," is behavioral rigidity. A child who does not differentiate the essential and nonessential parts of an object is thrown off balance whenever any part of the whole changes. So, for example, a young child may fail to recognize his parent in a new garment, new hairstyle, or with glasses, whereas an older child will be indifferent to these changes. The same rigidity applies to routines: The young child insists on eating in a certain chair, having a particular fork and plate, following the same nighttime routine each evening. For him, the act of eating includes food–chair–fork–plate, and going to bed is a single occurrence made up of pajamas–bed–book–coverlet. There can be no behavioral flexibility without an understanding that the whole—for example, going to bed—consists of a series of parts that can be separated, supplemented, substituted, reorganized, etc.

6. Werner describes syncretism as follows: "If several mental functions or phenomena, which would appear as distinct from each other in a mature state of consciousness, are merged without differentiation into one activity or into one phenomenon, we may speak of a *syncretic function* or a *syncretic phenomenon*" (1948, p. 53, italics in original).

Syncretism, although a juvenile attribute, enlivens and intensifies experiences. The gain with age in objectivity and analytic skills comes at the cost of a vivid impressionability. Egan (1988) suggests that one of the reasons childhood appears, in retrospect, clearer, brighter, and better recalled than later life, is because the events of early childhood are infused with emotion. Bruner argues that it is important for a culture "to keep them [thinking, perceiving, and feeling] related and together in those images, stories, and the like by which our experience is given coherence and cultural relevance" (1966, p. 69).

Although very much the minority, there are advocates of more integrated, authentic school experiences for the handicapped child. Poplin (1988a, 1988b) vigorously supports what she calls "holistic" (as opposed to "reductionistic") teaching because it recognizes that learning is personally motivated, child constructed, nonlinearly derived from prior knowledge, and life-like. (Also see Heshusius, 1986.)

7. "Schema" as noted by John Flavell (1963), a preeminent interpreter of Piaget, is a vague term that grows in comprehensibility when applied to a child's behavior. His own definition may or may not clarify the concept:

> A schema is a cognitive structure which has reference to a class of similar action sequences, these sequences of necessity being strong, bounded totalities in which the constituent behavioral elements are tightly interrelated . . . The first and most obvious thing to be said about schemas is that they are labeled by the behavior sequences to which they refer . . . *the schema of sucking,* the *schema of prehension* . . . Schemas come in all sizes and shapes. However, they all possess one general characteristic in common: the constituent behavior sequence is an organized totality. Thus, an action sequence, if it is to constitute a schema, must have a certain cohesiveness and must maintain its identity as a quasi-stable, repeatable unit. (pp. 52–54, italics in original)

Although, Flavell emphasizes, schemas must be supple and shifting in order to meet the demands of growth, they also must be repetitive in order to assimilate the environment. "In fact, only behavior patterns which recur again and again in the course of cognitive functioning are conceptualized in terms of schemas" (p. 55). The powerful pressure for schemas to repeat, seen in what Piaget calls "reproductive assimilation," is analogized by Flavell to a "repetition compulsion" (p. 55).

8. The belief in knowledge through action is fundamental to many modern theories of learning and, according to Piaget (1970), was accepted by all the great classical educators. Dewey (1897/1959, 1902/1959, 1938), although not a developmentalist, shared the Werner and Piaget emphasis on experience as the route to learning. Vygotsky also believed that thought arises from actions, and that language is initially the representation of familiar activities (Levina, 1979; Vygotsky, 1979). Bruner (1966) sounded the same trumpet when describing the path children take in representing the world: first through habitual action patterns ("enactive" representation), then through images relatively independent of actions ("ikonic" representation), and finally through language ("symbolic" representation). (See also Fisher & Farrar, 1987.)

9. Nelson (1988) found that even most normal 4-year-olds, when asked to associate items from different categories, used functional rather than categorical relationships. Function and movement, however, are not the only means by which children establish the meaning of words and

categories. Clark (1979), for instance, claims initial words are "percept-based." Two objects that look the same will be given the same name. Looking the same means sharing characteristics based on movement, shape, size, sound, taste, and actions. These perceptual groupings produce the under- and overextension of word meaning characteristic of early language (e.g., "car" is restricted to a moving car; "doggie" includes all four-legged animals). Whatever the criteria for anchoring word meaning, linguists seem to agree that concepts are constructed by, not given to, children (Bruner, 1983; Clark, 1973, 1979, 1983; Keil, 1988; Mervis, 1987).

10. Borrowing from Vygotsky, Tharp and Gallimore (1988) make the same objection to the instruction of young children in educational settings. "Everyday concepts," they point out, "are learned 'upward,' from sensory experience to generalization. Schooled concepts, however, are leaned 'downward,' from generalization to palpable example" (p. 107).

11. Bruner (1983) describes the complex, long developmental path involved in the seemingly simple matter of making a request. A child, before indicating *what* it is he wants, must know and indicate simply *that* he wants. His mother, using context clues, guesses what's on his mind. Then, in successive stages, the child reaches for a distant object, points to it, and lastly accompanies the gesture with a name. Context and redundant information are built into the usual requesting between mother and child: the request is usually expected, and the object is being used or wanted. A label given without all these context clues—a known and sought-for object, a familiar exchange format—is unlikely to stick.

12. While neo-Piagetians have debated the exact age at which various cognitive milestones are achieved, Piaget's major propositions and sequences have held up well. When tasks are simplified, many of the skills show up sooner than Piaget noted, but it is unclear whether reducing complexity and providing more support makes it easier for children to demonstrate superior reasoning or, instead, fundamentally changes the nature of the task. When investigators replicate Piaget's original tasks and techniques, his designated ages appear appropriate (Bidell & Fischer, 1989; Halford, 1989).

In the first flush of the Head Start movement, efforts were mounted to accelerate the passage through developmental stages (as well as to increase IQ). Probably the most famous was the Bereiter–Englemann programs (1966) based on intense didactic instruction in carefully sequenced academic tasks. It was Engelmann's assumption that it is not necessary to wait for the development of cognitive structures or for a child's independent discovery if, instead, you carefully teach children the relevant rules. In 1971, Kamii and Derman (1971) reexamined some children to whom Engelmann had taught relevant rules regarding specific gravity (what things float) and conservation of volume (amount remains constant even if container changes). They found that although the children knew the rules, they could apply them only superficially. For example, they could recite the rule that an object will float on water if it is lighter than a piece of water the same size, and sink if it is heavier than a piece of water the same size. However, when asked *why* a particular group of objects floated, they resorted to explanations based on the properties of the objects—light and heavy, big and small—not the relationship of objects to water. Generally absolute weight was determinative in children's explanations (6 years old) at the preoperational stage. The investigators concluded that no acceleration occurred; the children learned only rote applications.

Along the same lines, researchers have found that preschool children (ages 3 to 5) equated big with tall, rather than overall size, and so made persistent errors in big–little comparisons (Hobbs & Bacharach, 1990; Ravn & Gelman, 1984).

13. By changing the perceived locus of causality, intrinsic motivation and extrinsic reinforcement can work in opposition, rather than in concert, with each other. Experiments have shown that when reinforcement is given for an existing behavior (e.g., drawing) and then withdrawn, a child's level of performance may decline below prior nonreinforced levels. This does not mean that there is no place for reinforcement. Rewards induce a person to do something for which initially she has no appetite; and sometimes intrinsic interest may follow a behavior elicited under extrinsically reinforced conditions (Deci, 1975; Deci & Ryan, 1982; Fein & Kohlberg, 1987; Harter, 1978; Lepper, 1981).

14. Others call these social reciprocal occasions "routines." The repetitive activities familiar to both mother and child create a context for new words to be assimilated (Lucariello & Nelson, 1987; Snow, 1989; for a similar view see Brown, 1980; Cazden, 1983). Because the words are integral to the context and cannot be isolated from it, language is constrained initially to the here and now (Snow, 1983). The abstract word instruction in early intervention, where words are not added onto existing routines but selected from vocabulary lists, contradicts normal early speech development.

15. The impoverished conversational skills of children with Down syndrome is well documented (Brooks-Gunn & Lewis, 1982; Cardoso-Martins & Mervis, 1985; Crawley & Spiker, 1983; Cunningham, Reuler, Blackwell, & Derk, 1981; Davis, Stroud, & Green, 1988; Dunst & Trivelte, 1988; Fewell & Kaminsky, 1988; Girolametto, 1988; Hodapp, 1988; Kopp, 1990; Mahoney, 1988a, 1988b; Marfo, 1984; Marfo & Kysela, 1988; Maurer & Sherrod, 1987; Mervis, 1990; Odom, 1983; Tannock, 1988; Vietze, Abernathy, Ashe, & Faulstich, 1978). Recently, investigators have questioned

the previous sweeping condemnation of parental "directiveness" in language teaching. They have found that directiveness, sensitivity, and intrusiveness are independent variables (Crawley & Spiker, 1983). Some forms of directiveness possibly enhance, while other forms restrict, language production. It is possible for parents to prime their slow child through directions and still maintain mutual responsivity (Marfo, 1990; Marfo & Kysela, 1988; Tannock, 1988). On the other hand Cunningham et al. (1981) argue that directiveness and unresponsiveness are linked in an unfortunate spiral: the poor language in retarded children elicits directiveness in parents which then suppresses child language which then stimulates more parental directiveness.

The tendency of the impaired child to elicit excessive intrusion from parents has been elaborated by Bell and Harper (1977) in their "control theory" model. According to them, when a child reaches the "lower limit" of acceptable interaction, the parent tries hard to prime increased performance; when the child reaches the "upper limit" of acceptability, the parent works to reduce excessive behavior. It is only under optimal conditions—when children fit parental expectations—that permissiveness reins. It follows that parents of the retarded quite naturally pressure their children and, when their efforts are unsuccessful, raise the ante. "Natural," however, is not necessarily beneficial.

16. A concession of "defect" within the retarded population does not automatically translate into a cultural transmission skill-training model. One could just as well conclude that the existence of a defect is simply an obstacle teachers must confront when attempting to tap a child's initiative, not a justification for giving up (much as a limp gets in the way of, but does not preclude, walking). One gives up on appealing to a child's interests very, very reluctantly. As Sarason (1990) says, in discussing the controversy over teaching the subject versus the child:

> Learning is arid, unproductive, and stifling to the degree that it does not take into account the interests, curiosity, and questions of the learner. To the degree that classroom learning requires of children that they conform to what others say is important, learn it in ways that others say is the way to learn, and separate this learning from all other contexts of experience and learning children bring to school, the school then is remarkably and predictably effective in getting children to regard the classroom as an uninteresting place. (p. 159)

CHAPTER TEN

1. The reader may question whether outcome studies support a more progressive approach. The comparison of different intervention models is, of course, a narrower version of the general question—Does early

intervention help?—and even thornier to research. To do an adequate study, investigators must be sure that (a) programs are equally faithful to their model, (b) teacher personality has no specific effect, (c) the same measures are used across studies, and (d) extraneous variables—length of program, resources, place and manner of service, etc.—are equated (Peters et al., 1985; Rivlin & Timpane, 1975). This degree of control has not been achieved, so that the limited findings available are inconclusive.

What investigations suggest is that in programs for the disadvantaged, behavioral approaches may have the edge in securing preacademic attainments (e.g., arithmetic, letters, sentence production) but developmental programs may be more effective in other areas (e.g., curiosity, social interaction, inventiveness, problem-solving, and self-monitoring). Generally, no long-term differential effects have been documented (McKey et al., 1985; Miller & Dyer, 1975; Peters et al., 1985; Rivlin & Timpane, 1975; Schweinhart, Weikart, & Larner, 1986). However, Miller and Bizzell (1983) found that males from two nondidactic Montessori programs outperformed males from two didactic programs on achievement (not IQ) tests in Grades 6 through 8, and DeVries and Kohlberg (1987) conclude from their review of the literature that "a child-centered program with a self-conscious cognitive emphasis appears to be more effective on the whole in promoting lasting intellectual development than either traditional nursery school (romantic) or straight didactic teaching (cultural transmission). Also, less didactic and cognitive-developmental programs have more positive long-term effects" (p. 387).

In programs for the handicapped, the same difficulties of comparative evaluation are compounded by the lack of long-term investigations and the limited range of outcome measures. Most reviewers find no evidence for the superiority of one model over another, or for the advisability of matching model to child diagnosis (Farran, 1990; Fewell & Kelly, 1983; Guralnick, 1988). Duration and intensity may swamp any model effects (Casto, 1987; Dunst, Snyder, & Mankinen, 1989). Yoder (1990), in his review of various intervention approaches, concludes that efficacy of treatment is probably mediated by the degree of deficit, the age of the child, and the targeted area of function.

We have not heard the last word on this matter. Although it is very costly to research how different sorts of children best achieve different kinds of objectives under different teaching approaches, the work must be done if social science is to inform public policy.

I would argue that academic proficiency cannot be the sole criterion of success in this research. Even if the developmental–progressive model does not produce greater school achievement, a more child-led curriculum is justified if, as a result, retarded children have broader interests, show greater directed activity, make wiser decisions, develop a moral code, and resist as well as conform to external demands. That the handicapped are rather indifferent to self-expression and self-determination is suggested by one study (Arnold, 1984) that found while handicapped adolescents do not rank "freedom" as one of their three most important values, the nonhandicapped put it first. The present emphasis on submission to teacher direction encourages what Piaget (1970) called a "heteronomous," as opposed to an autonomous, morality; that is, good and bad are that which please adults, not the products of personal reflection.

2. The flexibility and informality of home may be more conducive to play than school. Malone and Stoneman (1990) found that the play of retarded children at home was more complex, constructive, imaginative, and lasted longer than their play in a mainstreamed class. They, too, suggest that the "home environment may well be the setting to lend direction to programming in other environments" (p. 484).

3. There is enormous disagreement among experts on how to treat autism, as might be expected, given how little we know about the disorder and its resistance to any intervention. In contrast to the behavioral methods of Lovaas (1987) and Strain (1990a; Strain et al., 1986) touched on in Chapter Three, there are those who believe that even with this disorder, the intervener takes her lead from the child. Jeanne Simons (Simons & Oishi, 1987), for example, advocates moving in on an autistic child slowly, observing and waiting until he can tolerate your presence before making a demand. A teacher might establish initial contact with a child simply by sitting in the same room; when he is comfortable with her presence, she could include the child's name in a song; after that, she might tentatively insert a foot into his "space," or mimic his actions. Each new initiative would be calibrated to the child's reaction.

Early intervention programs do not seem to have specific treatments for children with autism, beyond expecting them to participate in the general routines. The children characteristically refuse to do so and spend a great deal of time wandering or at odds with the instructor. It is, however, when an autistic child willingly cooperates and absorbs the classroom instruction, that the poor fit between his needs and the core curriculum may become clearest, as the following incident reveals.

> An autistic boy, upon being introduced to me at an early intervention center, insisted that I sit down and, handing me a box of crayons, follow his directions: "Draw an orange circle, draw a red square, draw a green triangle." I, preferring a more social game, suggested as a first step that we take turns. He became agitated, disregarded the interruption, and began again: "Make one green line, make two green lines, make three red lines." After each of my strokes, he checked for accuracy. Then, assuring himself that I had followed instructions, he jumped up and down gleefully, before issuing another directive, with no demurral allowed.

4. The architect Felix Drury has pioneered the design of flexible modular boxes as a basic structure for creating preschool settings. He and his colleague, Lois Rho, have built a remarkable environment for young children with special needs in Connecticut. For information on their work, contact Felix Drury at 85 Willow St., New Haven, CT 06511; or Lois Rho at the Stephen August Early Intervention Center, 1686 Waterbury Rd., Cheshire, CT 06410.

Early intervention programs are cheerful places filled with toys, but often the environment fits a 3- to 5-year-old better than a slow child functioning like a 1- to 2-year-old. The role of a setting in promoting development may be greater than conventionally appreciated. It has been found, for instance, that children do better (i.e., achieve Piagetian milestones) in settings that react to (are activated by) the initiatives of children and present opportunities for exploration, as opposed to those that are cluttered, confusing and noisy (Wachs, 1979).

CHAPTER ELEVEN

1. The philosopher Allan Bloom, in his introduction to *Emile* (1979), points to the fundamental contribution Rousseau made in distinguishing *amour de soi*, the natural unfettered love of self, from *amour-propre*, the love of self that comes from the approval of others. In a state of nature, where one individual does not compete with another for goods or attention, where man relies on himself alone, there is only *amour de soi*. But in a state of civilization, a child soon learns that even as an infant (through tears) he can control others. It is not long before control of others replaces doing-for-self; securing power replaces securing survival. From then on man's self-esteem is entirely dependent upon the recognition of others. The object of Rousseau's education is to stop this shift from occurring. Bloom agrees. The "doubling or dividing of self-love . . . is one of the few distinctively human phenomena (no animal can be insulted); and from it flow anger, pride, vanity, resentment, revenge, jealousy, indignation, competition, slavishness, humility, capriciousness, rebelliousness" (p. 11).

I am grateful to my colleague David Hogan for bringing Bloom's introduction to my attention.

References

Abeson, A., Burgdorf, R. L., Jr., Casey, P. J., Kunz, J. W., & McNeil, W. (1975). Access to opportunity. In W. Hobbs (Ed.), *Issues in the classification of children* (Vol. 2, pp. 270–292). San Francisco: Jossey-Bass.

American Psychiatric Association. (1987). *Diagnostic and statistical manual of mental disorders* (3rd ed., rev.). Washington, DC: Author.

Anastasiow, N. J. (1978). Strategies and models for early childhood intervention programs in integrated settings. In M. J. Guralnick (Ed.), *Early intervention and the integration of handicapped and nonhandicapped children* (pp. 85–111). Baltimore: University Park Press.

Arnold, J. (1984). Values of exceptional students during early adolescence. *Exceptional Children, 51*, 230–234.

Astman, J. A. (1984). Special education as a moral enterprise. *Learning Disabilities Quarterly, 7*, 299–308.

Bagnato, S. J., & Neisworth, J. (1981). *Linking developmental assessment and curricula: Prescriptions for early intervention.* Rockville, MD: Aspen.

Bagnato, S. J., Neisworth, J., & Munson, S. M. (1989). *Linking developmental assessment and early intervention: Curriculum-based prescriptions* (2nd ed.). Frederick, MD: Aspen.

Bailey, D. B., Jr., & Wolery, M. (1984). *Teaching infants and preschoolers with handicaps.* Columbus, OH: Merrill.

Ballard, K. D. (1987). The limitations of behavioral approaches to teaching: Some implications for special education. *Exceptional Children, 34*, 197–212.

Barr, M. W. (1899). The how, the why, and the wherefore of the training of feeble-minded children. *Journal of Psycho-asthenics, 3*, 205–212.

Barrett, M. J. (1990). The case for more school days. *The Atlantic Monthly, 266*, 78–106.

Baumrind, D. (1967). Child care practices anteceding three patterns of preschool behavior. *Genetic Psychology Monographs, 75*, 43–88.

Baumrind, D. (1968). Authoritarian versus authoritative parental control. *Adolescence, 3*, 255–272.

Baumrind, D. (1971). Current patterns of parental authority. *Developmental Psychology Monographs, 4*(1, Pt. 2), 1–103.

Baumrind, D. (1975). The contributions of the family to the development of competence in children. *Schizophrenic Bulletin, 14,* 12–37.

Bell, R. Q., & Harper, L. V. (1977). *Child effect on adults.* Hillsdale, NJ: Erlbaum.

Bereiter, C., & Englemann, S. (1966). *Teaching the culturally disadvantaged in the preschool.* Englewood Cliffs, NJ: Prentice-Hall.

Berkeley, T. R., & Ludlow, B. L. (1989). Toward a reconceptionalization of the developmental model. *Topics in Early Childhood Special Education, 9,* 51–66.

Berreuta-Clement, J. R., Schweinhart, L. J., Barnett, W. S., Epstein, A. S., & Weikart, D. P. (1984). Changed lives: The effects of the Perry Preschool Program on youth through age 19. *Monographs of the High Scope Educational Research Foundation* (Serial No. 8). Ypsilanti, MI: High Scope Press.

Berry, W. (1977). *The unsettling of America: Culture and agriculture.* San Francisco: Sierra Club Books.

Bidell, T. R., & Fischer, K. W. (1989). Commentary and reflections on 25 years of Piagetian cognitive developmental psychology, 1963–1988. *Human Development, 32,* 363–368.

Billig, M. (1982). *Ideology and social psychology: Extremism, moderation, and contradiction.* New York: St. Martin's Press.

Blake, W. (1803/1950). Auguries of innocence. In W. H. Auden & N. H. Pearson (Eds.), *Poets of the English language* (Vol. IV, p. 18). New York: Viking Press.

Bloom, A. (Ed. and Trans.). (1979). Introduction. In J. J. Rousseau, *Emile* (pp. 3–28). New York: Basic Books.

Bloom, B. (1964). *Stability and change in human characteristics.* New York: Wiley.

Bluma, S., Shearer, M., Frohman, A., & Hilliard, J. (1976). *The Portage Guide to Early Intervention.* Portage, WI: Cooperative Educational Service Agency.

Bornstein, M. H. (1985). Colour-name versus shape-name learning in young children. *Journal of Child Language, 12,* 387–393.

Bowden, J., Black, T., & Daulton, D. (1990). *Estimating the costs of providing early intervention and preschool special education services.* Chapel Hill, NC: University of North Carolina, National Early Childhood Technical Assistance System.

Bredekamp, S. (Ed.). (1987). *Developmentally appropriate practice in early childhood programs serving children from birth through age 8* (expanded ed.). Washington, DC: National Association for the Education of Young Children.

Brigance, N. H. (1978). *Brigance Diagnostic Inventory of Early Development.* North Billerica, MA: Curriculum Associates.

Brinker, R. P., & Lewis, M. (1982). Discovering the competent handicapped infant: A process approach to assessment and intervention. *Topics in Early Childhood Special Education, 2,* 1–16.

Brooks-Gunn, J., & Lewis, M. (1982). Affective exchanges between normal and handicapped infants and their mothers. In T. Field & A. Fogel (Eds.), *Emotion and early interaction* (pp. 161–188). Hillsdale, NJ: Erlbaum.

Brown, A. L. (1974). The role of strategic behavior in retardate memory. In N. R. Ellis (Ed.), *International review of research in mental retardation* (Vol. 7, pp. 55–111). New York: Academic Press.

Brown, R. (1973). *A first language.* Cambridge: Harvard University Press.

Brown, R. (1977). Preface. In C. E. Snow & C. A. Ferguson (Eds.), *Talking to children: Language input and acquisition* (pp. vii–x). London: Cambridge University Press.

Brown, R. (1980). The maintenance of conversation. In D. R. Olson (Ed.), *The social foundations of language and thought* (pp. 187–210). New York: Norton.

Brownell, C. A., & Strauss, M. S. (1985). Infant stimulation and development: Conceptual and empirical considerations. In M. Frank (Ed.), *Infant intervention programs: Truths and untruths* (pp. 109–130), New York: Haworth Press.

Bruner, J. S. (1966). On cognitive growth. In J. S. Bruner, R. R. Olver, & P. M. Greenfield (Eds.), *Studies in cognitive growth* (pp. 1–29). New York: Wiley.

Bruner, J. S. (1972). Nature and uses of immaturity. *American Psychologist, 8,* 687–707.

Bruner, J. S. (1983). *Child's talk: Learning to use language.* New York: Norton.

Bureau of the Census. (1990). *Statistical abstract of the United States* (110th ed.). Washington, DC: U.S. Government Printing Office.

Campione, J. C., Brown, A. L., & Ferrara, R. A. (1982). Mental retardation and intelligence. In R. J. Sternberg (Ed.), *Handbook of human intelligence* (pp. 392–490). New York: Cambridge University Press.

Cardoso-Martins, C., & Mervis, C. (1985). Maternal speech to prelinguistic children with Down syndrome. *American Journal of Mental Deficiency, 89,* 451–458.

Carr, J. (1988). Six weeks to twenty-one years old: A longitudinal study of children with Down's syndrome and their families. *Journal of Child Psychology and Psychiatry, 29,* 407–431.

Carta, J. J., Schwartz, I. S., Atwater, J. B., & McConnell, S. R. (1991). Developmentally appropriate practice: Appraising its usefulness for young children with disabilities. *Topics in Early Childhood Special Education, 11,* 1–20.

Casto, G. (1987). Plasticity and the handicapped child: A review of efficacy research. In J. J. Gallagher & C. T. Ramey (Eds.), *The malleability of children* (pp. 103–113). Baltimore: Brookes.

Casto, G., & Mastropieri, M. A. (1986). The efficacy of early intervention programs: A meta-analysis. *Exceptional Children, 52,* 417–424.

Casto, G., & White, K. (1985). The efficacy of early intervention programs with environmentally at-risk infants. In M. Frank (Ed.), *Infant in-*

tervention programs: Truths and untruths (pp. 37–50). New York: Haworth Press.

Cazden, C. B. (1983). Adult assistance to language development: Scaffolds, models, and direct instruction. In R. P. Parker & F. A. Davis (Eds.), *Developing literacy: Young children's use of language* (pp. 3–18). Newark, DE: International Reading Association.

Chapman, R. S. (1981). Mother–child interaction in the second year of life. In R. L. Schiefelbusch & D. D. Bricker (Eds.), *Early language: Acquisition and intervention* (pp. 201–250). Baltimore: University Park Press.

Cicchetti, D., & Beeghly, M. (1990). An organizational approach to the study of Down syndrome: Contributions to an integrative theory of development. In D. Cicchetti & M. Beeghly (Eds.), *Children with Down syndrome: A developmental perspective* (pp. 29–62). New York: Cambridge University Press.

Cicchetti, D., & Sroufe, L. A. (1976). The relationship between affective and cognitive development in Down's syndrome infants. *Child Development, 47,* 920–929.

Clark, E. (1973). What's in a word? On the child's acquisition of semantics in his first language. In T. E. Moore (Ed.), *Cognitive development and the acquisition of language* (pp. 65–110). New York: Academic Press.

Clark, E. (1979). *The ontogenesis of meaning.* Wiesbaden: Akademische Verlagsgesellschaft Athenaion.

Clark, E. (1983). Meanings and concepts. In P. H. Mussen (Series Ed.) & J. H. Flavell & E. M. Markman (Vol. Eds.), *Handbook of child psychology: Vol. 3. Cognitive development* (4th ed., pp. 787–840). New York: Wiley.

Clarke, A. M., & Clarke, A. D. B. (1976). *Early experience: Myth and evidence.* New York: Free Press.

Code of Federal Regulations. (1986). *Title 34, Chapter III, Office of Special Education and Rehabilitation Services* (Parts 300–399).

Cohen, D. J., Donnellan, A. M., & Paul, R. (Eds.). (1987). *Handbook of autism and pervasive developmental disorders.* New York: Wiley.

Cohen, L. (1981). Examination of habituation as a measure of aberrant infant development. In S. L. Friedman & M. Sigman (Eds.), *Preterm birth and psychological development* (pp. 241–253). New York: Academic Press.

Crawley, S., & Spiker, D. (1983). Mother–child interactions involving two-year-olds with Down syndrome: A look at individual differences. *Child Development, 54,* 1312–1323.

Cremin, L. A. (1976). *Public education.* New York: Basic Books.

Crombie, M., Gunn, P., & Hayes, A. (1991). A longitudinal study of two cohorts of children with Down syndrome. In C. J. Denholm (Ed.), *Adolescents with Down syndrome: Implications for parents, researchers and practitioners* (pp. 3 13). Victoria, BC: School of Child and Youth Care, University of Victoria.

Cunningham, C., Reuler, E., Blackwell, J., & Derk, J. (1981). Behavioral and linguistic development in the interactions of normal and retarded children with their mothers. *Child Development, 52,* 62–70.

Curtiss, S. (1977). *Genie: A psycholinguistic study of a modern-day "wild child."* New York: Academic Press.

Curtiss, S. (1981). Feral children. In J. Wortis (Ed.), *Mental retardation and developmental disabilities* (Vol. XII, pp. 129–161). New York: Brunner/Mazel.

Davis, H., Stroud, A., & Green, L. (1988). Maternal language environment of children with mental retardation. *American Journal of Mental Deficiency, 93,* 144–153.

de Villiers, J. G., & de Villiers, P. A. (1978). *Language acquisition.* Cambridge, MA: Harvard University Press.

Deci, E. L. (1975). *Intrinsic motivation.* New York: Plenum Press.

Deci, E. L., & Ryan, R. M. (1982). Curiosity and self-directed learning: The role of motivation in education. In L. G. Katz (Ed.), *Current topics in early childhood education* (Vol. IV, pp. 71–85). Norwood, NJ: Ablex.

DeVries, R., & Kohlberg, L. (1987). *Constructivist early education: Overview and comparison with other programs.* Washington, DC: National Association for the Education of Young Children.

Dewey, J. (1897/1959). My pedagogic creed. In M. S. Dworkin (Ed.), *Dewey on education: Selections* (pp. 19–32). New York: Teachers College.

Dewey, J. (1902/1959). The child and the curriculum. In M. S. Dworkin (Ed.), *Dewey on education: Selections* (pp. 91–111). New York: Teachers College.

Dewey, J. (1938). *Experience and education.* New York: Collier.

Dorris, M. (1989). *The broken cord.* New York: Harper Perennial.

Dunn, L. M., Chun, L. T., Crowell, D. C., Dunn, L. M., Alevy, L. G., & Yackel, E. R. (1976). *Peabody Early Experiences Kit: Teacher's Guide.* Circle Pines, MN: American Guidance Services.

Dunst, C. J. (1981). *Infant learning: A cognitive–linguistic intervention strategy.* Hingham, MA: Teaching Resources.

Dunst, C. J. (1985). Rethinking early intervention. *Analysis and Intervention in Developmental Disabilities, 5,* 165–201.

Dunst, C. J. (1986). Overview of the efficacy of early intervention programs. In L. Bickman & D. L. Weatherford (Eds.), *Evaluating early intervention programs for severely handicapped children and their families* (pp. 79–147). Austin, TX: Pro-Ed.

Dunst, C. J., Snyder, S., & Mankinen, M. (1989). Efficacy of early intervention. In M. Wang, M. Reynolds, & H. Walberg (Eds.), *Handbook of special education: Research and practice* (Vol. 3, pp. 259–293). New York: Elmsford.

Dunst, C. J., & Trivelte, C. M. (1988). Determinants of parent and child interactive behavior. In K. Marfo (Ed.), *Parent–child interaction and developmental disabilities* (pp. 3–31). New York: Praeger.

Edgar, E. (1987). Secondary programs in special education: Are many of them justifiable? *Exceptional Children, 53,* 555–561.

Egan, K. (1986). *Teaching as storytelling.* Routledge, IL: University of Chicago Press.

Egan, K. (1988). *Primary understanding: Education in early childhood.* New York: Routledge, Chapman, & Hall.

Eisner, E. W. (1985). *The educational imagination: On the design and evaluation of school programs* (2nd ed.). New York: Macmillan.

Elkind, D. (1988). *Miseducation: Preschoolers at risk.* New York: Knopf.

Emde, R. N., Katz, E. L., & Thorpe, J. K. (1978). Emotional expression in infancy. Early deviations in Down's syndrome. In M. Lewis & L. A. Rosenblum (Eds.), *The development of affect* (pp. 351–360). New York: Plenum Press.

Erikson, E. H. (1977). *Toys and reasons: Stages in ritualization of experience.* New York: Norton.

Farran, D. C. (1990). Effects of intervention with disadvantaged and disabled children: A decade review. In S. J. Meisels & J. P. Shokroff (Eds.), *Handbook of early childhood intervention* (pp. 501–539). New York: Cambridge University Press.

Fein, G. G. (1981). Pretend play in childhood: An integrative review. *Child Development, 52,* 1095–1118.

Fein, G. G., & Kohlberg, L. (1987). Play and constructive work as contributors to development. In L. Kohlberg with R. DeVries, G. Fein, D. Hart, R. Mayer, G. Noam, J. Snarey, & J. Wertsch (Eds.), *Child psychology and childhood education: A cognitive developmental view* (pp. 392–440). New York: Longman.

Fewell, R. R., & Kaminsky, R. (1988). Play skills development and instruction for young children with handicaps. In S. Odom & M. Karnes (Eds.), *Early intervention for infants and children with handicaps* (pp. 145–158). Baltimore: Brookes.

Fewell, R. R., & Kelly, J. F. (1983). Curriculum for young handicapped children. In S. G. Garwood (Ed.), *Educating young handicapped children: A developmental approach* (2nd ed., pp. 407–433). Rockville, MD: Aspen.

Fisher, K. W., & Farrar, M. J. (1987). Generalizations about generalization: How a theory of skill development explains both generality and specificity. *International Journal of Psychology, 22,* 643–677.

Fisher, K. W., Hand, H. H., Watson, M. W., VanParys, M. M., & Tucker, J. L. (1984). Putting the child into socialization: The development of social categories in preschool children. In L. G. Katz, P. J. Wagemaker, & K. Steiner (Eds.), *Current topics in early childhood* (Vol. 5, pp. 27–72). Norwood, NJ: Ablex.

Fivush, R. (1987). Scripts and categories: Interrelationships in development. In U. Neisser (Ed.), *Concepts and conceptual development: Ecological and intellectual factors in categorization* (pp. 234–254). New York: Cambridge University Press.

Flavell, J. H. (1963). *The developmental psychology of Jean Piaget.* Princeton, NJ: Van Nostrand.

Frank, A. R., Sitlington, P., Cooper, L., & Cool, V. (1990). Adult adjustment of recent graduates of Iowa mental disabilities programs. *Education and Training in Mental Retardation, 25,* 62–75.

Freeman, R. D. (1976). Some psychiatric reflections on the controversy over methods of communication in the life of the deaf. In *Methods of communication currently used in the education of deaf children* (pp. 110–118). Seminar proceedings conducted at Garnett College in Roehampton. London: Royal National Institute of the Deaf.

Froebel, F. (1826/1887). *The education of man* (W. N. Hailmann, Ed. and Trans.). New York: Appleton.

Furth, H. G. (1973). *Deafness and learning: A psychosocial approach.* Belmont, CA: Wadsworth.

Furuno, S., Inatsuka, T., O'Reilly, K., Hosaka, C., Zeisloft, B., & Allman, T. (1984). *Hawaii Early Learning Profile.* Palo Alto, CA: Vort.

Gallagher, J. J. (1972). The special education contract for mildly handicapped children. *Exceptional Children, 38,* 527–535.

Gallagher, J. J. (1989). A new policy initiative: Infants and toddlers with handicapping conditions. *American Psychologist, 44,* 387–390.

Gallagher, J. J., & Ramey, C. T. (Eds.). (1987). *The malleability of children.* Baltimore: Brookes.

Ganiban, J., Wagner, S., & Cicchetti, D. (1990). Temperament and Down syndrome. In D. Cicchetti & M. Beeghly (Eds.), *Children with Down syndrome: A developmental perspective* (pp. 63–100). New York: Cambridge University Press.

Gannon, J. (1981). *Deaf heritage: A narrative history of deaf America.* Silver Springs, MD: National Association of the Deaf.

Gard, A., Gilman, L., & Gorman, J. (1980). *A world of words.* Salt Lake City, UT: Wordmaking Productions.

Garden, R. A. (1987). The second IEA mathematics study. *Comparative Education Review, 31,* 47–68.

Garwood, S. G. (1982). (Mis)use of developmental scales in program evaluation. *Topics in Early Childhood Special Education, 1,* 61–69.

Garwood, S. G. (1983). Special education and child development: A new perspective. In S. G. Garwood (Ed.), *Educating young handicapped children: A developmental approach* (pp. 3–37). Rockville, MD: Aspen.

Gelman, R., & Cohen, M. (1988). Qualitative differences in the way Down syndrome and normal children solve a novel counting problem. In L. Nadel (Ed.), *The psychology of Down syndrome* (pp. 51–99). Cambridge, MA: MIT Press.

Girolametto, L. E. (1988). Developing dialogue skills: The effects of a conversational model of language intervention. In K. Marfo (Ed.), *Parent–child interaction and developmental disabilities* (pp. 145–162). New York: Praeger.

Gleitman, L. R., Newport, E. L., & Gleitman, H. (1984). The current status of the motherese hypothesis. *Journal of Child Language, 11,* 43–79.

Golden, C. J., & Wilkening, G. N. (1986). Neuropsychological bases of exceptionality. In R. T. Brown & C. R. Reynolds (Eds.), *Psychological perspectives in childhood exceptionality. A handbook* (pp. 61–90). New York: Wiley.

Goldstein, D. J., & Sheaffer, C. I. (1988). Ratio developmental quotients from the Bayley are comparable to later IQs from the Stanford–Binet. *American Journal of Mental Retardation, 92,* 379–380.

Goodman, J. F. (1990). Infant intelligence: Do we, can we, should we assess it? In C. R. Reynolds & R. W. Kamphaus (Eds.), *Handbook of psychological and educational assessment of children: Intelligence and achievement* (pp. 183–208). New York: Guilford.

Goodman, J. F., & Bond, L. (1990). *The individual educational program: A retrospective critique from an early intervention perspective.* Unpublished manuscript, University of Pennsylvania, Graduate School of Education.

Goodman, J. F., & Cameron, J. (1978). The meaning of IQ constancy in young retarded children. *Journal of Genetic Psychology, 132,* 109–119.

Goodman, J. F., Fox, A. A., & Glutting, J. J. (1986). Contributions of the Lock Box to preschool assessment. *Journal of Psychoeducational Assessment, 4,* 131–144.

Grossman, H. J. (1983). *Classification in mental retardation.* Washington, DC: American Association on Mental Deficiency.

Gruber, H. (1973). Courage and cognitive growth in children and scientists. In M. Schwebel & J. Ralph (Eds.), *Piaget in the classroom* (pp. 73–105). New York: Basic Books.

Guidelines for reporting and writing about people with disabilities (3rd ed.). (1990). Lawrence, KS, University of Kansas: Research and Training Center on Independent Living.

Gunn, P., Berry, P., & Andrews, R. (1981). The affective response of Down's syndrome infants to a repeated event. *Child Development, 52,* 745–748.

Guralnick, M. J. (1988). Efficacy research in early childhood intervention programs. In S. Odom & M. Karnes (Eds.), *Early intervention for infants and children with handicaps* (pp. 75–88). Baltimore: Brookes.

Halford, G. S. (1989). Reflections on 25 years of Piagetian cognitive developmental psychology, 1963–1988. *Human Development, 32,* 325–357.

Halpern, A. S. (1985). Transition: A look at the foundations. *Exceptional Children, 51,* 479–486.

Hanson, M. J., & Lynch, E. W. (1989). *Early intervention: Implementing child and family services for infants and toddlers who are at-risk or disabled.* Austin, TX: Pro-Ed.

Hanzlik, J., & Stevenson, M. (1986). Interaction of mothers with their infants who are mentally retarded, retarded with cerebral palsy, or nonretarded. *American Journal of Mental Deficiency, 90,* 513–520.

Harbin, G., Terry, D., & Daguio, C. (1989). *Status of the states' progress toward developing a definition for developmentally delayed as required by Public Law 99-457, Part H.* Chapel Hill, NC: Carolina Policy Studies Program.

Hardman, M., & McDonnell, J. (1987). Implementing federal transition initiatives for youths with severe handicaps: The Utah Community-Based Transition Project. *Exceptional Children, 53,* 493–498.

Haring, K. A., & Lovett, D. L. (1990). A follow-up study of special education graduates. *Journal of Special Education, 23,* 463–477.

Harter, S. (1978). Effectance motivation reconsidered: Toward a developmental model. *Human Development, 21,* 34–64.

Harter, S., & Zigler, E. (1974). The assessment of effectance motivation in normal and retarded children. *Developmental Psychology, 10,* 169–180.

Hasazi, S. B., Johnson, R. E., Hasazi, J. E., Gordon, L. R., & Hull, M. (1989). Employment of youth with and without handicaps following high school: Outcomes and correlates. *Journal of Special Education, 23,* 243–255.

Haskins, R. (1989). Beyond metaphor: The efficacy of early childhood intervention. *American Psychologist, 44,* 274–281.

Haywood, H. C., Meyers, C. E., & Switzky, H. N. (1982). Mental retardation. In M. R. Rosenzweig & L. W. Porter (Eds.), *Annual review of psychology* (Vol. 33, pp. 309–342). Palo Alto, CA: Annual Reviews.

Heshusius, L. (1982). At the heart of the advocacy dilemma: Mechanistic world view. *Exceptional Children, 49,* 6–13.

Heshusius, L. (1986). Pedagogy, special education, and the lives of young children: A critical and futuristic perspective. *Journal of Education, 168,* 25–38.

Hobbs, M., & Bacharach, V. R. (1990). Children's understanding of big buildings and big cars. *Child Study Journal, 20,* 1–17.

Hodapp, R. M. (1988). The role of maternal emotions and perceptions on interactions with their young handicapped children. In K. Marfo (Ed.), *Parent–child interaction and developmental disabilities* (pp. 32–46). New York: Praeger.

Hodapp, R. M., Burack, J. A., & Zigler, E. (1990). The developmental perspective in the field of mental retardation. In R. M. Hodapp, J. A. Burack, & E. Zigler (Eds.), *Issues in the developmental approach to mental retardation* (pp. 3–26). New York: Cambridge University Press.

Hodapp, R. M., & Zigler, E. (1990). Applying the developmental perspective to individuals with Down syndrome. In D. Cicchetti & M. Beeghly (Eds.), *Children with Down syndrome* (pp. 1–28). New York: Cambridge University Press.

Hohmann, M., Banet, B., & Weikart, D. P. (1979). *Young children in action: A manual for preschool educators.* Ypsilanti, MI: High Scope Press.

Holden, C. (1990). Headstart enters adulthood. *Science, 247,* 1400–1402.

Holt, J. C. (1964). *How children fail.* New York: Pittman.

Hunt, J. McV. (1961). *Intelligence and experience.* New York: Ronald.

Hunt, J. McV. (1965). Intrinsic motivation and its role in psychological development. In D. Levine (Ed.), *Nebraska symposium on motivation* (pp. 189–282). Lincoln, NE: University of Nebraska Press.

Ickes, W. J., & Kidd, R. F. (1976). An attributional analysis of helping behavior. In J. H. Harvey, W. J. Ickes, & R. F. Kidd (Eds.), *New directions in attribution research* (Vol. 1, pp. 311–334). Hillsdale, NJ: Erlbaum.

Itard, J. (1801/1962). *The wild boy of Aveyron* (G. Humphrey & M. Humphrey, Trans.). New York: Appleton-Century-Crofts.

Jacobs, L. M. (1989). *A deaf adult speaks out* (3rd ed.). Washington, DC: Gallaudet University Press.

James, W. (1892/1958). *Talks to teachers.* New York: Norton.

Johnson-Martin, N., Jens, K., & Attermeler, S. (1986). *Carolina Curriculum for Handicapped Infants and Infants at Risk.* Baltimore: Brookes.

Jones, E. E. (1979). The rocky road from acts to dispositions. *American Psychologist, 34,* 107–117.

Jones, O. H. M. (1978). A comparative study of mother–child communication with Down's syndrome and normal infants. In H. Schaffer & J. Dunn (Eds.), *The first year of life: Psychological and medical implications of early experience* (pp. 175–195). New York: Wiley.

Jones, O. H. M. (1980). Prelinguistic communication skills in Down's syndrome and normal infants. In T. M. Field, S. Goldberg, D. Stern, & A. M. Sostek (Eds.), *High-risk infants and children: Adult and peer interactions* (pp. 205–225). New York: Academic Press.

Kagan, J. (1976). Resilience and continuity in psychological development. In A. M. Clarke & A. D. B. Clarke (Eds.), *Early experience: Myth and evidence* (pp. 97–121). New York: Free Press.

Kamii, C., & Derman, L. (1971). The Engelmann approach to teaching logical thinking: Findings from the administration of some Piagetian tasks. In D. R. Green, M. P. Ford, & G. B. Flamer (Eds.), *Proceedings of the CTB/McGraw-Hill conference on ordinal scales of cognitive development* (pp. 127–147). New York: McGraw-Hill.

Kamii, C., & DeVries, R. (1977). Piaget for early education. In M. C. Day & R. K. Parker (Eds.), *The preschool in action: Exploring early childhood programs* (pp. 363–420). Boston: Allyn & Bacon.

Kanner, L. (1943). Autistic disturbances of affective contact. *Nervous Child, 2,* 217–250.

Kauffman, J. M. (1989). The regular education initiative as Reagan–Bush policy: A trickle-down theory of education of the hard-to-teach. *Journal of Special Education, 23,* 256–278.

Kegan, R. (1982). *The evolving self: Problem and process in human development.* Cambridge, MA: Harvard University Press.

Keil, F. C. (1988). Conceptual heterogeneity versus developmental homogeneity (on chairs and bears and others such pairs). *Human Development, 31,* 35–43.

Kelley, H. H. (1972). Attribution in social interaction. In E. E. Jones, D. E. Kanouse, H. H. Kelley, R. E. Nisbett, S. Valins, & B. Weiner (Eds.), *Attribution: Perceiving the causes of behavior* (pp. 1–26). Morristown, NJ: General Learning Press.

Kelley, H. H. (1973). The process of causal attribution. *American Psychologist, 28,* 107–128.

Kerachsky, S., & Thornton, C. (1987). Findings from the STETS transitional employment demonstration. *Exceptional Children, 6,* 515–521.

Kessen, W. (1965). *The child.* New York: Wiley.

Kohl, H. (1978). *Growing with your children.* Boston: Little, Brown.

Kohlberg, L. (1968). Early education: A cognitive-developmental view. *Child Development, 39,* 1013–1062.

Kohlberg, L., with DeVries, R., Fein, G., Hart, D., Mayer, R., Noam, G., Snarey, J., & Wertsch, J. (1987). *Child psychology and childhood education: A cognitive developmental view.* New York: Longman.

Kohlberg, L. & Mayer, R. (1972). Development as the aim of education. *Harvard Educational Review, 42,* 449–496.

Kopp, C. B. (1990). The growth of self-monitoring among young children with Down syndrome. In D. Cicchetti & M. Beeghly (Eds.), *Children with Down syndrome: A developmental perspective* (pp. 231–251). New York: Cambridge University Press.

Kopp, C. B., Krakow, J. B., & Johnson, K. L. (1983). Strategy production by young Down syndrome children. *American Journal of Mental Deficiency, 88,* 164–169.

Kopp, C. B., Krakow, J. B., & Vaughn, B. (1983). Patterns of self-control in young handicapped children. In M. Perlmutter (Ed.), *Minnesota Symposia on Child Psychology: Vol. 16. Development and policy concerning children with special needs* (pp. 93–128). Hillsdale, NJ: Erlbaum.

Kopp, C. B., & McCall, R. B. (1982). Predicting later mental performance for normal, at-risk, and handicapped infants. In P. B. Baltes & O. G. Brim (Eds.), *Life-span development and behavior* (Vol. 4, pp. 33–61). New York: Academic Press.

Krakow, J. B., & Kopp, C. B. (1983). The effects of developmental delay on sustained attention in young children. *Child Development, 54,* 1143–1155.

Lane, H. (1989). *When the mind hears: A history of the deaf.* New York: Vintage Books.

Lazar, I., & Darlington, R. (1982). Lasting effects of early education: A report from the consortium for longitudinal studies. *Monographs of the Society for Research in Child Development, 47*(2–3, Serial No. 195).

Lee, J., O'Shea, L. J., & Dykes, M. (1987). Teacher wait-time: Performance of developmentally delayed and non-delayed young children. *Education and Training in Mental Retardation, 22,* 176–184.

Leestma, R. (1987). *Japanese education today: A report from the United States Study of Education in Japan* (USDE Publication No. 87009176). Washington, DC: U.S. Government Printing Office.

Leifer, J., & Lewis, M. (1984). Acquisition of conversational response skills by young Down syndrome and nonretarded young children. *American Journal of Mental Deficiency, 88,* 610–618.

Lepper, M. R. (1981). Intrinsic and extrinsic motivation in children: Detrimental effects of superfluous social controls. In W. A. Collins (Ed.), *Aspects of the development of competence* (pp. 155–214). Hillsdale, NJ: Erlbaum.

Levina, R. E. (1979). L. S. Vygotsky's ideas about the planning function of speech in children. In J. V. Wertsch (Ed.), *The concept of activity in Soviet psychology* (pp. 279–299). New York: Sharpe.

Lewin, K. (1935). *A dynamic theory of personality.* New York: McGraw-Hill.

Lewis, M., & Brooks-Gunn, J. (1984). Age and handicapped group differences in infants' visual attention. *Child Development, 55,* 858–868.

Liben, L. S. (1978). *Deaf children: Developmental perspectives.* New York: Academic Press.

Lightfoot, S. L. (1983). *The good high school.* New York: Basic Books.

Linder, T. W. (1983). *Early childhood special education: Program development and administration.* Baltimore: Brookes.

Locke, J. (1690/1980). *Second treatise of government.* Indianapolis, IN: Hackett.

Locke, J. (1693/1927). *Some thoughts concerning education.* Cambridge, England: Cambridge University Press.

Lovaas, O. I. (1987). Behavioral treatment and normal educational and intellectual functioning in young autistic children. *Journal of Consulting and Clinical Psychology, 55,* 3–9.

Loveland, K. A. (1987). Behavior of young children with Down syndrome before the mirror: Finding things reflected. *Child Development, 58,* 928–936.

Lucariello, J., & Nelson, K. (1985). Slot-filler categories as memory organizers for young children. *Developmental Psychology, 21,* 272–282.

Lucariello, J., & Nelson, K. (1987). Remembering and planning talk between mothers and children. *Discourse Processes, 10,* 219–235.

Luria, A. R. (1966). *Higher cortical functions in man.* New York: Basic Books.

MacTurk, R., Vietze, P. M., McCarthy, M., McQuiston, S., & Yarrow, L. (1985). The organization of exploratory behavior in Down syndrome and non-delayed infants. *Child Development, 56,* 573–585.

Mahoney, G. (1988a). Enhancing the developmental competence of handicapped infants. In K. Marfo (Ed.), *Parent–child interaction and developmental disabilities* (pp. 203–219). New York: Praeger.

Mahoney, G. (1988b). Maternal communication style with mentally retarded children. *American Journal of Mental Deficiency, 92,* 352–359.

Mahoney, G., Finger, I., & Powell, A. (1985). Relationship of maternal behavioral style to the development of organically impaired mentally retarded infants. *American Journal of Mental Deficiency, 90,* 296–302.

Mahoney, G., Fors, S., & Wood, S. (1990). Maternal directive behavior revisited. *American Journal of Mental Deficiency, 94,* 398–406.

Mahoney, G., O'Sullivan, P., & Fors, S. (1989). Special education practices with young handicapped children. *Journal of Early Intervention, 22,* 261–268.

Malone, D. M., & Stoneman, Z. (1990). Cognitive play of mentally retarded preschoolers: Observations in the home and school. *American Journal on Mental Retardation, 94,* 475–487.

Marfo, K. (1984). Interactions between mothers and their mentally retarded children: Integration of research findings. *Journal of Applied Developmental Psychology, 5,* 45–69.

Marfo, K. (1990). Maternal directiveness in interactions with mentally handicapped children: An analytic commentary. *Journal of Child Psychology and Psychiatry, 31,* 531–549.

Marfo, K., & Kysela, G. M. (1988). Frequency and sequential patterns in mothers' interactions with mentally handicapped and nonhandicapped children. In K. Marfo (Ed.), *Parent–child interaction and developmental disabilities* (pp. 64–89). New York: Praeger.

Maurer, H., & Sherrod, K. B. (1987). Context of directives given to young children with Down syndrome and nonretarded children: Development over two years. *American Journal of Mental Deficiency, 91,* 579–590.

McKey, R. H., Condelli, L., Ganson, H., Barrett, B. J., McConkey, C., & Plantz, M. C. (1985). *The impact of Headstart on children, families and communities* (DHHS Publication No. OHDS 85-31193). Washington, DC: U.S. Government Printing Office.

McKnight, C. C., Crosswhite, F. J., Dossey, J. A., Kifer, E., Swafford, J. O., Travers, K. J., & Cooney, T. J. (1987). *The underachieving curriculum: Assessing U.S. school mathematics from an international perspective.* Champaign, IL: Stipes.

Meadow, K. P. (1980). *Deafness and child development.* Berkeley: University of California Press.

Medoff, M. (1980). *Children of a lesser God: A play in two acts.* Clifton, NJ: White.

Meisels, S. J. (1979). Special education and development. In S. J. Meisels (Ed.), *Special education and development: Perspectives on young children with special needs* (pp. 3–10). Baltimore: University Park Press.

Mervis, C. B. (1987). Child-basic object categories and early lexical development. In U. Neisser (Ed.), *Concepts and conceptual development: Ecological and intellectual factors in categorization* (pp. 201–233). New York: Cambridge University Press.

Mervis, C. B. (1988). Early lexical development: Theory and application. In L. Nadel (Ed.), *The psychobiology of Down syndrome* (pp. 101–143). Cambridge, MA: MIT Press.

Mervis, C. B. (1990). Early conceptual development of children with Down syndrome. In D. Cicchetti & M. Beeghly (Eds.), *Children with Down syndrome: A developmental perspective* (pp. 252–301). New York: Cambridge University Press.

Miller, L. B., & Bizzell, R. P. (1983). Long term effects of four preschool programs: Sixth, seventh, and eighth grades. *Child Development, 54,* 727–741.

Miller, L. B., & Dyer, J. L. (1975). Four pre-school programs: Their dimensions and effects. *Monographs of the Society for Research in Child Development, 40*(5–6, Serial No. 162).

Miller, S. A. (1988). Parents' beliefs about children's cognitive development. *Child Development, 59,* 259–285.

Miranda, S. B., & Fantz, R. L. (1974). Recognition memory in Down's syndrome and normal infants. *Child Development, 45,* 651–660.

Mirenda, P. L., & Donnellan, A. M. (1987). Issues in curriculum development. In D. J. Cohen & A. M. Donnellan (Eds.), *Handbook of autism and pervasive developmental disorders* (pp. 211–226). New York: Wiley.

Miyake, K., Campos, J. J., Kagan, J., & Bradshaw, D. L. (1986). Issues in socioemotional development. In H. Stevenson, H. Azuma, & K. Kakuta (Eds.), *Child development and education in Japan* (pp. 239–261). New York: Freeman.

Moore, M., Strang, E., Schwartz, M., & Braddock, M. (1988). *Patterns in special education service delivery and cost.* Washington, DC: Decision Resources.

Motti, F., Cicchetti, D., & Sroufe, L. A. (1983). From infant affect expression to symbolic play: The coherence of development in Down syndrome children. *Child Development, 54,* 1168–1175.

Mowder, B. A., & Widerstrom, A. H. (1986). Philosophical differences between early childhood education and special education: Issues for school psychologists. *Psychology in the Schools, 23,* 171–174.

Mundy, P., & Kasari, C. (1990). The similar-structure hypothesis and differential rate of development in mental retardation. In R. M. Hodapp, J. A. Burack, & E. Zigler (Eds.), *Issues in the developmental approach to mental retardation* (pp. 71–92). New York: Cambridge University Press.

Mundy, P., Sigman, M., Kasari, C., & Yirmira, N. (1988). Nonverbal communication skills in Down syndrome children. *Child Development, 59,* 235–249.

Naglieri, J. A. (1989). A cognitive processing theory for the measurement of intelligence. *Educational Psychology, 24,* 185–206.

Nash, E. (1901/1902). Special schools for defective children. *Journal of Psycho-asthenics, 6,* 42–48.

Neil, A. S. (1960). *Summerhill: A radical approach to child rearing.* New York: Hart.

Neisworth, J. T., & Bagnato, S. J. (1987). *The young exceptional child: Early development and education.* New York: Macmillan.

Neisworth, J. T., Willoughby-Herb, S. J., Bagnato, S. J., Cartwright, C. A., & Laub, K. W. (1980). *Individualized education for preschool exceptional children.* Germantown, MD: Aspen.

Nelson, K. (1973). Structure and strategy in learning to talk. *Monographs of the Society for Research in Child Development, 38*(1–2, Serial No. 149).

Nelson, K. (1983). The derivation of concepts and categories from event representations. In E. K. Scholnick (Ed.), *New trends in conceptual representation: Challenges to Piaget's theory* (pp. 129–149). Hillsdale, NJ: Erlbaum.

Nelson, K. (1988). Where do taxonomic categories come from? *Human Development, 31,* 3–10.

Newborg, J., Stock, J. R., & Wnek, J. A. (1984). *Battelle Developmental Inventory.* Allen, TX: LINC Associates, DLM Teaching Resources.

Newport, E. L., Gleitman, H., & Gleitman, L. R. (1977). Mother, I'd rather do it myself: Some effects and non-effects of maternal speech style. In C. E. Snow & C. A. Ferguson (Eds.), *Talking to children: Language input and acquisition* (pp. 109–149). London: Cambridge University Press.

Odom, S. L. (1983). The development of social interchanges in infancy. In S. G. Garwood & R. R. Fewell (Eds.), *Educating handicapped infants* (pp. 215–254). Rockville, MD: Aspen.

Office of Human Development Services, Department of Health and Human Services. (1989). §1304. Chapter XIII, 1–3.

Parshall, L. (1991). *Status of former handicapped students in Michigan including a review of national post-school studies.* Washington, DC: WESTAT.

Peters, D. L., Neisworth, J. T., & Yawkey, T. D. (1985). *Early childhood education: From theory to practice.* Monterey, CA: Brooks/Cole.

Piaget, J. (1951/1962). *Play, dreams and imitation in childhood.* New York: Norton.

Piaget, J. (1952). *The origins of intelligence in children.* New York: International Universities Press.

Piaget, J. (1954). *The construction of reality in the child.* New York: Basic Books.

Piaget, J. (1964). Cognitive development in children: Piaget, development, and learning. *Journal of Research in Science and Technology, 2,* 176–186.

Piaget, J. (1967). *Six psychological studies.* New York: Random House.

Piaget, J. (1970). *Science of education and the psychology of the child* (D. Cottman, Trans.). New York: Orion Press.

Piaget, J. (1971). The theory of stages in cognitive development. In D. R. Green, M. P. Ford, & G. B. Flamer (Eds.), *Proceedings of the CTB/ McGraw-Hill conference on ordinal scales of cognitive development* (pp. 1–12). New York: McGraw-Hill.

Piaget, J. (1976). *To understand is to invent: The future of education.* New York: Penguin Books.

Poplin, M. S. (1988a). The reductionistic fallacy in learning disabilities: Replicating the past by reducing the present. *Journal of Learning Disabilities, 21,* 389–400.

Poplin, M. S. (1988b). Holistic/constructivist principles of the teaching/ learning process: Implications for the field of learning disabilities. *Journal of Learning Disabilities, 21,* 401–416.

Price, M., & Goodman, L. (1980). Individualized education programs: A cost study. *Exceptional Children, 46,* 446–454.

Project Head Start Statistical Fact Sheet. (1991, January). Administration for Children, Youth and Families, Office of Human Development Services, Departmant of Health and Human Services, Washington, DC.

Public Law 94-142. (1975). *Education for All Handicapped Children Act of 1975, 89,* Stat. 773.

Public Law 99-457. (1986). *Education of the Handicapped Act, Amendments of 1986, 100,* Stat. 1145.

Public Law 101-476. (1990). *Education of the Handicapped Act, Amendments of 1990, 104,* Stat. 1103, pp. 1141–1142.

Ramey, C. T., & Suarez, T. M. (1985). Early intervention and the early experience paradigm: Toward a better framework for social policy. In M. Frank (Ed.), *Infant intervention programs: Truths and untruths* (pp. 3–13). New York: Haworth Press.

Ravn, K. E., & Gelman, S. A. (1984). Rule usage in children's understanding of "big" and "little." *Child Development, 55,* 2141–2150.

Reich, P. A. (1986). *Language development.* Englewood Cliffs, NJ: Prentice-Hall.

Reynolds, M. C., Wang, M. C., & Walberg, H. J. (1987). The necessary restructuring of special and regular education. *Exceptional Children, 53,* 391–398.

Rivlin, A., & Timpane, P. M. (Eds.). (1975). *Planned variation in education: Should we give up or try harder?* Washington, DC: Brookings Institute.

Robinson, H., & Robinson, N. (1964). *The mentally retarded child: A psychological approach.* New York: McGraw-Hill.

Rondal, J. A. (1988). Parent–child interaction and the process of language acquisition in severe mental retardation: Beyond the obvious. In K. Marfo (Ed.), *Parent–child interaction and developmental disabilities* (pp. 114–125). New York: Praeger.

Rosch, E. (1975). Cognitive reference points. *Cognitive Psychology, 7,* 532–547.

Rosch, E. (1977). Human categorization. In N. Warren (Ed.), *Studies in cross-cultural psychology* (Vol. 1, pp. 1–49). London: Academic Press.

Rosch, E., & Mervis, C. B. (1975). Family resemblances: Studies in the internal structure of categories. *Cognitive Psychology, 7,* 573–605.

Rosenberg, S. A., & Robinson, C. C. (1988). Interactions of parents with their young handicapped children. In S. Odom & M. Karnes (Eds.), *Early intervention for infants and children with handicaps* (pp. 159–177). Baltimore: Brookes.

Ross, L. (1981). The "intuitive scientist" formulation and its developmental implications. In J. H. Flavell & L. Ross (Eds.), *Social cognitive development: Frontiers and possible futures* (pp. 1–42). Cambridge, England: Cambridge University Press.

Rousseau, J. J. (1762/1969). *Emile* (B. Foxley, Trans.). London: Everyman's Library.

Rousseau, J. J. (1964). *His educational theories selected from Emile, Julie, and other writings* (R. L. Archer, Ed.). Woodbury, NY: Barron's Educational Series.

Rubin, K. H., Fein, G. G., & Vandenberg, B. (1983). Play. In P. H. Mussen (Series Ed.) & E. M. Hetherington (Vol. Ed.), *Handbook of child psychology: Vol. 4. Socialization, personality, and social development* (4th ed., pp. 693–774). New York: Wiley.

Rusch, F. R., & Phelps, L. A. (1987). Secondary special education and transition from school to work: A national priority. *Exceptional Children, 53,* 487–492.

Rutter, M., & Schopler, E. (Eds.). (1978). *Autism: A reappraisal of concepts and treatment.* New York: Plenum Press.

Sacks, O. (1989). *Seeing voices: A journey into the world of the deaf.* Berkeley, CA: University of California Press.

Salisbury, C. L., & Vincent, L. J. (1990). Criterion of the next environment and best practices: Mainstreaming and integration 10 years later. *Topics in Early Childhood Special Education, 10,* 78–89.

Sanford, A. R., & Zelman, G. (1981). *Learning Accomplishment Profile.* Chapel Hill Training Outreach Project. Winston Salem, NC: Kaplan Press.

Sarason, S. B. (1990). *The predictable failure of educational reform.* San Francisco: Jossey-Bass.

Scarr, S. (1982). On quantifying the intended effects of interventions: A proposed theory of the environment. In L. A. Bond & J. M. Joffe (Eds.), *Facilitating infant and early childhood development* (pp. 466–484). Hanover, NH: University Press of New England.

Scarr, S., & Arnett, J. (1987). Malleability: Lessons from intervention and family studies. In J. J. Gallagher & C. T. Ramey (Eds.), *The malleability of children* (pp. 71–102). Baltimore: Brookes.

Schafer, S. & Moersch, M. S. (1981). *Developmental Programming for Infants and Young Children* (5 vols.). Ann Arbor, MI: University of Michigan Press.

Scheerenberger, R. C. (1983). *A history of mental retardation.* Baltimore: Brookes.

Scheerer, M., Rothmann, E., & Goldstein, K. (1945). A case of "idiot savant": An experimental study of personality organization. *Psychological Monographs, 58* (Whole No. 269).

Schlesinger, H. S., & Meadow, K. P. (1972). *Sound and sign: Childhood deafness and mental health.* Berkeley, CA: University of California Press.

Schweinhart, L. J., Weikart, D. P., & Larner, M. B. (1986). Consequences of three preschool curriculum models through age 15. *Early Childhood Research Quarterly, 1,* 15–45.

Seguin, E. (1866/1907). *Idiocy: And its treatment by the physiological method.* New York: Columbia University Press.

Seibert, J. M., Hogan, A., & Mundy, P. (1984). Mental age and cognitive stage in young handicapped and at-risk children. *Intelligence, 8,* 11–29.

Senate Report. (1985). 99-315, 99th Congress, 2nd Session, Seventh Annual Report.

Shepperdson, B. (1988). *Growing up with Down's syndrome.* London: Cassell Educational.

Shonkoff, J. P., & Hauser-Cram, P. (1987). Early intervention for disabled infants and their families: A quantitative analysis. *Pediatrics, 80,* 650–658.

Simeonsson, R. J., Olley, J. G., & Rosenthal, S. L. (1987). Early intervention for children with autism. In M. J. Guralnick & F. C. Bennett, *The effectiveness of early intervention for at-risk and handicapped children* (pp. 275–296). Orlando, FL: Academic Press.

Simmons, C. (1990). *Growing up and going to school in Japan: Tradition and trends.* Buckingham, England: Open University Press.

Simons, J., & Oishi, S. (1987). *The hidden child: The Linwood method for reaching the autistic child.* Kensington, MD: Woodbine House.

Sizer, T. R. (1984). *Horace's compromise.* Boston: Houghton Mifflin.

Skinner, B. F. (1948/1976). *Walden Two.* New York: Macmillan.

Smith, S. W. (1990). Individualized education programs (IEPs) in special education: From intent to acquiescence. *Exceptional Children, 57,* 6–14.

Snow, C. E. (1983). Literacy and language: Relationships during the preschool years. *Harvard Educational Review, 53,* 165–189.

Snow, C. E. (1989). Understanding social interaction and language acquisition: Sentences are not enough. In M. H. Bornstein & J. S. Bruner (Eds.), *Interaction in human development* (pp. 83–103). Hillsdale, NJ: Erlbaum.

Snyder, M. (1976). Attribution and behavior: Social perception and social causation. In J. H. Harvey, W. J. Ickes, & R. F. Kidd (Eds.), *New directions in attribution research* (Vol. 1, pp. 53–72). Hillsdale, NJ: Erlbaum.

Spiker, D. (1990). Early intervention from a developmental perspective. In D. Cicchetti & M. Beeghly (Eds.), *Children with Down syndrome: A developmental perspective* (pp. 424–448). New York: Cambridge University Press.

Stevenson, H. W., & Lee, S. (1990). Contexts of achievement: A study of American, Chinese, and Japanese children. *Monographs of the Society for Research in Child Development, 55* (No. 221).

Stillman, M. (1990). The two-year-old. In N. Cunningham, D. F. Tapley, G. T. Subak-Sharpe, & D. M. Goetz (Eds.), *Columbia University College of Physicians and Surgeons complete guide to early childhood care* (pp. 123–135). New York: Crown.

Stipek, D. J., & Sanborn, M. E. (1985). Teachers' task-related interactions with handicapped and nonhandicapped preschool children. *Merrill-Palmer Quarterly, 31*, 285–300.

Strain, P. S. (1990a). Peer-assisted interventions: Early promises, notable achievements, and future aspirations. *Clinical Psychology Review, 10*, 441–452.

Strain, P. S. (1990b). LRE for preschool children with handicaps: What we know, what we should be doing. *Journal of Early Intervention, 14*, 291–296.

Strain, P., Jamieson, B., & Hoyson, M. (1986). Learning experiences—An alternative program for preschoolers and parents: A comprehensive service system for the mainstreaming of autistic-like preschoolers. In S. J. Meisel (Ed.), *Mainstreaming handicapped children: Outcomes, controversies, and new directions* (pp. 251–269). Hillsdale, NJ: Erlbaum.

Suransky, V. P. (1982). *The erosion of childhood.* Chicago: University of Chicago Press.

Tannock, R. (1988). Control and reciprocity in mothers' interactions with Down syndrome children and normal children. In K. Marfo (Ed.), *Parent–child interaction and developmental disabilities* (pp. 163–180). New York: Praeger.

Tharp, R. G., & Gallimore, R. (1988). *Rousing minds to life: Teaching, learning, and schooling in social context.* New York: Cambridge University Press.

Thiele, J. E., & Hamilton, J. L. (1991). Implementing the early childhood formula: Programs under Public Law 99 457. *Journal of Early Intervention, 15*, 5–12.

Tobin, J. J., Wu, Y. H., & Davidson, H. (1989). *Preschool in three cultures: Japan, China, and the United States.* New Haven, CT: Yale University Press.

Tredgold, A. F. (1908). *Mental Deficiency (Amentia)*. New York: Wood.

Tredgold, A. F., Tredgold, R. F., & Soddy, K. (1952). *A textbook of mental deficiency* (9th ed.). Baltimore: Williams & Wilkins.

Vernon, P. A. (1990). An overview of chronometric measures of intelligence. *School Psychology Review, 19*, 399–410.

Vietze, P. M., Abernathy, S. R., Ashe, M. L., & Faulstich, G. (1978). Contingent interaction between mothers and their developmentally delayed infants. In G. P. Sackett (Ed.), *Observing behavior: Theory and applications in mental retardation* (Vol. 1, pp. 115–132). Baltimore: University Park Press.

Volkmar, F., Burack, J., & Cohen, D. (1990). Deviance and developmental approaches in the study of autism. In R. M. Hodapp, J. A. Burack, & E. Zigler (Eds.), *Issues in the developmental approach to mental retardation* (pp. 246–271). New York: Cambridge University Press.

Vygotsky, L. S. (1979). The development of higher forms of attention in childhood. In J. V. Wertsch (Ed.), *The concept of activity in Soviet psychology* (pp. 189–240). New York: Sharpe.

Wachs, T. (1979). Proximal experience and early cognitive–intellectual development: The physical environment. *Merrill-Palmer Quarterly, 25*, 3–41.

Wang, M. C., Reynolds, M. C., & Walberg, H. J. (1988). Integrating the children of the second system. *Phi Delta Kappan, 70*, 248–251.

Warren, S. F., & Rogers-Warren, A. (1982). Language acquisition patterns in normal and handicapped children. *Topics in Early Childhood Special Education, 2*, 70–79.

Weber, E. (1984). *Ideas influencing early childhood education: A theoretical analysis*. New York: Teachers College Press.

Werner, H. (1948). *Comparative psychology of mental development*. New York: International Universities Press.

Werner, H., & Kaplan, B. (1963). *Symbol formation*. New York: Wiley.

White, K. R. (1986). Efficacy of early intervention. *Journal of Special Education, 19*, 401–416.

White, M. (1987). *The Japanese educational challenge: A commitment to children*. New York: Free Press.

White, M. I., & LeVine, R. A. (1986). What is an ii ko (good child)? In H. Stevenson, H. Azuma, & K. Hakuta (Eds.), *Child development and education in Japan*, (pp. 55–62). New York: Freeman.

White, R. W. (1959). Motivation reconsidered: The concept of competence. *Psychological Review, 66*, 297–333.

White, S. H., & Buka, S. L. (1987). Early education: Programs, traditions, and policies. In E. Z. Rothkopt (Ed.), *Review of research in education* (Vol. 14, pp. 43–91). Washington, DC: American Educational Research Association.

Whitehead, A. N. (1929/1959). *The aims of education and other essays*. New York: Macmillan.

Whitman, T. L. (1990). Self-regulation and mental retardation. *American Journal of Mental Deficiency, 94*, 347–362.

Will, M. C. (1986). Educating children with learning problems: A shared responsibility. *Exceptional Children, 52,* 411–415.

Willoughby-Herb, S. J. (1983). Selecting relevant curricular objectives. *Topics in Early Childhood Special Education, 2,* 9–14.

Willoughby-Herb, S. J., & Neisworth, J. T. (1983a). *HICOMP Preschool Curriculum.* New York: Harcourt Brace Jovanovich.

Willoughby-Herb, S. J., & Neisworth, J. T. (1983b). *HICOMP Preschool Curriculum: Developmental activities handbook.* Columbus, OH: Merrill.

Wilson, R. S. (1983). The Louisville twin study: Developmental synchronies in behavior. *Child Development, 54,* 298–316.

Wise, A. E. (1979). *Legislated learning: The bureaucratization of the American classroom.* Berkeley: University of California Press.

Wood, D. H., Bruner, J. S., & Ross, G. (1976). The role of tutoring in problem solving. *Journal of Child Psychology and Psychiatry, 17,* 89–100.

Wylie, A. R. (1901). Instincts and emotions of the feeble-minded. *Journal of Psycho-asthenics, 5,* 98–107.

Yoder, P. J. (1990). The theoretical and empirical basis of early amelioration of developmental disabilities: Implications for future research. *Journal of Early Intervention, 14,* 27–42.

Zigler, E. (1969). Developmental versus difference theories of mental retardation and the problem of motivation. *American Journal of Mental Deficiency, 73,* 536–556.

Zigler, E., & Balla, D. (1982). Introduction: The developmental approach to mental retardation. In E. Zigler & D. Balla (Eds.), *Mental retardation: The developmental–difference controversy* (pp. 3–8). Hillsdale, NJ: Erlbaum.

Zigler, E., Balla, D., & Hodapp, R. (1984). On the definition and classification of mental retardation. *American Journal of Mental Deficiency, 89,* 215–230.

Zigler, E., & Hodapp, R. (1986). *Understanding mental retardation.* New York: Cambridge University Press.

Zigler, E., & Seitz, V. (1980). Early childhood intervention programs: A reanalysis. *School Psychology Review, 9,* 354–368.

Index